YMCA
Water Fitness for Health

YMCA OF THE USA

EDITED BY MARY E. SANDERS, MS

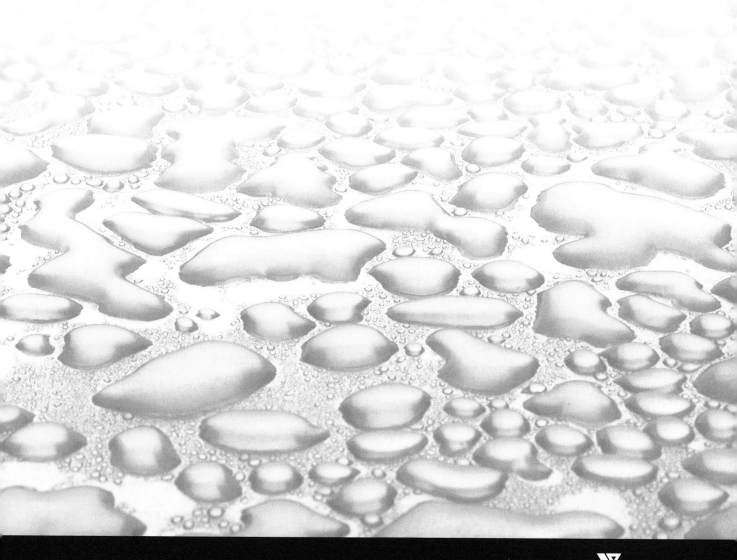

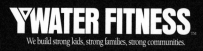
WATER FITNESS
We build strong kids, strong families, strong communities.

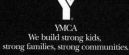
YMCA
We build strong kids,
strong families, strong communities.

Library of Congress Cataloging-in-Publication Data

Slane, Laura J.
    YMCA water fitness for health / [Laura J. Slane, Mary E. Sanders].
        p. cm.
    Includes bibliographical references and index.
    ISBN 0-7360-3246-0
1. Aquatic exercises—Study and teaching. I. Sanders, Mary E. II. Title.
    RA781.17 S53 1999
    613.7'16'071—dc21

Published for the YMCA of the USA
by Human Kinetics, Inc.

ISBN-10: 0-7360-3246-0
ISBN-13: 978-0-7360-3246-9
Copyright © 2000 National Council of Young Men's Christian Associations of the United States of America

YMCA STAFF CREDITS
Laura J. Slane

Acquisitions Editor: Pat Sammann
Managing Editor: Melinda Graham
Copyeditor: Don Amerman
Proofreader: Erin Cler
Indexer: Nancy Ball
Permission Manager: Cheri Banks
Book Design and Production: Studio Montage
Cover (background water image): Digital Vision, Ltd.
Interior Water Backgrounds: Digital Vision, Ltd.
Photographer (cover): Tracy Frankel
Photo Editor: Mary E. Sanders
Photographer (interior): Tracy Frankel—all photos except the following: Mary E. Sanders—p. 155, p. 176, upper left;
            David Madison (Courtesy of Northstar at Tahoe/Wave Aerobics)—p. 81, upper left, p. 112,
            bottom left; Andrea Randolph—pp. 54–59; Peter O. Whiteley—p. 114, 173.

Printer: Edwards Brothers

Printed in the United States of America
10   9   8   7

Copies of this book may be purchased from the YMCA Program Store, P.O. Box 5076, Champaign, IL 61825-5076
800-747-0089

The YMCA of the USA is a not-for-profit corporation that provides advice and guidance, but not rules of compliance, for
member associations of the National Council of YMCAs.

Contents

Preface

Water fitness is popular today, and rightly so. It's a great way for people to exercise no matter what kind of shape they're in. For those who are just starting, the water environment allows them to set their own pace and intensity and to rest when necessary, using the buoyancy of the water. For those who need a more intense workout, the resistance that water provides acts in all directions on one's muscles, no matter what the movement. In some ways water exercise is safer than land-based activity—falls don't carry the same threat of injury, and the stress of impact on joints is lessened. Furthermore, the water cools participants as they work out, so sweating is not a problem!

YMCA *Water Fitness for Health* is the text for training YMCA Water Fitness Instructors. It is meant to give you background information on human physiology and anatomy and on the properties of the water environment; specifics on how to design class workouts; and guidelines for how to run a safe, fun water fitness class. It also includes information on working with those who have medical problems that might require adaptations for participation. The manual is divided into five parts:

I. Program Development and Leadership

II. Healthy Lifestyle and Fitness Principles

III. Fundamentals of Water Exercise

IV. Water Fitness Class Design

V. Responsive Programs for Participants With Individual Challenges

Part I introduces the YMCA's water fitness program and covers issues related to leadership. The first chapter describes the YMCA, the YMCA's health and fitness and aquatics program areas, and the objectives for the water fitness program. Chapter 2 gives you, the instructor, some guidelines for teaching responsively and ethically. Chapter 3 describes some of your legal responsibilities to participants in regard to safety and how you can carry out your duties properly.

In part II, we turn to the principles of health and fitness. Chapter 4 explains the relationship between health and fitness and how water fitness is part of it. Chapter 5 provides you with basic concepts in fitness training, anatomy, and biomechanics.

It is in part III that we begin to discuss the specifics of the water environment and designing exercise programs that work in this environment. Chapter 6 is a review of the water exercise literature since 1993 and how it relates to water fitness class design. In chapter 7, we review the properties of water and how those properties affect movement. Chapter 8 offers some basic water exercise skills and principles for designing workouts for three different water depths. In chapter 9, the ACSM guidelines for fitness training are described and applied to water fitness.

Part IV covers the topic of water fitness class design. In chapter 10, we talk about how to put together a workout. Chapter 11 explains how you can teach responsively, responding to your participants' needs while keeping your own stress levels down. Chapter 12 gives you additional ideas for how to advance the level of your program once you and your participants have mastered the basics.

You may wish to purchase one or more of the videos that illustrate many of the concepts and exercises discussed in this section and referenced in the text: *The Introduction to the Speedo Aquatic Fitness System; The Golden Waves Program, Functional Water Training for Health, Videos I and II; Specificity of Training and Deep Water Program; Tidal Waves; Aquatic Step Program.* They are available through the YMCA Program Store.

The last part of the manual, part V, covers the use of water fitness with older adults and those who have medical problems. In chapter 13, we introduce the concept of functional training—water exercises that improve specific everyday movements on land, such as climbing stairs or getting up from a chair—and describe a sample program for functional training. Chapter 14 offers information regarding physical and mental changes that occur with aging, the benefits of exercise for older adults, and health and safety tips for working with an older population. In chapter 15, the emphasis is on various medical conditions, with specific information for each one relating to exercise design and safety. The last chapter, chapter 16, is an assessment you can use to determine the functional abilities of your participants.

Three appendixes offer you additional help with your water fitness classes. In appendix A, you can find program forms for use in screening participants prior to class and determining any medical conditions that may limit participation, as well as charts related to heart rate and body mass. Appendixes B and C both provide a number of ready-made workouts for you to

use or adapt as needed for your classes. Finally, a glossary defines the technical terms you need to understand as you read through the manual.

We think that this manual can give you both the technical background and the exercise design capabilities to create water fitness classes that meet your participants' needs. Water fitness is adaptable to almost every exerciser, from the most fit to the least fit, and it is especially good for those who have difficulty moving freely on land. Listen to what your participants say they want, and use what you learn in this manual to help them achieve it. Be a responsive instructor, and you'll find that your participants will respond positively to you and your classes.

Acknowledgments

The YMCA of the USA would like to acknowledge the contributions of the following people to YMCA *Water Fitness for Health*. Staff leadership for this project was coordinated by Laura J. Slane.

Shirley Archer, JD
Palo Alto YMCA
Stanford University,
Palo Alto, CA

Nancy Brattain
YMCA of Spartanburg
Spartanburg, SC

Donna Burch
Santa Rosa, CA

Jean Carmichael
Gardena YMCA
Gardena, CA

Mary Carter
Bethesda Chevy Chase YMCA
Bethesda, MD

Holly Colon
Countryside YMCA
Lebanon, OH

Paige Craig
M.E. Lyons Family Branch
YMCA
Cincinnati, OH

Mary Curry
College of St. Catherine
St. Paul, MN

Bethany Diamond
Marietta, GA

Debbie Miles-Dutton
University of California—
Santa Barbara
Santa Barbara, CA

Laura Fasano
Rochester YMCA
Rochester, NY

Diana Griffin
Reno YMCA
Reno, NV

Georgia Harrison
Crescenta-Canada YMCA
Flintridge, CA

Marcia Humphrey
J.M. Tull Branch/Gwinnett
YMCA
Lawrenceville, GA

Margery Johnson
YMCA of Collier County
Naples, FL

Dr. Ralph Johnson
North Greenville College
Greenville, SC

Terry Johnson
YMCA of Salina, Kansas
Salina, KS

Carol Kennedy, MS
Indiana University
Bloomington, IN

Suzanne King
St. Joseph YMCA
St. Joseph, MO

Dr. Karl Knopf
Fitness Educators of Older Adults
Sunnyvale, CA

Tatiana Kolovou, MBA
Indiana University
Bloomington, IN

Gayle Magee
Glenwood Park Branch YMCA
Erie, PA

Karen Mailen
Lebanon YMCA
Lebanon, PA

Tanya Marter
Portland YMCA
Portland, OR

Karen Martorano
YMCA of Greater Detroit
Detroit, MI

Kathy Mayan
Central Delaware Branch YMCA
Dover, DE

Cindy Gray McDermott
Waltham YMCA
Waltham, MA

Cathy Maloney-Hills, RPT
Courage Center
Golden Valley, MN

Tracey Mummert
Southeast YMCA
Woodbury, MN

Robyn Pendleton
Cleveland County YMCA
Norman, OK

Mary Sanders, MS
University of Nevada—Reno
Reno, NV

Laura J. Slane
YMCA of the USA
Chicago, IL

Mike Spezzano
YMCA of the USA
Chicago, IL

Dixie Stanforth, MS
University of Texas
Austin, TX

Jennifer Viets
Tuckahoe YMCA
Richmond, VA

Gigi Woodruff
YMCA of Metropolitan Houston
Houston, TX

Stephanie Young
Cleveland County YMCA
Norman, OK

We also would like to thank the following for their support of this project:

- Speedo International, Ltd., London, England
- Sanford Center for Aging, University of Nevada—Reno
- Speedo Authentic Fitness for their donation of attire and equipment for the photo shoot
- City of Reno Parks, Recreation and Community Services Department, Reno, Nevada for use of the pool during the photo shoot

- Reno Family YMCA Golden Waves™ class staff and members
- IDEA, The Health and Fitness Source for reprint permission on articles
- Tracy Frankel for her photos
- Water Fit/Wave Aerobics® for their educational materials and their personal time, energy, and support dedicated to this project

- A special thanks to Mary Sanders for her support for this project and for her hard work and dedication to helping people live better lives on land through quality water exercise

Mary Sanders would like to dedicate this book in memory of Michael Pollock, PhD (1937–1998), director of the Center for Exercise at the University of Florida since 1986. Dr. Pollock served as chair of the Position Stand Committee for the American College of Sports Medicine (ACSM), was a fellow of the American Heart Association, and published more than 275 articles, three books, and two monographs in the areas of exercise physiology, physical fitness, cardiac rehabilitation, and sports medicine. He helped provide the framework for health and fitness programs in America today. His enthusiastic care for people and his mission as an educator made it possible for us to do our work and learn from him as a person. Dr. Pollock was keenly interested in water fitness, especially as it related to older people and those with special conditions. Because of him, we can help others improve their lives and make each activity more joyous.

Credits

Information throughout this book adapted from Sanders, M. and Rippee. 1994. *Speedo aquatic fitness system, instructor training manual.* London: Speedo International Ltd.

Chapter 2

"Being Ethical," pp. 11 to 15, adapted, by permission, from Sanders, M. and D. Mast. 1995. A question of ethics. *IDEA Today* (March): 44–46. Adapted with permission of IDEA, The Health and Fitness Source, 800-999-IDEA or 619-535-8979.

Chapter 3

This chapter adapted, by permission, from Archer, S. 1998. Water exercise liability. *IDEA, The Health and Fitness Source* (February): 71-77. Adapted with permission of IDEA, The Health and Fitness Source, 800-999-IDEA or 619-535-8979.

Chapter 5

Figure 5.2 reprinted, by permission, from Borg, G. 1998, *Borg's Perceived Exertion and Pain Scales* (Champaign, IL: Human Kinetics), 31.

Figures 5.12 through 5.17 drawn by Marie Dauenheimer.

"Exercise Science and Training Principles of Cardiorespiratory Endurance Training," pp. 32 to 42, adapted, by permission, fromWilmoth, S.L. 1988. *Y's way to better aerobics: Leader's guide.* Champaign, IL: Human Kinetics.

"Anatomy and Biomechanics," pp. 43 to 45 and 60 to 61, adapted, by permission, from Franks, B.D. and E.T. Howley. 1989. *Fitness leader's handbook.* (Champaign, IL: Human Kinetics), 183–190.

Text of figure 5.18 adapted from material by Elizabeth W. Chicado.

Chapter 6

Material from the following sections, "Water Exercise and Cardiorespiratory Conditioning," "Monitoring Exercise Intensity in the Water," "Improving Body Composition With Water Exercise," "Improving Muscular Strength and Flexibility With Water Exercise," pp. 65 to 68, adapted, by permission, from Rippee, N. and M. Sanders. 1994. Get into water fitness. *IDEA Today* (October): 92. Adapted with permission of IDEA, The Health and Fitness Source, 800-999-IDEA or 619-535-8979.

Material on pp. 64 to 73 adapted, by permission, from Rippee, N. and M. Sanders. 1994. Probing the depths of water fitness research. *IDEA Today*, August: 49–60. Adapted with permission of IDEA, The Health and Fitness Source, 800-999-IDEA or 619-535-8979.

"Water Exercise and Weight Management," pp. 78 to 80 adapted, by permission, from Evans, E. 1996. Can water exercise tip the scale? *IDEA Today* (May): 27–31. Adapted with permission of IDEA, The Health and Fitness Source, 800-999-IDEA or 619-535-8979.

"Review of Water Exercise Literature From 1994 to 1998," pp. 73 to 77 and "Functional Exercise," pp. 80 to 83, adapted, by permission, from Sanders, M. and C. Kennedy. 1998. Water research update. *IDEA, The Health and Fitness Source* (June): 32–39. Adapted by permission of IDEA, The Health and Fitness Source, 800-999-IDEA or 619-535-8979.

Chapter 7

Table 7.1 adapted, by permission, from Kennedy, C. and M. Sanders. 1995. Strength training gets wet! *IDEA Today* (May): 24–30. Reprinted with permission of IDEA, The Health and Fitness Source, 800-999-IDEA or 619-535-8979.

Chapter 9

Illustrations on pp. 136–139 by Nancy L. Dunn.

Material for ACSM Guidelines on pp. 123 to 124, 130, 140, 143, and 148 adapted, by permission, from two ACSM articles, as indicated by text references: American College of Sports Medicine. 1998a. The recommended quantity and quality of exercise for developing and maintaining cardiorespiratory and muscular fitness, and flexibility in healthy adults. *Medicine and Science in Sports and Exercise.* 30(6): 975–991; American College of Sports Medicine. 1998b. Exercise and physical activity for older adults. *Medicine and Science in Sports and Exercise.* 30(6): 992–1008.

Information on pp. 131–134, adapted, by permission, from Kennedy, C. and M. Sanders. 1995. Strength training gets wet! *IDEA Today* (May): 24–30. Adapted with permission of IDEA, The Health and Fitness Source, 800-999-IDEA or 619-535-8979.

"Sample Muscular Endurance and Strength Training Progression," pp. 135–139, adapted, by permission, from Sanders, M. 1999 Cross over to the water. IDEA, The Health and Fitness Source (March). Adapted with permission of *IDEA, The Health and Fitness Source*, 800-999-IDEA, or 619-535-8979.

Chapter 11

"Choosing a Teaching Method," pp. 174–178 adapted, by permission, from Sanders, M. 1999. *WaterFit™ Instructor Training and Speedo's Aquatic Fitness System* (2nd ed.). Reno, NV: WaterFit International/WaveAerobics®.

"Responsive Teaching," pp. 178–183 adapted, by permission, from Sanders, M. 1999. *WaterFit™ Instructor Training and Speedo's Aquatic Fitness System* (2nd ed.). Reno, NV: WaterFit International/WaveAerobics®.

Chapter 12

"Water Fitness During Recovery From Injuries," pp. 203–204 adapted, by permission, from Kennedy, C. and M. Flegel. 1994. In the swim: How water fitness professionals can work with the medical community (pp. 56–57). In article by Rippee, N. and M. Sanders., Probing the depths of water fitness research. *IDEA Today* (August): 49–52, 55–60. Adapted with permission of IDEA, The Health and Fitness Source, 800-999-IDEA or 619-535-8979.

Chapter 13

This chapter adapted, by permission, from Sanders, M. and C. Maloney-Hills. 1999. *The Golden Waves™ program, functional water training for health, aging adults leadership course.* Reno, NV: WaterFit™/Wave Aerobics® and Sanders, M. and C. Maloney-Hills. 1999. *Responding to selected medical conditions and sports injuries.* Reno, NV: WaterFit™/ Wave Aerobics®.

Chapter 14

This chapter adapted, by permission, from Sanders, M. and C. Maloney-Hills. 1999. *The Golden Waves™ program, functional water training for health, aging adults leadership course.* Reno, NV: WaterFit™/Wave Aerobics® and Sanders, M. and C. Maloney-Hills. 1999. *Responding to selected medical conditions and sports injuries.* Reno, NV: WaterFit™/ Wave Aerobics®.

"Physical Changes Due to Aging," pp. 222–227, "The Unique Benefits of Water Programs for Older Adults," and "Exercise Modifications for Older Adults," pp. 229–237, and "Health Screening," pp. 239–240 adapted, by permission, from Hooke, A.P. and M.B. Zoller. 1992. *Active older adults in the YMCA: A resource manual.* Champaign, IL: Human Kinetics.

Chapter 15

This chapter adapted, by permission, from Sanders, M. and C. Maloney-Hills. 1999. *The Golden Waves™ program, functional water training for health, aging adults leadership course.* Reno, NV: WaterFit™/Wave Aerobics® and Sanders, M. and C. Maloney-Hills. 1999. *Responding to selected medical conditions and sports injuries.* Reno, NV: WaterFit™/ Wave Aerobics®.

"Your Role as a Water Fitness Instructor," pp. 243–244 adapted, by permission, from Tilden, H.M. Aquatic Exercise Instructor. In Norton, C. and L. Jamison (eds.) *A team approach to the aquatic continuum of care.* Woburn, MA: Butterworth-Heinemann. (in press).

Appendix B

Illustrations on pp. 300–304, and 308–313 by Nancy L. Dunn.

The following illustrations on pp. 316–317 are by the Corel Corporation: anemone fish, mute swan, sea otter, pelican, flamingo, sea horse, lobster, star fish, angel fish, octopus, squid, and crab.

The following illustrations on pp. 316–317 are by Peter Vine: fan worm, feather star, and shrimp from *Red Sea Invertebrates*.

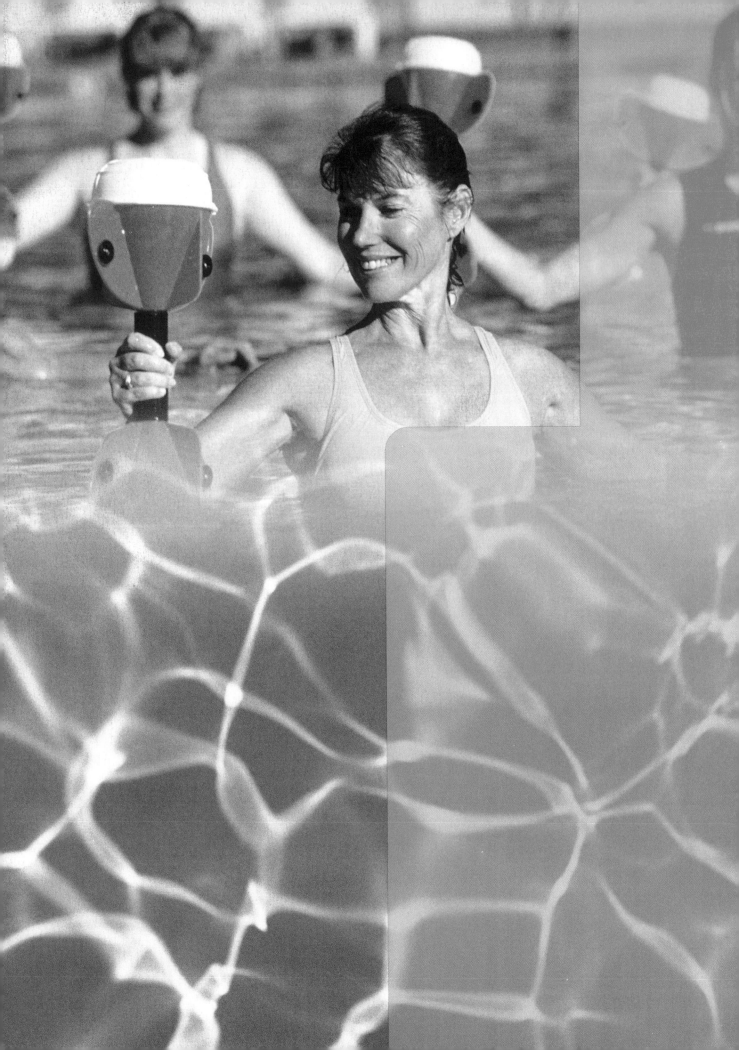

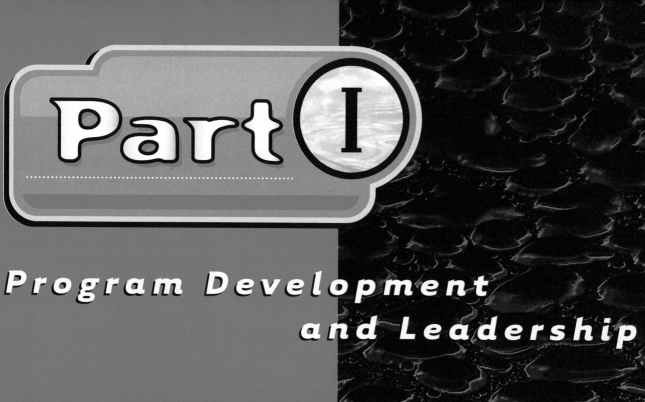

Part I

Program Development and Leadership

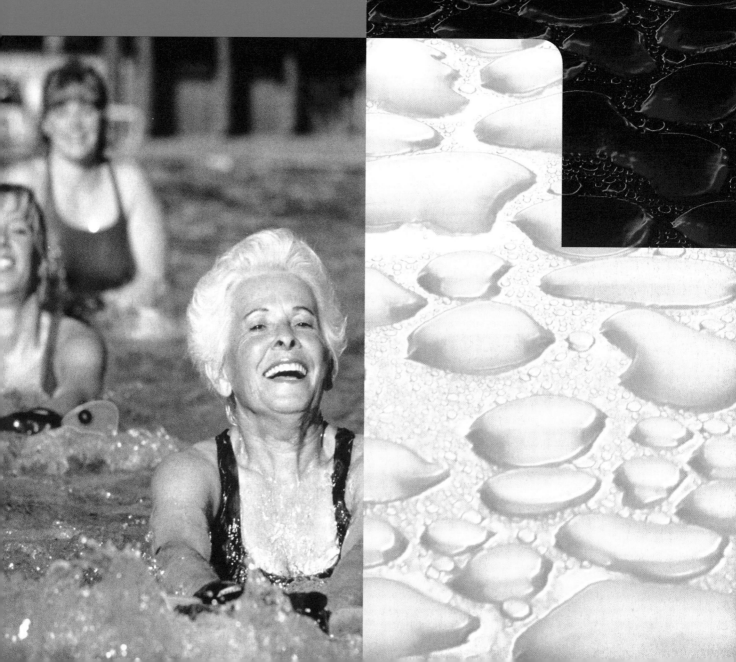

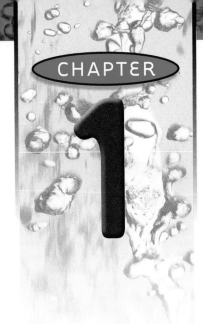

CHAPTER 1

Overview of the YMCA and the Water Fitness Program

Objectives:

◎ To describe the purpose, history, and organization of the YMCA

◎ To explain the YMCA program objectives and the integration of character development into Y programs

◎ To briefly describe the YMCA health and fitness and aquatic programs

◎ To list the objectives of the YMCA Water Fitness Program that develop the spirit, mind, and body

---

The YMCA Water Fitness Program draws on the Y's long tradition of excellence in both health and fitness and aquatic programming. It also incorporates the Y's mission and objectives in its activities. The following chapter gives you some insight into what the YMCA is and does. It explains how Y programs differ from those of other organizations and describes the YMCA health and fitness and aquatic program areas. Finally, it outlines the objectives for the water fitness program.

What Are YMCAs?

YMCAs are community-based, volunteer-led groups that build strong kids, strong families, and strong communities. YMCAs are often leaders in solving neighborhood problems and meeting community needs. They have been seen as building healthy spirit, mind, and body for more than 150 years, since the beginning of the movement in 1844. At the beginning of 1999, 2,283 YMCAs in the United States were serving more than 16 million people.

Impressive as that may seem, YMCAs often say they care little for national numbers, which have no practical use for them. Ys are intensely self-directed in control, outlook, financing, and services. This approach has proved so effective that today Ys are found in 130 nations worldwide.

Ys try to include everybody: people of all faiths, races, abilities, ages, and incomes. Half of those served are 17 or younger, and half are women.

A major source of strength is the way Ys bring together people from all walks of life in pursuit of common goals. They do so by subsidizing those who cannot pay full membership costs. For example, almost all youth activities are subsidized. Ys are both accessible and affordable.

While YMCAs are independent, they are active collaborators, working with other agencies in the community to combine resources and avoid duplication of efforts. It can be as simple as having a Leaders Club project involve volunteering at a Red Cross blood drive, or as complex as running all of a city's parks and recreation operations or combining with many other organizations to run comprehensive services for low-income children and families.

YMCAs are committed to four core values—caring, honesty, respect, and responsibility—and develop them both by creating programs that foster these values and by demonstrating them at every level of the organization.

Much of the YMCAs' work is done in small groups such as classes, clubs, committees, task groups, teams, support groups, and families. Such work builds leadership skills, the ability to give and take, and the sense of community that is central to YMCAs.

Now that we know what YMCAs are, let's look at how they started and how they're organized today.

History of the YMCA

The first YMCA was founded in London, England, in 1844 by George Williams and a dozen or so friends who lived and worked as clerks in a drapery, a forerunner of dry goods and department stores. Their goal was to save fellow live-in clerks from the wicked life on the London streets. The first members were evangelical Protestants who prayed and studied the Bible as an alternative to vice.

The first U.S. YMCA started in Boston in 1851, the work of Thomas Sullivan, a retired sea captain who was a lay missionary. Ys spread quickly and soon were serving boys and older men as well as young men. After World War II, U.S. YMCAs admitted women and girls to full membership and participation, and they have continued to expand to serve entire families.

The organization's original Protestant Christian goals also broadened over the years, and for the last 25 years, Ys have been formally required to serve and welcome all ranks within the associations: people of all faiths or no faith at all. Christian emphasis today remains most prominently in the values Ys put forward in their programs and actions.

The Organization of the YMCA

Each Y is incorporated under state law, meeting requirements of Section 501 (c)(3) of the U.S. Tax Code as a charitable not-for-profit organization. More than 500,000 charitable not-for-profits exist in the United States. Besides YMCAs, other examples are churches, private schools and colleges, private hospitals, social service groups, charitable foundations, nongovernment libraries, museums, and symphony orchestras.

Because they are corporations, all YMCAs are legally required to have a board of directors. And because Ys are not-for-profits, the board members are unpaid volunteers. A medium-sized YMCA with no branches might have 2,000 members, a full-time paid professional staff of five, and 25 policy-making volunteers on its board and committees.

But this same Y would have another, much larger number of unpaid volunteers—maybe 125—working in programs as leaders, coaches, referees, instructors, camp workers, group leaders, and every other unpaid job, plus another 10 or 15 full-time hourly rated employees and at least as many part-time staff members.

It is difficult to generalize about the U.S. movement because of the vast differences between the larger YMCAs in New York, Chicago, and Los Angeles and the smaller ones such as those in Little Falls, New York; Boone County, Iowa; and Bogalusa, Florida. While annual revenues for the Y in New York City are more than $80 million, Boone County's are approximately $40,000. That, plus their independence, which is guaranteed under the YMCA's national constitution, make it difficult to say many things for sure about all YMCAs.

This much is sure. The Y movement is self-governing. Each Y belongs to a geographical unit called a cluster, which in turn sends representatives to one of the four field committees. They in turn appoint 30 of the 50 members of the National Board of YMCAs. The national headquarters, called the YMCA of the USA, is in Chicago, with field offices in California, Pennsylvania, Georgia, and Minnesota and 18 Management Resource Centers across the country.

YMCAs in the United States are part of a worldwide movement, the World Alliance of YMCAs. It is a nonbinding organization of independent YMCA national movements from more than 100 countries, with headquarters in Geneva, Switzerland.

YMCA Programs

Ys nationwide offer hundreds of organized activities, called programs. These range widely, from swimming lessons to shelters for the homeless. The possibilities are just about endless.

YMCAs are best known for more than a century of health and fitness leadership. Healthy Lifestyles are still a major concern of the Y movement. So are camping, child care, aquatics, teen leadership, sports, older adults, community development, and families.

Y programs are practical, important, and fun. They vary from place to place and tend to concentrate more on preventing a problem than on treating those affected by it. Often they do both. They are always grounded in an atmosphere of caring and respect.

There is no central menu of programs that all YMCAs must follow. Each decides what its own community needs and wants. What is similar is that all Ys operate using the same set of principles and that program involvement provides youth with the developmental assets they need.

Three elements that are part of every Y program are YMCA program objectives, character development, and membership development.

YMCA Program Objectives

Because many organizations offer programs, the question may arise: What is different about YMCA programs? What makes them different is this: Many organizations offer their programs as an end in themselves, but the YMCA uses programs as a vehicle to deliver its unique mission of putting Christian principles into practice to build a healthy spirit, mind, and body for all. It is the activities within the programs that make the difference for Y members and participants.

The goal of all YMCA programs is to help people grow spiritually, mentally, and physically. To accomplish this goal, YMCA programs address seven specific objectives.

YMCA Objectives

GROW PERSONALLY:

Build self-esteem and self-reliance.

★ **Develop self-esteem.** People who are involved in YMCA programs gain a greater sense of their own worth. They learn to treat themselves and others with respect. High self-esteem helps people of all ages to build strong, healthy relationships and overcome obstacles in life so that they can reach their full potential.

TEACH VALUES:
Develop moral and ethical behavior based on Christian principles.

★ **Develop character.** The YMCA has been helping people develop values for 150 years. Founded originally to bring men to God through Christ, it has evolved into an inclusive organization that helps people of all faiths or none develop values and behavior that are consistent with Judeo-Christian principles. The YMCA believes the four values of caring, honesty, respect, and responsibility are essential for character development. Emphasis is on building a core set of values shared by the world's major religions and by people from all walks of life.

IMPROVE PERSONAL AND FAMILY RELATIONSHIPS:

Learn to care, communicate, and cooperate with family and friends.

★ **Support families.** YMCAs embrace families of all kinds and are more flexible in responding to their needs. Not only do Ys strengthen families through their own programs, but YMCA staff are increasingly being trained to help families in need or in crisis to find other community supports that can help.

YMCAs plan programs and events with today's busy, sometimes frantic, families in mind. Families also get involved in helping plan and run Y family programs. The idea is to program with families, not just for them.

APPRECIATE DIVERSITY:

Respect people of different ages, abilities, incomes, races, religions, cultures, and beliefs.

★ **Reflect the diversity of the community.** The country's diversity can be seen in terms of religion, race, ethnicity, age, income, abilities, and lifestyle. YMCAs must assess their membership to see whether it reflects the diversity of their communities. Diversity is a source of strength. The YMCA fosters an environment where everyone is treated with respect and is able to contribute to the larger community. Diversity should be celebrated, not merely tolerated.

BECOME BETTER LEADERS AND SUPPORTERS:
Learn the give-and-take necessary to work toward the common good.

★ **Promote leadership development through volunteerism.** The YMCA is driven by volunteer leadership, and it emphasizes providing meaningful volunteer opportunities for all kinds of people, especially youth and families. People are encouraged to move from program participation to deeper levels of involvement, including volunteer leadership. Volunteer leadership will enrich their lives, their YMCAs, and their communities.

DEVELOP SPECIFIC SKILLS:
Acquire new knowledge and ways to grow in spirit, mind, and body.

★ **Build life skills.** YMCA programs help people succeed in their daily lives through programs that build self-reliance, practical skills, and good values. Such programs include employment programs for teens and programs that support activities of daily living for seniors.

HAVE FUN:

Enjoy life!

Fun and humor are essential qualities of all programs and contribute to people feeling good about themselves and the YMCA.

In addition to the preceding objectives, programs should also meet the following goals:

- **Respond to demographic trends and social issues.** YMCAs are called to reach out and do more to help make their communities better places in which to live, work, and grow up. The vision is that the YMCA will be the country's leader in prevention and development programs for children and families and a leader in community development, bringing community resources to bear on social problems.

- **Develop cross-cutting programs.** The days of narrowly defined programs in the Y are gone. Programs must take advantage of the expertise of the staff in all program areas and combine that expertise into cross-cutting programs. One program area may be the focus, but many others are incorporated in some way.

- **Collaborate internally and externally.** From diverse staff groups meeting together to the YMCA working with other community organizations, the question must always be "How can we or our YMCA bring our resources to the table to make this program or initiative a success?" Staff at all levels need to learn the skills required for successful collaborative efforts, including planning, commitment, and implementation.

Character Development

Another part of all Y programs is character development. The Y's stated mission is "to put Christian principles into practice through programs that build healthy spirit, mind, and body for all." If we define principles as "a code of conduct, a basis for action" and Christian principles as "positive values," then challenging people to accept and demonstrate positive values is how we put them into practice. This is how YMCAs develop character.

Values are cornerstones that make our society safe and workable. They are the principles of thought and conduct that help distinguish right from wrong and provide a foundation for decision making. Values, which are sometimes referred to as character, are the basis of who we are, how we live, and how we treat others. The values we try to impart through character development are these four:

Caring: to put others before yourself, to love others, to be sensitive to the well-being of others, to help others

Honesty: to tell the truth, to act in such a way that you are worthy of trust, to have integrity, to make sure your actions match your values

Respect: to treat others as you would have them treat you; to value the worth of every person, including yourself

Responsibility: to do what you should do, to be accountable for your behavior and obligations

Living with and acting on good values contribute to the development of a healthy self-esteem and overall personal happiness. The Y defines self-esteem as the positive valuing of oneself. The Y helps children and adults to develop self-esteem by providing opportunities for them to become more capable and worthy. By *capable* we mean having practical abilities and competencies. The more capable a person is, the more confident that person is in his or her ability to think and to cope with life's basic challenges. By *worthy* we mean being able to act in a manner that is consistent with those principles a person has been taught are important, such as doing one's best or doing the right thing. As a person becomes more worthy, he or she also becomes more confident of the right to be successful and happy. It makes the person feel more deserving and entitled to assert his or her needs and wants, achieve his or her values, and enjoy the fruits of his or her efforts.

The YMCA Water Fitness Program is a part of our mission to help people develop character and a positive sense of self-worth. By helping people exercise to the degree that they are capable, we are setting the foundation for the development of character and self-esteem. Through this changing process participants will learn a great deal about themselves and other people that will contribute in many ways to their health and human development.

Membership Development

The YMCA is an association of people with a common purpose and mission: to put Christian principles into practice through programs that build healthy spirit, mind, and body for all. Membership in the YMCA is at the heart of the mission. It is about building relationships, and it goes beyond any single program. Everyone who crosses the threshold of a YMCA should be treated like a member, in a relationship based on the YMCA values of caring, honesty, respect and responsibility.

As part of YMCA staff, keep the following ideas about membership in mind:

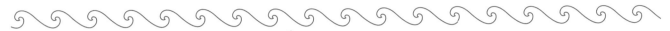

- It's an attitude, not a department.
- It is everybody's job.
- It is mission work. It is not just about units and dollars and center. It's about people.
- It is relationship development.
- It all begins with the way we treat people, staff and volunteers.

Make it part of your job to get members more involved by building relationships with them and promoting relationships among volunteers and members. When possible, get members involved with the Y by defining meaningful roles for them, asking them to get involved, and planning for their involvement. For example, create new adult fitness or aquatics volunteer opportunities, and ask your class members to volunteer in areas of interest to them.

YMCA Health and Fitness and Aquatics Programs

The following programs have resources and certification training available from the YMCA of the USA:

HEALTH AND FITNESS

- Fitness assessment
- Group exercise classes
- **Strength training**
- Youth fitness
- Healthy back
- Prenatal exercise
- Fitness walking
- Weight management
- Active Older Adults exercise

AQUATICS

- The YMCA Swim Lessons Programs: The Youth and Adult Aquatic Program and The Parent/Child and Preschool Aquatic Program
- YMCA Lifeguard
- YMCA Water Fitness for Health
- Arthritis Foundation/YMCA Aquatic Program
- YMCA Aquatics for Special Populations
- YMCA Synchronized Swimming
- YMCA Wetball (Water Polo)
- YMCA Scuba, Snorkeling, and Skin Diving
- YMCA Competitive Swimming and Diving

Details on certification training for each of these programs can be found in the YMCA course catalog, available by calling the YMCA of the USA Certifications Department at 1-800-441-9648.

Both the health and fitness programs and aquatics programs have been around for more than 100 years. Some of the key dates and developments are shown in figure 1.1, shown on page 8–9. Let's look more closely at each of the two program areas.

Health and Fitness

The YMCA takes the wellness, or holistic, approach to health and fitness: Its programs, which are organized around the principle that there is a oneness of spirit, mind, and body, focus on prevention.

All of what Ys do is aimed at promoting a long and productive life and having fun living it. That's the way the YMCA approaches exercise. It's not something just for the body. It's a way of life that requires education in good nutrition, proper exercise, avoidance of drug and alcohol abuse, dealing with stress, and structuring life to lessen problems posed by chronic ailments such as arthritis, cancer, and heart disease.

Today, emphasis on prevention stretches from the fields of medicine to insurance. People understand how important their daily actions can be for long-term health. The YMCA is a major provider of affordable health and fitness programs, which encourage self-improvement.

A variety of national training and certification programs are available to Y staff members. YMCA standards generally meet or exceed those required by local and state licensing boards. Since the 1880s the Y has been a leader in the field. Its own health and fitness professionals number in the thousands. It has also been a training ground for recreation and physical education professionals outside the Y, for the health club industry, and for corporate wellness programs.

It was in 1891 that a YMCA physical education leader created the now-familiar red triangle. To this day it symbolizes the association's commitment to helping people build healthy lives, healthy families, and healthy communities.

YMCA members and participants have a wide range of exercise alternatives from which to choose. Working out with weights or keeping step in group exercise classes helps many stay in shape. Others want more, to train for a competitive fitness event, perhaps. And some want less, just the strength to move from the couch to the jogging path. Whatever the goal, a Y staff member will help the individual draw up a realistic plan to achieve it, offer encouragement along the way, and help map out a new direction when the goal is reached.

The YMCA strives to recognize the unique needs of individuals who join its organization. The mission of the Y comes alive for each individual when it helps that person reach his or her unique potential through its programs and services. In helping people improve their health, it can recognize their uniqueness by

- assessing their current health status,
- discussing their personal goals,
- discussing their areas of interest,
- discussing roadblocks to achieving goals,
- setting realistic short- and long-term goals based on their interests and activities, and
- getting them involved in programs designed to meet their personal goals.

Aquatics

For more than 110 years, the YMCA has been a leader in aquatics and water safety. Aquatics has continued to be an important program area over this time because it has several benefits:

- It serves the need of communities for a resource that teaches people water safety. Today, many Americans do not know how to swim, even though water recreation activities are on the increase, and thousands of people drown annually. Offering education in water skills and safety is even more important now that public schools have cut back on physical education and aquatic course offerings.
- It offers a means for people of all ages to learn skills that build self-confidence and esteem. From preschoolers to adults, overcoming fears of the water and developing water and swimming skills are rewarding.
- It provides a fun activity that children and families can share and enjoy.
- It promotes better health as a **physical activity** that can be performed throughout life.

YMCA Water Fitness Program Objectives

As in all YMCA programs, the ultimate goal of the YMCA Water Fitness Program is to develop the whole person spiritually, mentally, and physically. In order to achieve this, you, as an instructor, should have a basic understanding of and respect for the individuality and uniqueness of each participant. The teaching methods recommended for use throughout the program are participant centered. They are designed to help develop each participant's human potential, to encourage participants' awareness of safety in all aspects of the program, and to assist participants in improving their health and fitness to the best of their ability.

Spiritual Development

As an instructor, you are an important role model for your classes. When you relate to participants and to other instructors with sensitivity, you'll probably find that they also become more sensitive. The Water Fitness Program should serve as a context for putting the Golden Rule into practice: Treat participants (and other instructors) as you would like to be treated.

Values form an integral part of the YMCA Water Fitness Program, with special attention being given to the potential moral growth of each participant. The YMCA of the USA has chosen four core values to promote: caring, honesty, respect, and responsibility. As a water fitness instructor, you are responsible for character development. You will actively teach, model, and reinforce the core values throughout your classes.

Mental Development

The YMCA Water Fitness Program includes teaching styles that challenge and develop participants' cognitive abilities. By explaining why certain exercises are used and how those exercises affect our bodies, Y instructors help participants learn how to develop their own fitness. Participants who are challenged and who meet those challenges know they have accomplished a great deal. Instructors also should continuously educate participants about health and fitness issues and self-development through handouts and discussion

Providing recognition, guidance, and enthusiasm are essential, as is creating an atmosphere of love and trust. Encourage participants to set their own mental, as well as physical, goals. Allow each participant to develop individually, competing against himself or herself rather than against others.

Physical Development

In the YMCA Water Fitness Program, health and **physical fitness** are used as a springboard for building self-confidence and for practicing the Golden Rule. As participants learn about the properties of water and understand how to help themselves in the water to achieve the workout they need, they also learn to help others, to work jointly, and to strive for excellence.

1851 The first YMCA in the United States opens in Boston, Massachusetts.

1856 A bowling alley is installed at the Brooklyn, New York, YMCA, giving the YMCA its first physical education program.

1860 At a national convention, YMCAs unanimously agree "that the establishment of gymnasiums is both desirable and expedient." By this time, Ys in New York City and Charleston, South Carolina, were already offering "gymnastics" programs, which today we would call calisthenics and strength training.

1876 Robert J. Roberts begins work as the "gymnasium superintendent" at the Boston YMCA. Roberts later coins the phrase "body building" to describe his program of exercises and drills with dumbbells.

1885 The first YMCA swimming pool is built in the Brooklyn YMCA in New York.

1891 Luther H. Gulick, a physician and professor at the YMCA Training School (later Springfield College), creates an enduring symbol for the YMCA, the triangle. Each side of the triangle stands for one aspect of human development—spirit, mind, and body.

The sport of basketball is invented by James Naismith, a teacher working for Dr. Gulick, at the YMCA Training School in Springfield, Massachusetts.

1895 The sport of volleyball is invented by William Morgan at the Holyoke, Massachusetts, YMCA.

1904 The first YMCA lifesaving corps is organized in 1904 at Camp Dudley in upstate New York.

1910 George Corsan uses group teaching methods instead of teaching individuals. He teaches crawl stroke first, contrary to the practice of the day.

1912 The National YMCA Lifesaving Service is organized.

1916 There are now 911 YMCAs in the United States conducting exercise and athletic programs with 735 gyms and 250,000 members. The YMCA is recognized as the leading physical education organization in the United States.

1923 The first YMCA swimming championships are held at the Brooklyn YMCA.

1938 The new YMCA aquatics program is published. Swimmers at varying degrees of ability are known as Minnows, Fish, and Sharks.

1950 By this time, women are admitted to nearly all YMCAs. Within a few years, all restrictions of gender, race, age, or religion have disappeared completely.

1956 The YMCA introduces the idea of "Learn to Swim Month."

1959 The YMCA Scuba program is developed.

1963 The YMCA publishes *The YMCA Guide to Adult Fitness*, a handbook for "every man or woman who cares about life-long fitness."

1964 The National YMCA Aquatic Conference adopts the Porpoise and Springboard Diving programs.

1968 Jogging programs are in full force at YMCAs all over the country as people flock to the Y to "get in shape."

1970 A woman named Jackie Sorenson begins teaching a new kind of dance exercise to music at the Towson, Maryland, YMCA. She goes on to fame and fortune as the creator of aerobic dancing.

1971 The first "National YMCA Consultation on Physical Fitness," a gathering of YMCA fitness leaders, is held in Philadelphia, Pennsylvania. A proposed new program model, the "Y's Way to Physical Fitness," is presented at this conference. Other consultations follow in 1975, 1982, and 1990, with 600 to 1,000 attendees each.

1972 The YMCA publishes the first edition of *Y's Way to Physical Fitness*. The protocol described in the text becomes the standard for adult physical fitness testing and programs. *Y's Way to Physical Fitness* is subsequently revised twice and is used by colleges and universities throughout the country.

The Progressive Swimming and Springboard Diving Program manual is published. The new program uses the "whole-part" rather than the "part-whole" method of instruction. Activities are pupil-centered rather than teacher-centered, and problem solving is emphasized rather than skill instruction and drills.

Tadpoles, a preschool program, is introduced. Polliwog and Flying Fish are added to the Progressive Swimming program. A synchronized swimming program is also introduced.

1973 The YMCA begins its first national emphasis on aquatic activities for the disabled.

1974 Working with Dr. Hans Kraus, Al Melleby, the director of physical fitness at the New York City YMCA, develops "Y's Way to a Healthy Back," the first nationally standardized exercise program for people with back pain. Over 300,000 people have since enrolled in the program.

1975 The National YMCA Swimming and Diving Championship becomes the largest swimming championship in the world, with more than 1,500 participants.

1981 A new level of the progressive swim system, Guppy, is introduced.

1982 The National Physical Fitness Through Water Exercise and the Arthritis programs are launched. The Aquatic Facility Manager course is adopted as a certification course.

1986 The YMCA of the USA introduces the "YMCA Fitness Leaders" course, a standard program for training and certifying leaders of fitness classes.

1987 The YMCA of the USA adopts the Pool Operator on Location course. The manual is published in 1989.

1988 *Y's Way to Water Exercise* is released as a new manual and specialty instructor course certification.

1992 The first YMCA "Healthy Kids Day" is conducted, a national event celebrating the Y's programs and activities designed to enhance the healthy development of youth and to advocate increased attention to youth health issues. More than 1,200 YMCAs across the country sponsor events and activities for kids and their families on this now-annually celebrated event.

The YMCA operates over 1,700 pools. The YMCA of the USA maintains records of over 25,000 lifeguards and instructors.

1994 *On the Guard II: The YMCA Lifeguard Program* is introduced. This edition emphasizes the decision-making skills needed to prevent accidents and how to safely and most effectively perform rescues. Aquatic Safety and Aquatic Personal Safety and Survival are two programs included in the lifeguard program to be used when teaching a variety of groups about water safety and accident prevention.

YMCA Synchronized Swimming Instructor and YMCA Wetball (Water Polo) Instructor/Coach are introduced through the cooperation of the U.S. Olympic Committee and the national governing bodies of the sports.

New training designs for instructor certification programs are released for Principles of Aquatic Leadership, YMCA Water Exercise, YMCA Progressive Swimming, and Y Skippers.

1995 A revised series of Health and Fitness certification courses is introduced by the YMCA of the USA. More than 35,000 Health and Fitness certifications have been issued by the YMCA.

The 12th National Aquatic Conference is held in Ft. Lauderdale to celebrate the 110th anniversary of YMCA swimming.

The YMCA Walk Reebok certification course, developed in collaboration with Reebok International, is introduced nationwide.

1996 YMCA community-based learn-to-swim program *Splash!* is released. This program's purpose is to help people of all ages, especially children and families, learn some basic swimming skills and water-safety practices.

1997 The third edition of *On the Guard II* is released.

1998 The YMCA introduces a new program developed in collaboration with IDEA, The Health and Fitness Source, titled *YMCA/IDEA Get Real Weight Management*.

The YMCA Personal Fitness Program is launched, an innovative new program for introducing inactive people to exercise.

1999 The Progressive Swimming Program and Skippers is replaced by the YMCA Swim Lessons Program. Instruction is student centered and allows students to discover the best methods of swimming for themselves. Program manuals include *Teaching Swimming Fundamentals, The Parent/Child and Preschool Aquatic Program Manual, The Youth and Adult Aquatic Program Manual,* and *YMCA Swim Lessons Administrator's Manual.* There is a revised instructor training program.

The YMCA Group Exercise Instructor certification course is offered, a new training program for leaders of exercise classes.

The instructor training manual for the new YMCA Water Fitness program, *YMCA Water Fitness for Health* is released.

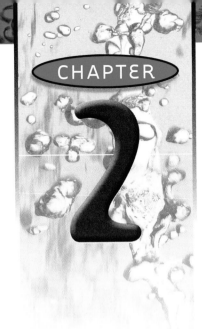

Leadership Principles for Instructors

MARY E. SANDERS

Objectives:

○ **To explore some components of an effective and healthy teaching philosophy**

○ **To introduce the concept of being a responsive instructor**

○ **To describe ethical behavior within the health and fitness field**

To prepare ourselves as professional instructors, we need to not only study bones, muscles, and great moves, but also to examine closely our personal motivations for becoming instructors and how they affect every person we touch with our skills.

We need to act in ways that are responsive to our participants' needs, and we also need to behave ethically among ourselves.

Developing a Positive Teaching Philosophy for Life and Health

The characteristics of a good instructor include traits such as being educated, compassionate, a good listener, and an effective responder. Your job basically is to motivate others to change their own lives. You'll want to develop your own teaching philosophy, one that inspires your participants and nurtures you. Every person you meet provides you with an opportunity to develop your unique style. Relationships are everything. If you fill each one with care, honesty, and hope, you'll discover everyone's greatness, including your own.

In an effort to improve the health of our community, a primary goal is to get people moving purposefully by teaching them why and how water exercise improves living on land. By your influence, participants are empowered with skills and knowledge so they can make exercise a component of their lives even when you aren't there to guide them personally.

Every class provides us with the gift of being an instructor, the honor of being in the company of participants, and the privilege to be woven into so many people's lives. If you see participants as your greatest teachers, if you observe, listen, and work together with them, your relationships will provide a continuing education program for life.

Recognize and create teaching moments. Seize them to make a difference, for a moment missed is an opportunity lost. A casual conversation in the grocery store can provide an opportunity to help someone learn a tip on proper nutrition. A participant's question or comment can create a learning and teaching moment for the entire class. For example, Dottie mentions that her hands were stiff after the last workout using resistance bands. Find out who else had a similar response, look for a probable cause, and make modifications for the next time. Include your participants in the solutions, and they then take charge of their own program! If you cannot solve the challenge, call an associate or expert who can help. But seek a solution.

Because every situation, facility, and participant population—and each of us—are unique, teaching methods need to meet our own needs. We will examine in detail teaching methods that can be adapted to your own program, but for now you should think about your personal philosophy of being an instructor. Why do you teach? Many instructors hope to make a difference in other people's lives, to make them happier and healthier. To know you have done

---

Part of this chapter reprinted with permission of IDEA, The Health and Fitness Source. (800) 999-IDEA or (619) 535-8979. See page x for complete source information.

this is an accomplishment powerful enough to nurture you for a long time. But there is something else. To help others, while keeping your own life in balance, is to celebrate not only your participants' lives, but your own as well. Balance for instructors means nurturing our own need for exercise, nutrition, family, and time to ourselves for fun, growth, and dreaming. Always remember to be a participant yourself. Take care of the greatest gift you can give to your participants . . . YOU!

Being a Responsive Instructor

Instructors are called "responsive" when they care for people by listening, observing, and then offering specific modifications or tips when necessary, and when they allow people to work at their own pace. To empower people with the skills that will make fitness a lifetime activity and improve the quality of their lives, instructors must be flexible and ready to respond to the needs of a wide variety of individuals. The YMCA Instructor Code of Ethics (shown in figure 2.1) lists some of the actions that a responsive instructor should take. We'll examine more specific responsive teaching methods later in chapter 11.

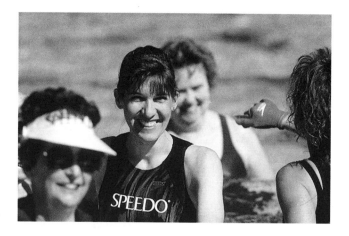

Being Ethical

Communication between instructors and participants is critical for professional success. But the way we communicate with each other affects how successfully our profession will grow. The fitness profession is still fairly young, and as it develops, questions about what is ethical or professional begin to surface. Most professions have ethical standards that are broad based and can serve as guidelines when situations arise.

Figure 2.1   **YMCA Instructor Code of Ethics**

I understand the purpose of the YMCA and its programs, which goes beyond skills and involves the spiritual, mental, and physical well-being of our participants.

I understand the YMCA program objectives, and I will strive to make sure they are incorporated into my classes.

I will teach the Y's values to participants by modeling those values, celebrating them and holding them up as what is right, and asking participants to practice those values. I will consistently reinforce participants for behaviors that support the values, and I will consistently confront participants whose actions are inconsistent with the values without devaluing those participants.

I will set a good example in appearance, speech, and attitude.

I will be reliable, prompt, and prepared.

I will be a good role model for my participants, and I will not use alcohol, tobacco, or illegal drugs.

I will speak clearly and use words whose meaning is clear to my participants. I will not use profanity.

I will create a good learning atmosphere.

I will be encouraging, respectful, and considerate to participants and instructors regardless of race, religion, or culture.

I will always be conscious that the safety of my participants comes first.

I am committed to keeping my certification and training up to date, and I will take part in learning opportunities to remain an effective instructor.

I believe I am free of psychological or physical conditions that might adversely affect others' health, including significant fever or contagious conditions.

I will follow the Golden Rule.

I will remember how intimidating a pool can be to a nonswimmer.

I will report any suspected child abuse or molestation according to the proper procedures

I will refrain from socializing or associating with program participants or members under the age of 18 outside of YMCA activities.

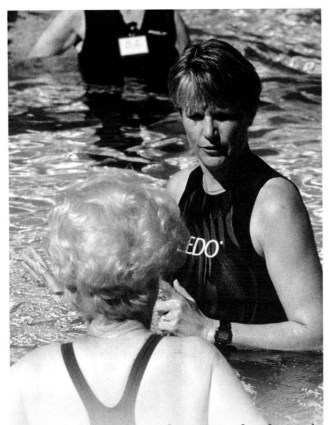

However, ethical behavior for a group of professionals begins with each individual making decisions based on standards of morality, fairness, and honesty.

Let's start by examining some situations that may help you define those virtues that lead to ethical behavior and virtuous professionalism:

- Imagine that you walk into a workshop and watch while your professional associate presents the program that you researched and developed, then claims it is his or her own work.

- Imagine that you agree to teach a workshop and at the conclusion you are not reimbursed according to the agreement in a timely manner. Other projects are delayed or canceled due to lack of funds.

- Imagine that you commit to developing a program that will benefit many, and the associates working with you (also professing to be committed to the success of the project) communicate with you in a manner that is condescending, angry, critical, and downright nasty.

- Imagine that you receive a workshop evaluation from an associate that reads, "Loser, go home."

Imagine how you would feel if you were in any of these situations.

In all of these interactions among professionals, the result was intimidation; disruption of service; and creation of distrust, fear, and anger among colleagues, weakening the individuals involved and ultimately damaging the fitness of our profession. While the message of fitness professionals to the public is that fitness helps people live healthy and balanced lives, that message is contradicted by such negative interactions among fitness professionals.

Psychologists and experts tell us that how we treat others is a reflection of how we feel about ourselves. Perhaps, in a profession that promotes health and wellness for others, we need to turn our view inward and examine our own behavior and motivations, in order to better understand the consequences that our behavior creates and the responsibility that we have to establish ethical practices.

Integrity is defined by Webster as *completeness; soundness; honesty and sincerity.* Part of integrity in fitness is setting objectives for our classes, telling our participants what those objectives are, and doing our best to meet those objectives.

In our complex world, integrity is often laughed at or, worse, scorned outright by some as a sign of being weak and naive. However, James F. Hind writes that "a high quality of integrity . . . gives people a stronger ethic and motivation to do their work well" (Hind, 1989).

The Golden Rule advises us to "treat others as you wish to be treated." In a letter from physicians to their patients, the physicians attribute the origin of many illnesses to relationship problems, stating, "Man is a whole, and our body registers in its own way the fluctuations, the joys, the missing elements in our relationships with others and ourselves" ("Open letter," 1993). By nurturing others, instead of seeking to destroy their fragile belief in themselves, we begin to build relationships based on cooperation rather than competition, expanding ourselves and our profession in a healthy direction.

A sphere is a complete, encompassing body that offers safety and wholeness to those housed within it. Within a sphere of integrity, we are able to nurture others by applying the virtues described by the YMCA character development values:

Caring: to love others; to be sensitive to the well-being of others

Honesty: integrity; to tell the truth; to act in such a way that you are worthy of trust

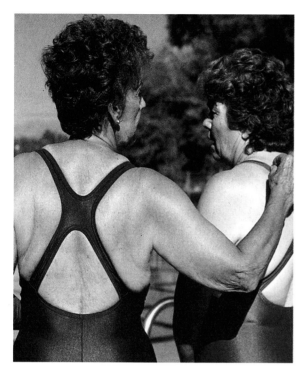

It is important for each of us to stay focused on our goals and values.

Physicians' prescription for the health of their patients includes "more mercy . . . clarify the situation without anger . . . forgive and turn away from self, working for the greater good" ("Open letter," 1993).

By applying virtuous professionalism to the previous example situations, we can see the positive interactions that help build our sphere of integrity:

The Cooperation Equation, 1+1=3. Your associate uses your idea and combines it with his or her own original idea or interpretation to create a third unique idea. If he or she shows respect for your contribution through proper referencing, you both can share the credit for the new development. Colleagues appreciate each other's efforts, participants admire the loyalty and cooperation between instructors, and everyone benefits from cooperative growth and learning. "Each instructor reaches members in a way that is uniquely his or her own…it may not be your way, but none of us will ever be the right instructor for everyone," IDEA 1995 Fitness Instructor of the Year award winner Kari Anderson advises. "Celebrate in our differences and give your honest support, with no ulterior motives, to your colleagues."

Respect: regard; to treat others as you would have them treat you; to value the worth of every person, including yourself

Responsibility: duty; to do what you should; to be accountable for your behavior and obligations

Expanding, rather than diminishing, the sphere of integrity to encompass all those within our profession provides a safe environment for growth and expression. Likening virtues to a diamond, we find within these virtues a purity, strength, clarity, and brilliance that cannot be hidden or destroyed, not only within ourselves, but within each person we deal with daily.

We, as fitness professionals, may get caught up in the glamour of our field, but it is important for each of us to stay focused on our goals and values. If each of us makes a commitment to teach and reflect the diamond virtues, the sphere of integrity will surround us all, allowing us to be tough (pliable, but not easily broken) without ever having to resort to meanness to protect ourselves. Perhaps the greatest investment that each of us can make in this profession is the development of ethical practices.

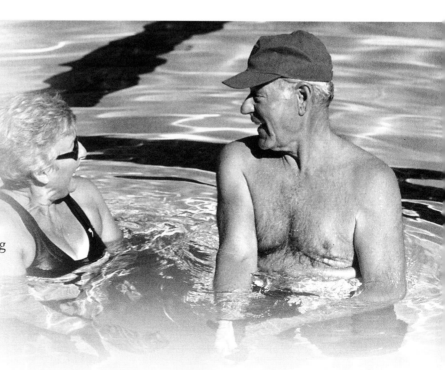

The Virtuous Contract. Honesty and responsibility are essential in contractual agreements, allowing professionals to meet their own obligations and to have the resources to continue providing new services. When basic needs are met, professionals can continue to grow without having to sacrifice or struggle to make ends meet. When people meet their obligations, instructors have the security to pursue personal fulfillment within the profession without having to seek income elsewhere.

Faithful Communication. Successful group interactions require communication based on respect, compassion, responsibility, honesty, and perseverance. When these virtues are present, a comfortable environment emerges, allowing individuals to freely explore and express their ideas to the group without fear of criticism or detraction from their personal endeavors. Many professionals choose to avoid people who are not "faithful communicators," and many projects lose valuable insight. It's simply more fun to work with people who are supportive!

Compassionate Assessment. The evaluation process is designed to "find the value" of a presentation. Objective assessment, based on reasonable criteria and written responsibly, stimulates growth by providing valuable insight from knowledgeable professionals. Honest, tactful feedback allows presenters to improve their skills and more effectively contribute to our profession. Take a walk in your associates' sneakers or water shoes and admire the courage it takes to stand before strangers and give them a part of yourself.

The sphere of integrity is a domain where each person's greatness sparkles, and the consequence is a healthy and fit group of human beings who radiate the joy of life. The cost to join is the investment of the virtuous work we perform not by our living, but rather, *with* our living.

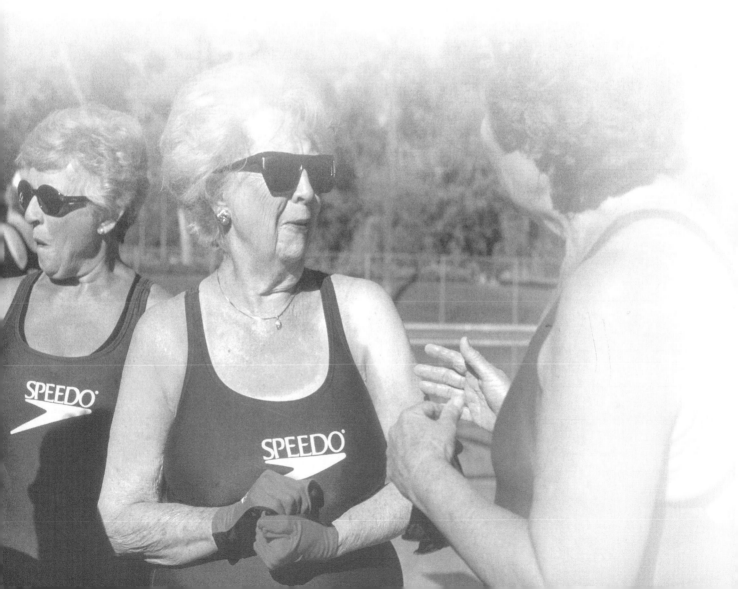

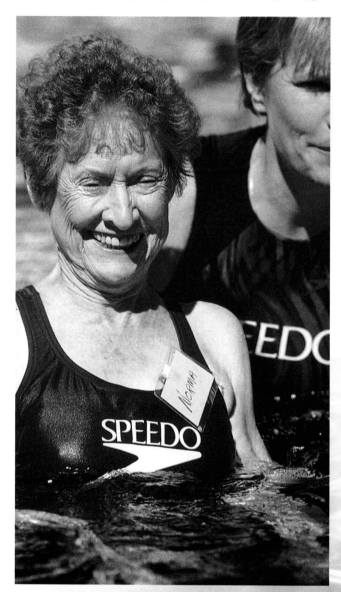

When we develop a healthy teaching philosophy based on caring for both our participants and ourselves, the difference in people's lives can be significant. By applying ethical behavior to our relationships, we ensure that the quality of our work matches the quality of life we hope to achieve both personally and professionally.

Bibliography

Dyer, W.W. 1991. *You'll see it when you believe it.* Nightingale-Conant Audio.

Hind, J.F. 1989. *The heart and soul of effective management.* Wheaton, IL: Victor Books.

Open letter from physicians to their patients. 1993. *Le lien des cellules de priere.* (July-September).

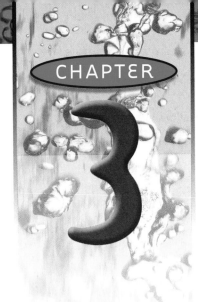

Water Exercise Program Safety

SHIRLEY ARCHER

Objectives:

To make pool owners or managers, aquatic directors, and water fitness instructors aware of the following:

- Pools are highly regulated by state, county, and city statutes, as are lifeguard and emergency services.

- Duty of care determines what responsibilities water fitness instructors have for their participants' safety.

- Negligence per se may be part of lawsuit considerations if all pool regulations have not been followed.

- Following pool safety and health guidelines, as laid out in the checklists in this chapter, can help ensure participants' well-being and protect you in case of a lawsuit.

- Liability risks can be reduced by having participants sign informed consent and waiver forms and by obtaining personal liability insurance.

Aquatic exercise is rapidly becoming a popular choice for many exercise enthusiasts. As a facility owner or manager, program director, trainer, or group fitness instructor, you can diversify your career or programming by offering or conducting water fitness training sessions or classes. However, you must be able to offer these programs *responsibly*.

As aquatic activities pose special risks, local and state governments extensively regulate pool operations, particularly in areas that involve the greatest potential for public harm. Legal liability with consequent financial costs occurs when this responsibility to protect public safety is not met or a person suffers injury or death as a direct result of this failure. Before getting wet, therefore, all fitness professionals should fully understand the risks involved and their responsibility to take preventive measures. This knowledge not only will minimize the likelihood of legal liability, but it may also save lives.

This chapter provides an overview of the legal responsibilities pertaining to water fitness instruction. Topics covered include government regulations and the legal standard of care owed to participants; the role of safety procedures in meeting this standard of care; safety checklists for facility owners, manager, trainers, and instructors; waivers, informed consent forms, and liability insurance; and incident reports.

Local rules and regulations governing pool operations, definitions of standards of care, and the acceptability of informed consent forms and waivers of liability vary from state to state, county to county, and even city to city. The information in this chapter is therefore general. This discussion is not intended to be legal advice and should not be considered to be a substitute for legal counsel on specific liability issues pertaining to your individual situation.

Pool Regulatory Environment

State and local laws specify health and safety standards that govern in detail the construction, design, maintenance, and management of public swimming pools. The regulations help ensure these pools are sanitary, healthful, and safe. Although the specific definition may vary from one jurisdiction to another, any pool available for use by members of the public is generally considered to be a "public swimming pool." This classification applies even if members pay for admission. Accordingly, pools in YMCAs, public parks, and hotels and motels all are subject to these

This chapter adapted with permission of IDEA, The Health and Fitness Source. (800) 999-IDEA or (619) 535-8979. See page x for complete source information.

regulations, which may be set forth in building, fire, electrical, administrative, bathing, and health and safety codes. In residential complexes and private homes, pools are considered "public" if people pay to use them.

YMCA facility managers or aquatic directors who are responsible for managing a swimming pool should review copies of these codes and implement procedures to ensure compliance; otherwise they risk pool closure, fines, and/or imprisonment. Regulated aspects of pool operation include design safety; electrical wiring; the bacteriological and chemical quality and clarity of the water; cleanliness and maintenance, including the condition of the deck, rest rooms, dressing rooms, and showers; the health of employees and patrons; lifesaving; first aid; and control of people using the pool.

Health and safety inspectors may periodically visit your YMCA to ensure these standards are enforced. Persons violating bathing codes may be found guilty of a misdemeanor and be subject to a fine (the amount of which varies from state to state) and/or imprisonment for up to six months. Each day of a violation may be considered to be a separate offense. If, in the opinion of the enforcing agent, pool operations create an unhealthful, unsafe, or unsanitary condition, the pool may be closed and may not reopen until the appropriate corrections are made and approved by the enforcing agent.

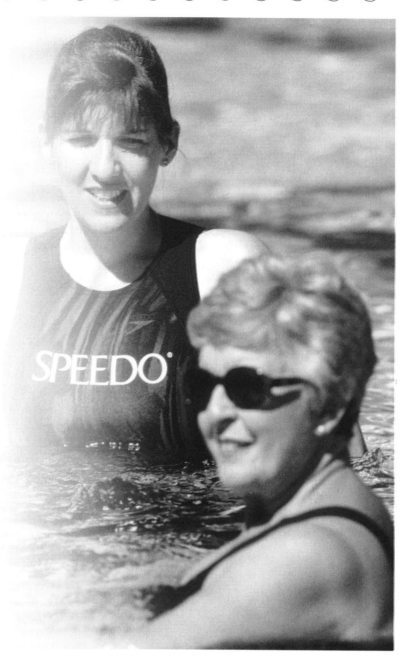

Lifeguard Guidelines

Regulations also provide guidelines for lifeguard services and safety and rescue procedures. In almost all states, lifeguard services are required in pools where a direct fee is charged for use or any organized activity is conducted. Although codes may not specifically address water exercise activities for which a direct fee is charged, lifeguard services are generally required whenever organized activities such as swimming instruction are conducted in a pool. Accordingly, some hotel and residential complex pools may not require a lifeguard for recreational swimming, but adding a fee-based class may trigger the requirement.

Enough lifeguards should be present to adequately supervise the number of people in the pool. The number of lifeguards is based on several factors:

- Activity or activities in the pool area (on deck and in the water)
- The size and shape of the pool
- Equipment in the pool area (slides, inflatable objects, and so on)
- The bather load
- The skill level of the swimmers
- Changes in glare from sunlight

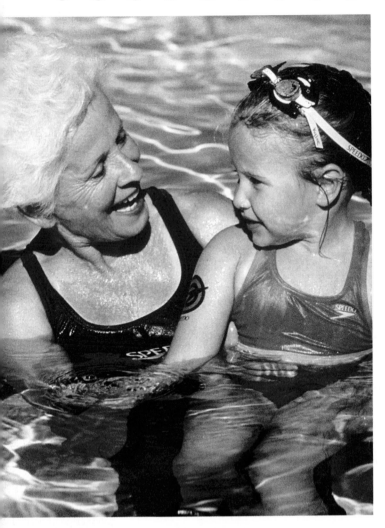

Furthermore, any violation of code requirements may be deemed a violation of the standard of care or "negligence per se." (See the following section for further discussion.) Such a violation renders the fitness professional liable for accidents or injuries resulting directly from the violation.

Duty of Care

In the event of an accident or injury to a participant, the question of whether a fitness professional is liable is determined by an examination of the duty of care. *Duty of care* relates to how much responsibility the fitness professional has for participant safety. How this question is analyzed varies from state to state. In general, the legal standard is reasonable care under the circumstances, and the factual details of the accident or injury are examined by a jury. Failure to meet the standard of reasonable care may be deemed negligence, rendering everyone from the instructor to the owner liable to the participant.

In extreme cases, failure to meet the standard of care may be considered willful or wanton misconduct or gross negligence. For example, consider a case in which a father and his son both drowned in a motel pool that had no signage warning that a lifeguard was not present. In this case, health inspection reports stating that the pool did not have the required lifesaving and safety equipment were admissible as evidence of willful and wanton misconduct.

- High-use areas
- Ability to handle emergencies in a proper and effective manner
- Meeting or exceeding compliance with applicable state and local codes

The YMCA of the USA recommends having an appropriate number of lifeguards on duty whenever there is activity in the pool area.

In addition, the lifeguard's sole duty should be to supervise participant safety. In other words, the instructor or trainer *should not* function as both instructor and lifeguard, even if a facility is short staffed.

To maximize pool safety, facility managers and program directors must weigh the *quantity* of program offerings against their *quality*. What if classes are in high demand but staff and budget are short? It's better to have a reputable program, with certified lifeguards and competent staff, that serves a smaller population than a larger program with substandard safety procedures.

Negligence per Se

Another aspect of the duty of care is the concept of *negligence per se*. According to *Black's Law Dictionary*, negligence per se is "conduct, whether of action or omission, [that] may be declared and treated as negligence without any argument or proof as to the particular surrounding circumstances" (p. 1035), usually because the conduct violates a statute or municipal ordinance.

As swimming pools are subject to extensive regulation by local codes, many water safety cases have been based on negligence per se. What this means is that, if your pool is in violation of health and safety or building codes and your violation results in an injury to a person who falls within the class of persons the code was designed to protect, you will be deemed negligent per se, without any additional fact investigation by the court. For example, when the father and son drowned in the motel pool, the motel operators were deemed negligent per se because no lifeguard was present, no sign advised guests that no lifeguard was present, the various water depths and breaks in the pool's slope were not marked, and no sign warned that children were not to use the pool without an adult in attendance. Accordingly, if a water exercise participant were to drown in a pool in a locality where regulations required a lifeguard to be present and no lifeguard was present, this could be considered negligence per se.

If you are in complete compliance with pertinent regulations and an accident or injury occurs, negligence per se will not apply.

Safety Procedures and Prevention

The first step to limit your liability is to implement all reasonable safety measures and operational procedures. Figure 3.1 is a sample checklist you can use to ensure the safety of participants and protect yourself from liability. The checklist will need to be modified based on your facility, your program policy, and your local and state codes.

If you observe the safety procedures outlined in these checklists, the likelihood of injuries occurring at your pool will be greatly reduced.

Through your training as a YMCA Aquatic Safety Assistant or YMCA lifeguard, you learned about emergency procedures. It's important to keep up with your skills and to practice them on a regular basis.

Other Risk Reducers

Here are some additional ways to reduce your risk of liability:

- **Informed consent.** This type of form documents that the participant fully understands the risks involved in an activity and knowingly and voluntarily accepts these risks as well as the possibility of any injuries resulting from them. An informed consent form should describe the nature of the activity and the potential risks of harm resulting from participation.

- **Waivers.** You might also ask each participant to sign a waiver (follow your association's procedures in this matter). A waiver is a contract that attempts to limit some of the responsibility of one party toward another party. As the law generally does not support limitations of responsibility, waivers must meet specific requirements to be considered valid. Again, the rules of law governing the specific requirements that must be adhered to in order for courts to uphold waivers of liability vary from state to state. Courts have upheld YMCA waivers that are clear and unambiguous concerning the intent to hold harmless the owner and employees for any injuries or damages caused by owner/employee negligence. To ensure that your informed consent form and waiver comply with relevant laws in your jurisdiction, you must discuss your documents with a local attorney.

- **Liability insurance.** Purchasing liability insurance is another way to limit your personal and professional liability. Depending on the policy, liability insurance may provide coverage to business owners and certified trainers and instructors for accidents, injuries, and legal defense fees. For an annual premium, the insurer will pay up to a specified amount per occurrence, not to exceed a set annual amount. The insurer will cover these costs even if the court finds the fitness professional negligent.

To maximize pool safety, facility managers and program directors must weigh the quantity of program offerings against their quality.

Figure 3.1 **Sample safety checklist for instructors**

Instructors and trainers should take the following preventive measures to protect themselves and participants.

_____ Keep current certification through the YMCA Aquatic Safety Assistant or YMCA Lifeguard course.

_____ Maintain certification in standard first aid and CPR.

_____ Review the pool's emergency action plan, introduce yourself to the lifeguards, and understand how to communicate with rescue staff in an emergency.

_____ Know the location of the rescue equipment and first-aid station.

_____ Do not simultaneously serve as a lifeguard and an instructor.

_____ Understand proper incident reporting.

_____ If your participants include nonswimmers, know who they are and be able to teach them recovery to a stand and how to float in the water.

_____ Learn how to spot signs of panic, active drowning, and passive drowning. Unless you're a trained and certified lifeguard, do not attempt to rescue a drowning person yourself; instead, notify the lifeguards.

_____ As panic often contributes to drowning, encourage people who do not know how to swim to enroll in basic swimming lessons.

_____ Prior to the training session or class, check the decks and pool access for any hazards; also make sure you can easily see the pool bottom and are aware of any "drop-offs" to deeper levels.

_____ Immediately report any hazards you may notice. If a hazard cannot be removed and will interfere with the safety of class participants, do not conduct your training session or class.

_____ Foster open communications with participants to encourage feedback.

_____ Inform participants of the importance of proper footwear: It provides support, protects the soles of the feet, and prevents slipping.

_____ If participants need to wear corrective vision glasses in the pool to see you, encourage them to do so. (**Note:** In some states, glasses made of glass are not allowed. Be sure to check the code in your area.)

_____ If outdoors, have participants face away from the sun so they can see you, and advise them to wear sunscreen, hats or visors, and sunglasses.

_____ Know the policies and procedures for outdoor and indoor pool closure due to inclement weather.

_____ Encourage participants to wear appropriate exercise attire, drink plenty of water, maintain good posture, and work at their own pace.

_____ On deck, use safe demonstration techniques to minimize impact.

_____ Develop good visual cueing skills to spare your voice.

_____ Understand how to use electrical outlets. Stay informed about electrical safety issues and be aware of the danger of electrical shock. (Electrical outlets should be at least 10 feet from the pool.)

_____ Attend in-service training sessions, and practice emergency procedures.

Ensuring Participants' Safety

Although the specter of liability seems threatening, pool standards exist to guarantee public safety and well-being. Making sure that your participants are safe is a very important part of your career as a fitness professional. Understanding the risks and safety issues associated with working in a pool will help you guarantee this safety. Water activity is fun and beneficial, but can be deadly. An ounce of prevention may save a life.

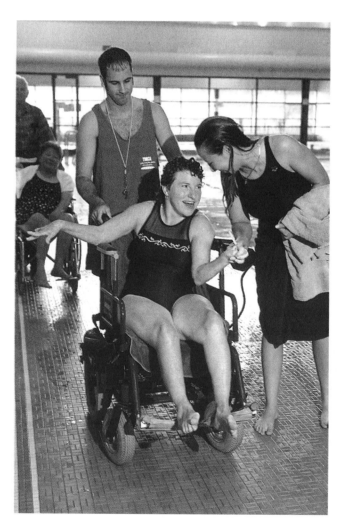

Bibliography

Aerobics and Fitness Association of America. 1994. *Home study program for aqua fitness.* Sherman Oaks, CA: Aerobics and Fitness Association of America.

American Jurisprudence. 1990. *American jurisprudence.* 2nd ed. 62A. Supplement issued April 1997. Rochester, NY: Lawyers Cooperative Publishing.

American Law Reports. 1965. 1. *American law reports.* 3rd ed. Supplements issued August 1997. Rochester, NY: Lawyers Cooperative Publishing and San Francisco: Bancroft-Whitney.

American Law Reports. 1990. 79. *American law reports.* 4th ed. Supplement issued September 1997. Rochester, NY: Lawyers Cooperative Publishing.

American Red Cross. 1993. *CPR for the professional rescuer.* St. Louis, MO: Mosby Lifeline.

American Red Cross. 1995. *Lifeguarding today.* St. Louis, MO: Mosby Lifeline.

Black, H.C. 1990. *Black's law dictionary.* 6th ed. St. Paul, MN: West Publishing.

Champion, W.T. 1990. *Fundamentals of sports law.* Cumulative supplement. Deerfield, IL: Clark Boardman Callaghan.

Champion, W.T. 1996. *Fundamentals of sports law.* Cumulative supplement. Deerfield, IL: Clark Boardman Callaghan.

Diamond, B. 1997. Training water fitness instructors. *IDEA Today* 15(4): 25–29.

Friedman, G.R., and K.J. Worthington. 1992. Accidents in swimming facilities. *Trial* 28: 44.

Official California Appellate Reports. 1993. Vol. 17, 4th series.

Osinski, A. 1996. Playing it safe in the pool. *IDEA Today* 14(3): 39-43.

Sanders, M., and N. Rippee. 1994. *Speedo aquatic fitness system, instructor training manual.* London: Speedo International.

West's Pacific Reporter. 1996. Vols. 478 and 903 Pacific, 2nd series. St. Paul, MN: West Publishing.

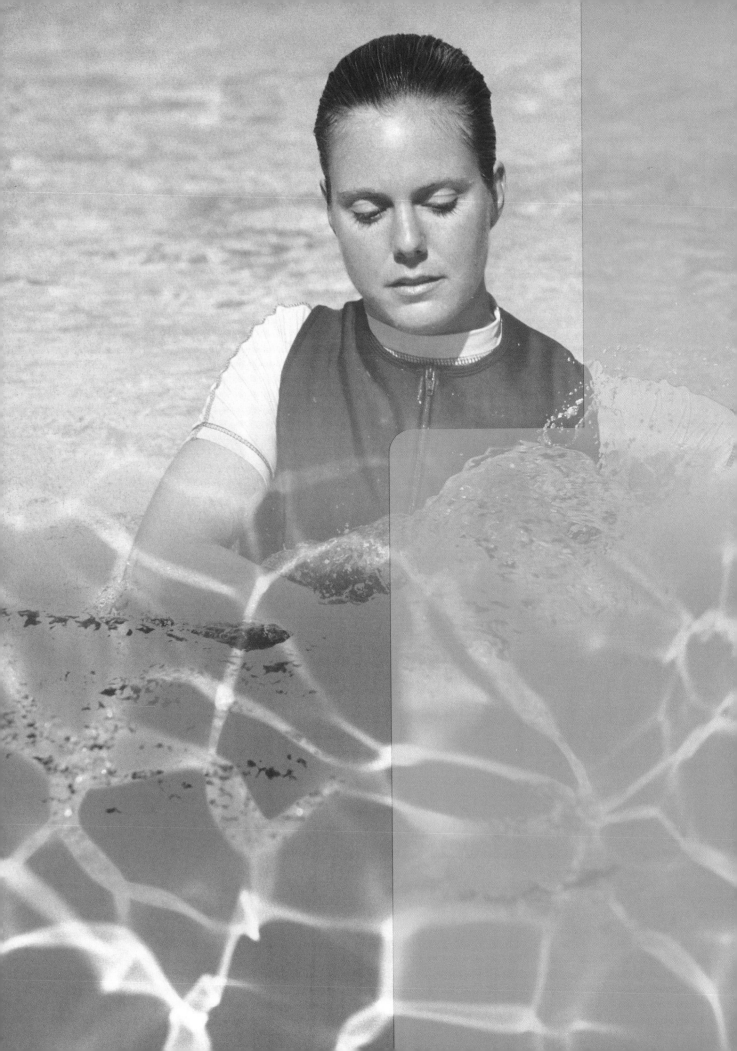

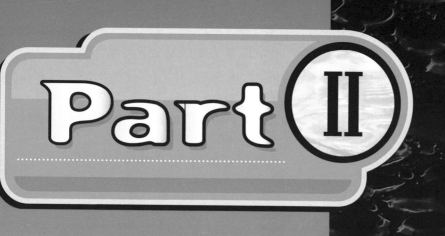

Part II

Healthy Lifestyle and Fitness Principles

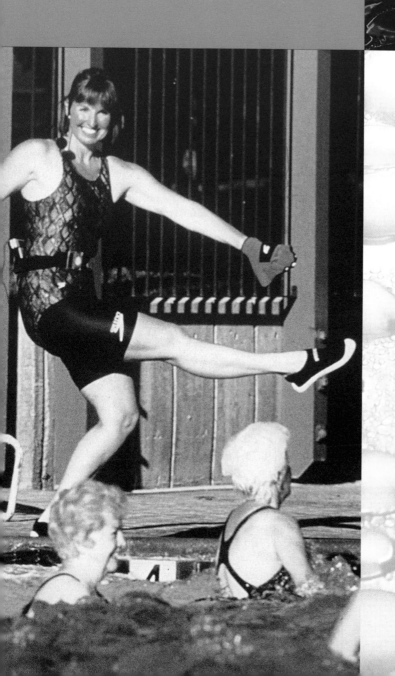

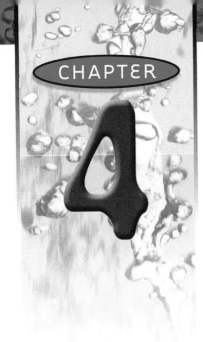

Healthy Lifestyle Principles

CAROL KENNEDY

Objectives:

◎ **To examine the relationship between medical care and wellness education**

◎ **To review present exercise recommendations by the American College of Sports Medicine**

◎ **To identify where water exercise fits in the health care continuum**

◎ **To explore how instructors can project positive body images for their participants**

In order to make a difference in the health and wellness of our participants, we need to have a better understanding of what constitutes a "healthy lifestyle." In the last 10 years, we have heard a great deal of discussion on how much exercise is enough and what the difference is between physical activity and fitness. We also have seen the medical community and businesses become more involved in wellness education. Some people have made fitness a part of their lifestyles, while others have chosen not to. The fitness movement, however, is only a small part of a much larger "wellness revolution" that is occurring in the United States.

This wellness revolution is driven by economics and our quest for a better quality of life. We know it is cost effective to keep people healthy rather than to take care of them when they are sick. Containing medical costs will become even more of a priority as our population ages. The population of the United States, for example, is getting older. It is estimated that by the year 2005, individuals aged 65 and older in the United States will rise to 13 percent of the total population, Japan's to 17 percent, and Germany's to 19 percent. We will continue to have many people in need of medical care. Our job as fitness educators will continue to be that of enhancing quality of life through exercise.

Unfortunately, medical education and training do not tend to emphasize health promotion and wellness. Our physicians are trained in disease treatment, with little emphasis on disease prevention. This is

why it's important for you to be knowledgeable about what constitutes a healthy **fitness program**. You may actually give more advice about fitness than a physician does, because physicians often do not have time to get into the specifics of how to develop a healthy lifestyle. A recommendation by the U.S. Preventive Services Task Force stated that

> the most effective interventions available to clinicians for reducing the incidence and severity of the leading causes of disease and disability in the United States are those that address the personal health practices of patients. Primary prevention as it relates to such risk factors as smoking, physical inactivity, poor nutrition, and alcohol and other drug abuse holds generally greater promise for improving overall health than many secondary preventive measures such as routine screening for early disease. (U.S. Preventive Services Task Force, 1994)

Physicians clearly need more training in the areas of exercise, nutrition, and healthy lifestyles. However, many physicians see their role as one of referring patients to local programs that are already providing preventive health care. This includes your water exercise program; establish a link with your local medical providers so they know that you exist and want to help their patients develop a healthy lifestyle. Becoming partners with medicine is certainly the future of wellness services. Neiman (1999, p. 22) reminds us of some of the positive facts associated with the current wellness revolution:

- **Life expectancy is increasing.** Life expectancy in 1995 was 75.8 years, the highest in our history.

- **Death rates for heart disease are declining.** Between 1950 and 1995 the American death rate for stroke fell 70 percent and for heart disease, 55 percent.

- **Diets are improving.** Americans now consume less fat than at any other time in history.

- **Cigarette consumption is falling.** In 1965, 52 percent of men and 33 percent of women smoked. Now only 25 percent of all Americans smoke.

- **Alcohol consumption is falling.** Alcohol consumption is down due to the public's awareness of the dangers of alcohol.

- **Death rates for the elderly are falling.** In 1984, 12 percent of the population was elderly; by the year 2030 it will be close to 18 percent.

- **The prevalence of high blood pressure and high cholesterol is falling.** The proportion of Americans with these two risk factors is falling.

Neiman (1999, p. 23) also reminds us that even though we have come a long way, we still have a long way to go. He lists the following health promotion concerns for the future:

- **Stress levels are high.** About 60 percent of adults report that they experience moderate to high levels of stress.

- **Cancer death rates are rising.** Although second to heart disease, cancer is a very close second and is related to lifestyle.

- **Too many Americans are obese.** About 35 percent of the adult population is 20 percent or more above desirable body weight.

- **Too many Americans have high blood pressure.** Fifty million Americans suffer from high blood pressure.

- **Too many Americans have high blood cholesterol.** One out of five Americans has blood cholesterol levels above 240 mg/dl.

- **Too many Americans still smoke.** One out of four Americans still smokes, especially those with little education or blue-collar workers.

- **Too few Americans exercise regularly.** Only 15 percent of American adults exercise vigorously.

In the United States we have a great need to improve the integration of wellness into medicine. Currently, reimbursement for preventive services is limited, but when a patient has an illness, the illness is completely covered. Hence, many physicians do not tend to spend a lot of time advising patients on how to improve their lifestyles, as they are usually too busy dealing with illness and getting their patients back to the not ill (sedentary) zone.

As you can see from figure 4.1, there is certainly a great deal more to the continuum than just reaching the not ill, or sedentary, zone. Our job as fitness educators is to try to encourage the right side of the health care continuum. Much of the education on

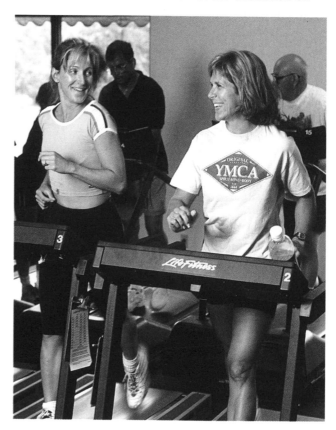

Figure 4.1 *Health care continuum*

Illness·········· Not ill (sedentary)	Physically active ··········· Physically fit ·········· Athletes
(Physicians)	(Fitness educators)

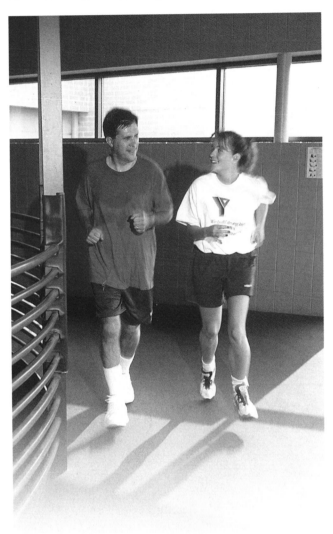

area of fitness/wellness. Our future programming and organizational missions ought to strive to include the 78 percent we may be missing and thus truly impact the health and well-being of our population. Water exercise is an opportunity to bring back many of the 78 percent who have not been able to enjoy exercise. If we want to be recognized for our contribution to the health and wellness of our participants, we need to look at fitness in a broader, more comprehensive way than we ever have.

In 1998, ACSM put forth the following exercise recommendations (ACSM, 1998):

Frequency: Three to five days per week

Intensity: 55/65 percent to 90 percent of maximum heart rate or 40/50 percent to 85 percent of maximum oxygen uptake reserve (otherwise known as maximum heart rate reserve)

Duration: 20 to 60 continuous minutes or 10-minute bouts accumulated throughout the day to equal 20 to 60 minutes

Mode: Walking, running, rowing, stair climbing, aerobics

Resistance: One set of 8 to 12 reps for people under 50 years old; 10 to 15 reps for people over 50 years old

Flexibility: Major muscle groups two to three times a week

Franks, Welsch, and Wood (1997) suggest that guidelines for intensity should differ according to the current activity status of individuals. They recommend that less active individuals or persons with special health or medical needs should start with lower-intensity exercise. For these individuals, the intensity of activity is much less important and should receive little emphasis in recommendations for health and fitness goals. The emphasis for these individuals is to begin and continue regular physical activity at levels that will be included as part of their lifestyles. Increased intensity is recommended for individuals seeking to improve their fitness status or prepare for sport performance.

It's amazing how many more studies there have been in the last 10 years on the benefits of an exercise program. These studies have educated us all and taught us that not only is cardiorespiratory fitness important, but so too is musculoskeletal fitness. In the next segment, we will discuss how these changes have had an impact on water fitness classes.

health and wellness is up to us as we are usually the ones who motivate our participants to enhance their quality of life and not accept the not ill/sedentary zone. Therefore, we will spend some time discussing the current guidelines for fitness for healthy living so you will be better prepared to answer questions on how much exercise is enough for improved health benefits.

Exercise for Healthy Living Recommendations

The *Healthy People 2000* report (Public Health Service, 1991) tells us that fitness programming may only be reaching 22 percent of the population. Therefore, we need to rethink our current program offerings in order to reach a broader group of participants in the

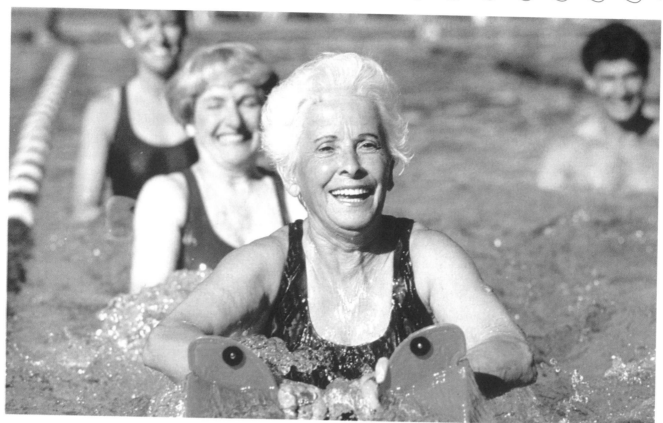

Water Exercise and the Health Care Continuum

Where does water fitness fit in the health care continuum, and why is water exercise increasing in popularity? Many of the health-related components of fitness are enhanced in a water exercise class. The resistance of the water creates appropriate overload for muscular strength and endurance training. The effect of buoyancy and the lack of gravity help enhance flexibility, and moving in the water benefits the cardiorespiratory system. With a land group exercise session, participants need to use external resistance devices such as weights and machines to provide muscular overload and must sit down to stretch effectively so gravity doesn't interfere. Beginners can easily lose motivation because weight-bearing exercise can be difficult for those who are not used to exercising. Therefore, water exercise is an effective and efficient way to improve both health and fitness. In a one-hour session, participants get more quality experiences with movement that will cross over into their daily living activities (Sanders and Maloney-Hills, 1998).

The overall benefits of water exercise lie in the fact that exercise effectiveness is enhanced because partici-

pants are in an upright functional mode. Also, the muscles that are assisted by gravity in daily living are resisted by buoyancy in the water. For example, if on land a person abducts the arms against gravity, the shoulder muscles (deltoids) contract to perform the movement. The middle back (latissimus dorsi) muscles perform adduction but are assisted by gravity so they perform little work. Therefore, the shoulder muscles (deltoids) eccentrically contract against gravity in shoulder adduction. In the water, if a person moves up against the water's resistance and abducts the arms, the shoulder muscles (deltoids) will contract on the abduction phase. If that person moves down with this same movement, the middle back muscles (latissimus dorsi) will contract against buoyancy. Therefore, weaker muscles are automatically worked more in the water. The lack of gravity allows for more muscle balance overall. Even if you don't know all the muscle groups, you will teach a more muscularly balanced class.

Many water exercise movements utilize the stabilizers (abdominals, lower back, and hip and gluteal muscles) of the body as assistors, since almost all movements are performed in an upright position. This functional training helps participants cross over the movements in the water to movements on land.

Improving body image involves changing how we think about our bodies.

For example, if a participant uses a variable resistance weight machine to perform a biceps curl exercise, he or she usually performs the exercise in a seated position. This strengthens the biceps but not the stabilizers. While the participant will get stronger biceps, his or her back may go out because the back muscles have not been trained to assist with the movement. Since water exercise is performed in an upright position, the stabilizers are engaged in all activities.

Now that you have a better understanding of how water fitness instructors play a role in the health care continuum, let's review one other important health issue—body-image acceptance. We, as fitness instructors, have extra pressure to maintain a certain body image because of the nature of our positions. We need to understand how this affects our ability to teach.

Body Image and the Exercise Experience

A survey at a large water fitness national conference (Evans and O'Connor, 1995) on the body-image perceptions of water fitness instructors revealed some of the following statistics: 48 percent of instructors agreed that they constantly worry about being or becoming fat, 36 percent had taken diet pills to control or lose weight, and 83 percent answered yes to the question, "Have you ever restricted your food intake due to concerns about your body size or weight?" Body image is definitely a topic that warrants more discussion by fitness instructors.

In another article by Evans and Kennedy (1993), results of an informal research study of female fitness instructors showed that their average body fat was 20 percent, but 46 percent of them indicated they felt they were very or somewhat overweight. A study (Nardini, Raglin, and Kennedy, 1999) of 148 female fitness instructors found that 64 percent of instuctors perceived an ideal body as one that was thinner than their current body. Olson, Williford, Richards, Brown, and Pugh (1996) also studied female aerobic instructors and found that 40 percent of the instructors indicated a previous experience with eating disorders. This study suggested that aerobic dance instructors possessed scores on the Eating Disorder Inventory suggesting behavior and attitudes consistent with female athletes whose sports emphasize leanness and comparable to those who have eating disorders such as anorexia and bulimia.

Freeman (1988) reminds us that body image is quite independent of physical characteristics. One can feel plain or homely when he or she is really attractive. Because body image and self-esteem are *perceptions*, changing our bodies will not improve our body image or self-esteem unless the physical changes are accompanied by changing perceptions. Improving body image involves changing how we think about our bodies. Changed perceptions must precede physical changes if these changes are to be made in a healthy, loving manner.

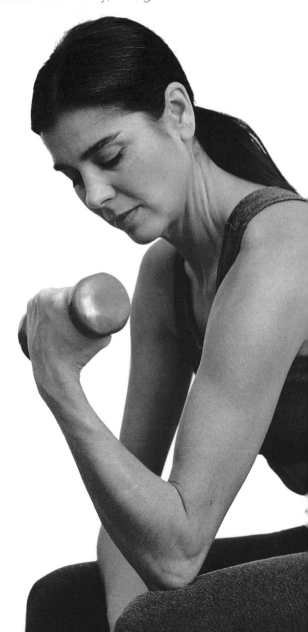

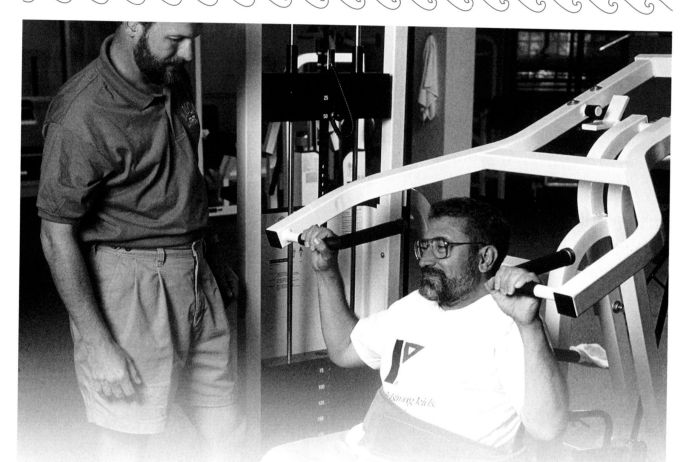

Davis (1994) studied physical activity in the development and maintenance of eating disorders and found that, for a number of anorexic women, sport or exercise is an integral part of the progression toward self-starvation. She suggests that overactivity be viewed as a primary and not secondary symptom for eating disorders. It's important as instructors that we not teach several classes in one day. We will be indirectly telling our participants that overexercising is healthy.

It's easier for us as fitness instructors to overexercise to maintain our weight, but we also often look to dieting as a way to change our body image. Consumer Reports (1993) reviewed all the diets on the market and found that no program is very effective. Dieting to achieve the "ideal fitness instructor" norm could prove to be more harmful than good. A study of the Framingham population (Lissner et al., 1991) found that people who experience frequent weight fluctuations due to dieting have a greater risk for coronary heart disease and death than do people with stable weight.

Gaesser (1997) reminds us that exercising and improving our health are far more important than weighing ourselves on a scale. He encourages us to throw away our scales and put fitness first. McDonald and Thompson (1992) assessed samples of physically active males and females for eating disturbances, body dissatisfaction, self-esteem, and reasons for engaging in exercise. Their results indicate that women's motivation for exercise is more often related to weight and tone than is the case for men. However, exercising for health is positively associated with self-esteem for both sexes.

Bain, Wilson, and Chaikind (1989) performed a research study on overweight women in an organized exercise program. They found that 35 percent of the overweight and only 7 percent of the normal-weight participants dropped out. They noted that although factors such as safety, comfort, and quality of instruction affected the women's exercise behaviors, the most powerful influences seemed to be the social circumstances of the exercise setting, especially concerns about visibility, embarrassment, and judgment by others. We spend a great deal of time on how to effectively format our water exercise sessions. We also need to think about how comfortable our participants are in our environment, as well as how comfortable we are with our own body image. If we are comfortable, we will be able to make our students comfortable. If we mention how unhappy we are with our body images, this will most certainly affect our participants as well.

Evans (1993) recommends the following methods for enhancing participant and instructor body-image perceptions:

- Wear professional instructor attire; for example, wear a one-piece suit with tights, which is less intimidating than a two-piece bathing suit.
- Display body-image educational materials at strategic locations.
- Use positive motivational strategies. For instance, promote participants' independence and responsibility for themselves by encouraging activity outside of class.
- Choose class music that sends a positive message.

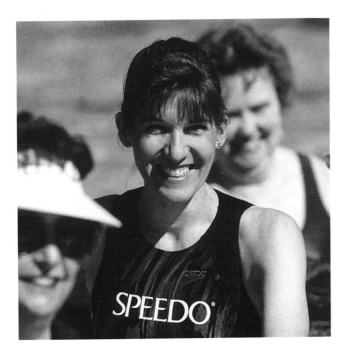

We live in a culture in the United States in which a thin and toned body is seen as the ideal. According to Ibbetson (1996), we all accept the "thinness-is-beauty" ideal to the point that body-image dissatisfaction is remarkably high. Some researchers indicate that body-image disturbance is so prevalent that it can be considered a normal part of the female experience (Silberstein, Striegel-Moore, and Rodin, 1987). It is definitely our choice; we can choose to either buy into the media and societal pressures or portray a normal, healthy example to our participants.

Bibliography

ACSM (American College of Sports Medicine). 1998. The recommended quantity and quality of exercise for developing and maintaining cardiorespiratory and muscular fitness and flexibility in healthy adults. *Medicine and Science in Sports and Exercise* 30(6): 975–991.

Bain, L., T. Wilson, and E. Chaikind. 1989. Participant perceptions of exercise programs for overweight women. *Research Quarterly* 60(2): 134–143.

Blair, S., H. Kohl, C. Barlow, R. Paffenbarger, L. Gibbons, and C. Macera. 1995. Changes in physical fitness and all-cause mortality. *JAMA* 273(14): 1093–1098.

Consumer Reports. 1993. Losing weight: What works and what doesn't. *Consumer Reports* (June): 343–357.

Davis, C. 1994. The role of physical activity in the development and maintenance of eating disorders. *Psychological Medicine* 24: 957–967.

Dishman, R. 1982. Compliance/adherence in health-related exercise. *Health Psychology* 1: 237–267.

Evans, E. 1993. Body image: Programming for a healthy perspective. *NIRSA Journal* (Fall): 46–51.

Evans, E., and C. Kennedy. 1993. The body image problem in the fitness industry. *IDEA Today* (May): 50–56.

Evans, E., and O'Connor, P. 1995. Body image of water aerobics instructors. *Medicine and Science in Sports and Exercise* 27(5): Abstract 852.

Feigenbaum, M., and M. Pollock. 1997. Strength training: Rationale for current guidelines for adult fitness programs. *Physician and Sports Medicine* 25(2): 44–64.

Franks, D., M. Welsch, and R. Wood. 1997. Physical activity intensity: How much is enough? *ACSM Journal Health & Fitness* 1(6): 14–19.

Freeman, R. 1988. *Bodylove: Learning to like our looks and ourselves.* New York: Harper-Collins.

Gaesser, G. 1997. *Big fat lies.* New York: Fawcett Columbine.

Godin, G., P. Valois, R.J. Shephard, and R. Desharnais. 1987. Prediction of leisure-time exercise behavior: A path analysis (LISREL V) model. *Journal of Behavioral Medicine.* 10: 145–158.

Haskell, W. 1994. Health consequences of physical activity: Understanding and challenges regarding dose-response. *Medicine and Science in Sports and Exercise* 26(6): 649–660.

Ibbetson, J. 1996. Body image and self-esteem: Factors that affect each and recommendations for fitness professionals. *NIRSA Journal* (Fall): 22–27.

Lissner, L., P. Odell, R. D'Agostino, J. Stokes, B. Kreger, A. Belanger, and K. Brownell. 1991. Variability of body weight and health outcomes in the Framingham population. *The New England Journal of Medicine* 324: 1839–1844.

McDonald, K., and J.K. Thompson. 1992. Eating disturbance, body image dissatisfaction, and reasons for exercising: Gender differences and correlational findings. *International Journal of Eating Disorders* (11)3: 289–292.

Nardini, M., J. Raglin, and C. Kennedy. 1999. Body image, disordered eating, obligatory exercise and body composition among women fitness instructors. *Medicine and Science in Sports and Exercise* 31(5): Supplement, S297, 1472.

Neiman, D. 1999. *Fitness and sports medicine, a health-related approach.* 4th ed. Mountain View, CA: Mayfield Publishing.

Olson, M., H. Williford, L. Richards, J. Brown, and S. Pugh. 1996. Self-reports on the Eating Disorder Inventory by female aerobic instructors. *Perceptual and Motor Skills* 82: 1051–1058.

Pate, R., M. Pratt, S. Blair, W. Haskell, C. Macera, C. Bouchard, D. Buchner, W. Ettinger, G. Heath, A. King, A. Kriska, A. Leon, B. Marcus, J. Morris, R. Paffenbarger, K. Patrick, M. Pollock, J. Rippe, J. Sallis, and J. Wilmore. 1995. Physical activity and public health: A recommendation from the Centers for Disease Control and Prevention and the American College of Sports Medicine. *JAMA* 273(5): 402–407.

Public Health Service, U.S. Department of Health and Human Services. 1991. *Healthy People 2000: National health promotion and disease prevention objectives.* Washington, DC: U.S. Printing Office, DHHS Publication No. (PHS) 91-50212.

Sallis, J., M. Hovell, and C. Hofstetter, 1989. A multivariate study of determinants of vigorous exercise in a community sample. *Prev Med.* 18: 20–34.

Sanders, M., and C. Maloney-Hills. 1998. Aquatic exercise for better living on land. *ACSM's Health & Fitness Journal,* 2(3): 16–23.

Silberstein, L.R., R.H. Striegel-Moore, and J. Rodin. 1987. *Feeling fat: A woman's shame.* Hillsdale, NJ: Lawrence Erlbaum Associates.

U.S. Preventive Services Task Force. 1994. *Guide to clinical preventive services.* Alexandria, VA: International Medical Publishing.

5

Fitness Principles

Objectives:

◎ **To identify exercise science and training principles of cardiorespiratory endurance training**

◎ **To define key terms and concepts relating to anatomy and biomechanics**

I n order to respond to our students' desire to improve their health and fitness, we need to understand how the body works, whether we are training on the land or in the water. This chapter introduces some basic concepts of exercise science and training for cardiorespiratory endurance, as well as anatomy and biomechanics, so you can better understand how to help your participants train safely and effectively. Becoming familiar with the terminology related to each body system also helps you understand fitness information and communicate with your participants.

Exercise Science and Training Principles of Cardiorespiratory Endurance Training

All **aerobic** or **cardiorespiratory endurance** activities have the following common elements:

- They place a demand on the cardiorespiratory (cardio = heart; respiratory = lungs) system.
- They use large muscle groups.
- They predominantly use the aerobic (with oxygen) energy system (see later section on energy systems).
- They are rhythmic in nature.
- They can be safely performed at a moderate level of intensity.

Examples of aerobic activities include swimming, walking, jogging (on the land and in the water), running, cycling, stair climbing, and aerobic dance/ group exercise.

If performed continuously for 20 minutes or more, aerobic activities prompt adaptations, or **training**

responses, within the cardiorespiratory, muscular, energy, and nervous systems. Understanding how these systems adapt can help you

- realize the importance of individualized fitness,
- plan safe and beneficial workouts,
- understand training benefits gained from aerobics classes,
- answer questions concerning exercise, and
- react logically to injuries or emergencies.

Before you can understand how a system responds to exercise, you need a basic understanding of how that system functions at rest; otherwise, you may misinterpret some of the physiological changes it undergoes. For example, during moderate exercise, the heart beats around 150 beats per minute (bpm). This heart rate may sound dangerously high to someone who does not know that the average **resting heart rate** is around 68 to 72 bpm. At a moderate level of exercise, the amount of blood pumped through the heart per minute (cardiac output) increases to 15 liters (15.9 quarts), which

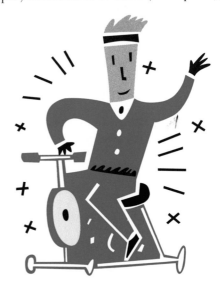

is three times the cardiac output at rest. The demands placed on these systems during exercise are much greater than those placed on them at rest.

The body's adaptations to exercise can be studied at three general levels:

- Changes at the cellular (biochemical) level, for example, the changes within the muscle cells during different types of exercise. Understanding these responses provides insight about energy production and other chemical processes.

- Changes in the body's systems, for example, the amount of blood being pumped per minute to various sites in the body.

- Other considerations, for example, the influence of environmental factors (such as exercising in the heat and cold) or changes in body composition (fat weight versus lean weight).

To relate every known or probable response to aerobics at each of these levels would take volumes. Your task is to select those pieces of information from exercise physiology that are most applicable to designing your program. Not gathering enough information may mean that you will not offer the best program possible or that you will fail to adjust the level of exercise to each individual's needs. Yet if you tried to learn everything known about exercise, you would not have time left to lead your classes. A fair compromise, then, is to become familiar with how the major body systems function at rest as well as during fitness classes.

The next section examines the resting functions of the major body systems most involved in exercise. Let's begin by looking at the cardiorespiratory system.

Cardiorespiratory System

The cardiorespiratory system is actually comprised of two systems—the heart and its vessels (the cardiovascular system) and the lungs (the respiratory system). Let's take a look at each component.

Cardiovascular System

The heart's function is to pump blood through the body. The pressure of the heartbeat forces the blood to flow in a continuous, traceable route. This path is shown in figure 5.1. Blood enters the right atrium

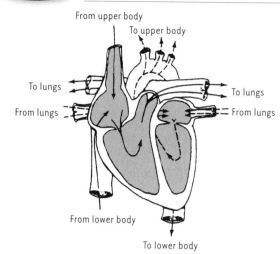

Figure 5.1 **Path of blood flow through the heart**

(RA), which is a thin-walled storage compartment that receives blood returning to the heart. The blood is forced by atrial contraction through the tricuspid valve into the right ventricle (RV). The ventricles are the heart's pumping chambers and comprise most of the heart's muscle mass. The right ventricle pumps blood through the pulmonary valve into the pulmonary artery and to the lungs. After oxygen and carbon dioxide have been exchanged in the lungs, the blood returns to the left atrium (LA) through the pulmonary veins. Left atrial contraction forces blood through the mitral valve into the left ventricle (LV). From the left ventricle, blood is pumped through the aortic valve and on through the body.

Cardiac Output

The volume of blood the heart pumps per minute is referred to as the cardiac output. This volume is expressed in liters (L) or milliliters (ml) of blood pumped per minute (min). The symbol $\dot{Q}$ is often used to represent cardiac output in scientific literature or in tables of data. Cardiac output is calculated as the stroke volume (SV, the amount of blood pumped out of the left ventricle in one beat) times the heart rate (HR):

$$\dot{Q} \text{ (ml/min)} = SV \text{ (ml/beat)} \times HR \text{ (beats/min)}$$

Your cardiac output changes in proportion to the degree of your activity. The average cardiac output of a person lying down in a state of complete rest is approximately 5 L/min. Walking would raise the cardiac output to about 7.5 L/min. Strenuous exercise might raise it to as much as 25 L/min or as high as 35 L/min in a highly trained athlete (Guyton, 1974).

The heart has a maximum rate at which it can pump. Within physiological limits, the heart pumps all of the blood that flows into it at a rate that prevents excessive damming of the blood in the veins. The amount of blood that the heart can pump each minute depends on two major factors: the heart's pumping effectiveness and the ease with which blood can flow through the body and return to the heart.

Blood Pressure

As the heart's left ventricle contracts, blood is forced into the systemic arteries, creating pressure. This pressure can be measured in the larger arteries of the body. Blood pressure varies from person to person and from one measurement to the next in the same person. For example, your blood pressure is higher when you stand than when you sit, and it is much higher during aerobic exercise than when you are at rest.

Despite individual variations, there is a range of normal values for blood pressure. In a blood pressure ratio reading, such as 120/80 (read "120 over 80"), the top number is the systolic pressure. This number (in this case, 120) represents the pressure resulting from the force of ventricular contraction as blood is pumped out of the heart. The bottom number of the ratio (80 in this example) is the diastolic pressure, which represents the pressure in the arteries during the filling of the atria. The example of 120/80 is an average value for normal blood pressure. Mild hypertension is considered to be between 140/90 and 160/95. High blood pressure, or hypertension, is defined by a value greater than 160/95. Regular aerobic exercise may help reduce elevated blood pressure.

Redistribution of Blood Flow

The body has a priority system for the amount of blood each of its parts receives. When the body is at rest, the major organs receive the most blood (see table 5.1). During exercise, however, there is a shift of priorities, or a redistribution, to supply adequate blood to the large muscle groups of the arms and legs.

Heart Rate

During rest, the average heart beats 68 to 72 times a minute. This value would be lower, however, for a regular participant in exercise class. Heredity and age are additional factors that influence heart rate. A higher aerobic capacity (i.e., ability to perform continuous exercise) can be genetically determined; also, as a person gets older, aerobic capacity begins to decrease at a rate that correlates with fitness level.

Each person in your class may be at a different level of aerobic fitness. Sometimes you can designate the level of instruction (e.g., beginning, intermediate, or advanced) for a class. More likely, though, your class will include individuals with a wide range of cardiorespiratory fitness levels. (Even if you do offer specialized classes based on fitness levels, participants do not always evaluate their levels of fitness accurately.) Your job, then, becomes one of challenging the fit person while at the same time pacing the less experienced beginner. Old-timers, on the one hand, in advanced fitness categories may be overachievers who tend to push their bodies too far. Beginners, on the other hand, may have cardiorespiratory capabilities that have not been stressed for a long time. To maintain safety, you need to help all participants monitor their heart rate responses to your workouts so that they do not attempt too much or too little in trying to achieve the desired training benefits.

In order to handle the increased workload that vigorous physical activity places on the heart, participants

Table 5.1   Approximated Shift of Blood Flow From Rest to Exercise

Site	% of flow during rest	% of flow during exercise
Skin	5	10
Bone	5	1
Brain	15	6
Heart	5	5
Liver, stomach, and intestines	30	5
Kidneys	25	3
Skeletal muscles	15	70

Note: Data from *Textbook of Work Physiology* (3rd ed., p. 152) by P.O. Åstrand and K. Rodahl, 1986, New York: McGraw-Hill. Copyright 1986 by McGraw-Hill.

Figure 5.2 — Borg perceived exertion scale

6	No exertion at all
7	
8	Extremely light
9	Very light
10	
11	Light
12	
13	Somewhat hard
14	
15	Hard (heavy)
16	
17	Very hard
18	
19	Extremely hard
20	Maximal exertion

Borg RPE scale
© Gunnar Borg, 1970, 1985, 1984, 1998

must slowly begin to train the heart to progressively handle a little more work each time they exercise. This gives it time to adapt to pumping faster and to supplying larger amounts of blood to the needed areas. Eventually, each participant's heart will be able to perform at an increased workload with ease. This gradual progression in performance and in giving the heart (and lungs) time to adapt to the added stress is what becoming aerobically fit is all about.

Using heart rates in water as we do on land to determine exercise intensity is difficult. Land rates and methods do not translate directly to water. In chapter 6, we'll discover that research indicates that water heart rates do not accurately predict exercise intensity. It's difficult to take an accurate heart rate in water due to wide variations in water depth and temperature. For these reasons, we'll focus attention on other methods that are more accurate.

An alternative method of determining exercise intensity that has been shown to be accurate in the pool is the rating of perceived exertion (RPE) scale. Based on a subjective determination of how hard they are working, participants rate their efforts on a scale of 6 to 20. This scale, originally developed in 1970 and then revised in 1984, 1985, and 1998 by Gunnar Borg, has proved to be both valid and reliable. The scale is shown in figure 5.2.

RPE can be used either alone or in combination with a heart rate monitor to assess exercise intensity. It is particularly valuable for participants who take medication that affects their heart rate.

Another method of checking the level of exercise intensity is the "talk test." This simply means that an exerciser should be able to talk easily to someone during a workout. If the exerciser can't because of lack of breath, the level of intensity is too high and should be lowered.

If participants still want to use heart rate as an additional indicator of exercise intensity, they can use a heart rate monitor. Participants can easily determine their predicted land rate by using the chart included with the monitor, then adjust it for water. Research suggests that the land range rates be adjusted to deep water rates by decreasing the numbers 12 to 15 beats per minute. In shallow water (navel to nipple depth), when water temperatures are approximately 84 degrees F (29 degrees C), the land rates on the monitor chart can be used without modification.

Table 5.2 shows the advantages and disadvantages of using heart rate, RPE, and the talk test for monitoring water fitness exercisers.

Respiratory System

The cardiovascular system is only half of the cardiorespiratory system; the lungs are the other half. The lungs' main function is to aerate blood. During exercise, as well as during rest, carbon dioxide and oxygen are continually exchanged between the tiny air sacs of the lungs and the capillaries of the cardiovascular system. This exchange route can be traced as follows.

Air is inhaled through the nose or mouth and

Figure 5.3 — The tubular structure of the lungs

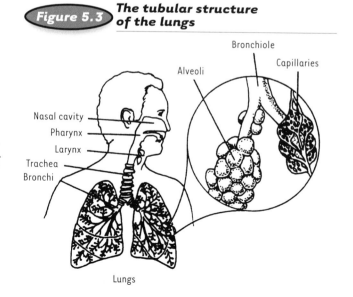

Bronchiole
Capillaries
Alveoli
Nasal cavity
Pharynx
Larynx
Trachea
Bronchi
Lungs

Table 5.2   *The Pros and Cons of Using THR, RPE, and the Talk Test*

THR—Target heart rate (using a heart rate monitor)

Pros

1. Indicates a definite increase in workload or heart rate (as long as it is linked to a metabolic load, that is, an aerobic activity).
2. Is the most accurate method for land exercise: a 10-s pulse count is accurate within 6 beats per minute (bpm). For water, a 6-s pulse count may be more accurate due to rapid heart rate changes because of cool water temperature.
3. May work better for inexperienced exercisers especially if heart rate monitors are used.

Cons

1. External factors, such as temperature and buoyancy, may affect heart rate.
2. Heart rate may not accurately reflect intensity. Lower rates may "push" participants to overwork.
3. Concepts may not be easily explained or understood. A heart rate chart with adjusted rates should be easily accessible for reference.

RPE—Rate of perceived exertion

Pros

1. Concept is easy to understand and explain based on the 6 to 20 scale.
2. Continuity of exercise need not be interrupted.
3. Is appropriate for experienced exercisers.
4. Provides effective means of determining anaerobic threshold.
5. Trains exercisers to become aware of how they feel while exercising.

Cons

1. Untrained exercisers may perceive effort at a higher rate than their heart rate would indicate.
2. Measurement is subjective.
3. Requires practice.

Talk Test

Pros

1. Can easily identify personal threshold.
2. Stimulates social interaction.
3. Puts exercisers in touch with how they feel.

Cons

1. Measurement is subjective.
2. Is least accurate (best when used in combination with THR and/or RPE methods).

Source: Liz Chicado

travels down an elaborate system of elastic tubing (see figure 5.3). The trachea divides into bronchi that, in turn, branch into smaller tubes. These tubes (bronchioles) continue to branch until they become microscopic air sacs known as alveoli, which are surrounded by capillaries. The alveoli are extremely thin-walled structures that allow a rapid exchange of oxygen (O_2) and carbon dioxide (CO_2).

As you saw in figure 5.1, the vascular arrangement between the heart and lungs is quite simple. The right ventricle pumps blood into the pulmonary artery. The blood then flows through the pulmonary artery, finally arriving at the pulmonary capillaries that surround the alveoli. The exchange of gases takes place due to the high concentration of these gases in the alveoli and in the surrounding capillaries. The alveoli have a high concentration of oxygen, whereas the capillaries (because they are carrying blood that has already circulated and delivered oxygen throughout the body) have a high concentration of carbon dioxide (see figure 5.4). After the gases are exchanged, the blood flows back

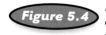

Figure 5.4 *Exchange of carbon dioxide and oxygen between the alveoli and capillaries*

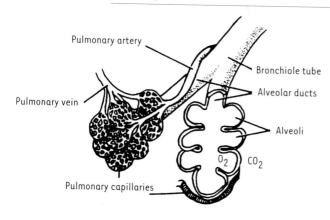

through the pulmonary veins and eventually back into the left atrium. From there the blood flows into the left ventricle to the aortic valve and on through the body. The blood delivers oxygen to all body cells, and carbon dioxide is blown off with every exhalation in the lungs.

Aerobic training improves the ability of the heart and lungs to perform this teamwork task of taking in oxygen and delivering it to the working muscles during exercise.

Effectiveness of Aerobic Training

Participants in group exercise classes are often curious as to how aerobically fit they are compared with participants in other activities. Research has shown that aerobics is a legitimate training method to increase aerobic capacity. Understanding oxygen consumption will help you begin to see what aerobic fitness is all about. The term for the quantity of oxygen used by the body is oxygen consumption. Of the many factors that affect oxygen consumption, three of the most important are the following:

- **Oxygen transport.** This is how much oxygen the blood can carry.
- **Oxygen delivery.** This is how much oxygen can get to the active cells.
- **Oxygen use.** This is how much oxygen the cells can extract from the blood passing by them.

The amount of oxygen being used per minute by an exerciser is another way (such as monitoring the heart rate) of determining the intensity at which a person is working out. Oxygen consumption, or $\dot{V}O_2$ as it is symbolically written, is traditionally measured in liters of oxygen consumed per minute

(a dot above the V denotes a per-minute measurement). $\dot{V}O_2$ comparisons can be made among persons of different sizes, as $\dot{V}O_2$ measurements are divided by body weight.

A $\dot{V}O_2$ measurement, therefore, is expressed as milliliters of oxygen per kilogram (1 kg = 2.2 lb) of body weight per minute, or ml/kg/min. The amount of oxygen being consumed at rest (for example, by sitting and reading this book) is approximately 3.5 to 4.5 ml/kg/min. Depending on the pace or intensity of the exercise being performed, this resting value can increase to 42 ml/kg/min or more. To determine the intensity of exercise for an individual based on $\dot{V}O_2$, his or her **maximal oxygen consumption** ($\dot{V}O_2$max) must also be known. $\dot{V}O_2$max—the maximal amount of oxygen that can be used per minute—is usually determined in a laboratory setting by a maximal stress test. A typical test involves walking, jogging, or running (depending on the individual's level of fitness) on a treadmill under the supervision of a team led by an exercise physiologist. Once a person's $\dot{V}O_2$max is known, his or her $\dot{V}O_2$ during exercise can be calculated as a percentage of the $\dot{V}O_2$max.

While maximal oxygen consumption increases as one's level of fitness rises, it is also influenced by age and heredity. For example, after the age of 30, there is a slow but progressive loss of aerobic capacity—by the age of 65 it may have declined 35 percent. Also, some individuals inherit larger aerobic capacities and therefore are able to train at higher performance levels.

Linear Relationship Between Heart Rate and Oxygen Consumption

Measuring the amount of an exerciser's oxygen use per minute is obviously not as convenient as measuring his or her heart rate per minute. However, research on aerobic exercise has shown that the two values increase and decrease as a pair. In other words, as the heart rate goes up, so does the amount of oxygen being consumed. This linear relationship makes many aerobic fitness measurement calculations possible. For example, if you are working at a certain heart rate during aerobic exercise, it is possible to estimate the amount of oxygen you are using even without the elaborate equipment necessary to measure oxygen consumption. For example, a heart rate of 100 beats per minute (light work) is accompanied by a $\dot{V}O_2$ of approximately 10 ml/kg/min, while a heart rate of 135 (moderate work) denotes a $\dot{V}O_2$ of approximately 20 ml/kg/min

The linear relationship between heart rate and oxygen consumption for aerobic exercises

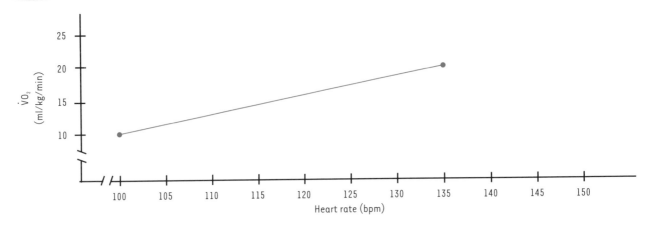

(see figure 5.5). This linear relationship is not true, however, for anaerobic exercise (such as weightlifting or sprinting), in which the heart rate may increase much more than the $\dot{V}O_2$.

To convert a liter of oxygen to ml/kg/min, you need to know the person's body weight. For the sake of standardizing examples, exercise physiologists have created and use what are known as the reference man and reference woman. The reference man weighs 70 kg and the reference woman, 58 kg. So, a $\dot{V}O_2$ of 20 ml/kg/min with a heart rate of 135 can be converted for a woman to 1,160 ml/min (i.e., 20×58) or 1.16 L/min and for a man to 1,400 ml/min (i.e., 20×70) or 1.4 L/min.

Caloric Cost of Aerobics

Another interesting physiological relationship is between oxygen consumption and the number of calories (kcal) expended during exercise. Elementary math teaches us that certain units of measurement can be converted into others; for example, 12 inches equal 1 foot, and 3 teaspoons equal 1 tablespoon. Likewise, the amount of oxygen being consumed during exercise can be converted into the amount of calories being used per minute. For example, when 1 liter of oxygen is used, approximately 5 kcal are expended. Hence, a woman exercising at a moderate pace with a heart rate of 135 beats per minute, using approximately 20 ml/kg/min (1.16 L/min), would expend approximately 5.8 kcal a minute. A man using approximately 1.4 L/min would expend about 7.0 kcal per minute.

Exercise physiologists use this energy conversion to calculate the approximate number of calories expended in aerobic exercise. Most studies confirm

that working out at a moderate intensity in your training heart rate range will expend between six and eight calories per minute during aerobic exercise. Table 5.3 shows an estimated caloric expenditure for some water and land fitness activities.

Muscular System

Regardless of how well the cardiorespiratory system might function, no one could move were it not for the muscles and their phenomenal ability to contract. Each muscle has tough, fibrous ends called *tendons* that attach the muscles to bone. The middle (belly) of the muscle is thick. If you cut through the belly of the muscle and look inside, you would see something similar to what is depicted in figure 5.6.

Skeletal muscle is comprised of millions of individual contractile fibers that are bound together in groups called *bundles*. Each muscle fiber is wrapped in connective tissue called the *endomysium*. Just inside and attached to the endomysium is the *sarcolemma*, or cell membrane.

Estimated Caloric Expenditure for Selected Land and Water Activities

Activity	Calories/min
Aquatic exercise	5.7–6.5
Aerobic dance on land	6.2–6.6
Running 11 min/mile on land	8.0
Deep water walking	8.8
Deep water running	11.5

Source: Kravitz, L., and Mayo, J. 1997. Aquatic exercise: A review. AKWA *Letter.* October/November.

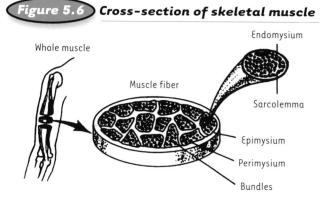

Figure 5.6 *Cross-section of skeletal muscle*

Whole muscle

Muscle fiber

Endomysium

Sarcolemma

Epimysium

Perimysium

Bundles

The bundles of fibers are encased in a sheath (*perimysium*) of connective tissue that could be compared to plastic wrap wrapped snugly around a piece of meat. Encasing all of the bundles, and hence the whole muscle, is another sheath known as the *epimysium*. The muscle fibers are richly supplied with capillaries that weave in and out of them much like the threads in cloth.

It is within the microscopic muscle fiber (cell) that the vital functions of contraction, the exchange of oxygen and carbon dioxide with the capillaries, and energy production take place. The fibers' ability to perform these functions is enhanced by regular aerobic activity.

Muscular Fitness

Muscular fitness has three subcomponents:

- strength,
- endurance, and
- flexibility.

Muscular strength is defined as the maximum force a muscle or muscle group can exert for a brief period of time. The result of strength exercises is an increase in the size of the muscle or muscle group. The enlargement of a muscle group is known as *hypertrophy*. This increase in size results mostly from an increase in the size of the muscle fibers themselves. In some animals that have been trained with weights, researchers have noted an increase in the number of fibers comprising the muscle, but this observation has yet to be substantiated in humans.

Muscular endurance is the ability of a muscle or muscle group to continue to exert force without fatiguing. Endurance is increased by gradually increasing the repetitions (more than 10) of an exercise. For example, performing 25 sit-ups demonstrates endurance of the abdominal muscles. You can help participants increase their strength and endurance by including the proper type and number of repetitions of calisthenic exercises during the warm-up and cool-down.

The body's ability to bend and stretch is its flexibility, which can be increased by gradual stretching of the muscles and tendons. Most instructors teach participants to perform flexibility exercises *statically*, by reaching and holding a stretch for 10 to 30 seconds or so, rather than *ballistically*, by reaching and bouncing for a shorter count of 8 or 10. The preferred method according to exercise scientists is static stretching. The bouncing movement of ballistic stretching can result in a reflexive action of the muscle that causes it to tighten. This, of course, defeats the purpose of a nice, slow, full stretch. Bouncing may also cause microscopic tears in muscle tissue. So please, do not bounce to the beat while stretching. Select music for your stretching exercises that doesn't encourage moving to a beat. Remind your class to relax, to stretch, to hold, to breathe, but *not* to bounce.

Stretching in cool water can be challenging. When water temperatures are too cool to maintain body warmth during static stretching, try including controlled dynamic stretches. *Dynamic stretching* consists of rhythmic actions that mimic an activity, such as walking. Each movement is gradually increased from small to larger motions, such as starting with small steps and gradually increasing their size. In water, these movements can be controlled because of buoyancy and resistance, reducing the risk of injury that might be a problem on land. Enlarging a movement gradually with control can improve dynamic flexibility and improve participants' range of motion during movements.

Another cool water option is to coordinate upper- and lower-body movements to increase body heat. For example, if the participants are holding a static stretch for the upper body, have them jog or walk gently to keep warm. During a lower-body stretch, have participants scull with their arms to generate heat. To balance body warmth, have participants alternate upper-body stretches and jogging with static lower-body stretches.

Do not ask participants to stretch when they feel chilled. If necessary, they can warm up by getting into a whirlpool or taking a warm shower, then stretch on land.

Individuals in your class will probably vary greatly in their degrees of flexibility. The amount of flexibility at

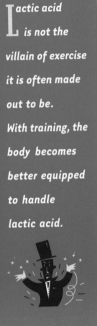

a joint is a reflection of the joint capsule, the muscle, the tendons, and the ligaments that comprise the joint. Encourage safe (static) or gentle range-of-motion stretching practices and individual achievement.

Teach participants a series of total stretching exercises that they can use any time. Doing stretching exercises can be a welcome relief from long hours of sitting.

Energy Production Systems

For some, energy is a rather abstract word. Everyone has it, makes it, and uses it, but we often describe it differently. All of the energy in our solar system originates from the sun. Solar energy reaches the Earth as sunlight. The millions of green plants that grow on the Earth store some of that solar energy as chemical energy and use it to produce their food. Unfortunately, people cannot produce their own food in such a manner, and we must eat plants and animals for our energy supply. The food we eat does not supply the energy we need directly. Instead, it is changed chemically into usable nutrients. These nutrients are distributed throughout the body, with some being stored as an energy compound in cells. This energy-rich compound stored within the muscle cells is adenosine triphosphate, commonly referred to as ATP.

The energy that muscles use for contraction is made within the muscle cells. How the energy is made and how fast it is produced depend on the type of activity being performed and on the person's level of physical fitness.

Anaerobic Energy Production

During rest, as well as exercise, movement can occur as long as ATP is available at the site of muscle contraction. ATP, however, is available only in very limited amounts, so it must continually be broken down and resynthesized within the muscle cells. Three different energy systems that are capable of resynthesizing ATP have been identified in the body. Two of these systems do not require oxygen to be present to produce ATP. They are called **anaerobic** energy-producing systems and include the ATP-PC and the lactic acid systems. These systems supply energy for short-term, high-intensity exercise. A slower system requiring oxygen to be present is the aerobic energy system. All three systems

actually go into operation during muscle contraction. The amount of energy needed to sustain an activity and the activity's duration denote which system will produce the predominant amount of energy to sustain that activity.

As you begin to work out vigorously, there is a temporary shortage of oxygen being delivered to the working muscles. The energy for the first 2 to 3 minutes of a workout is predominantly supplied anaerobically. The skeletal muscles are prepared to produce energy for approximately 2 to 3 minutes without oxygen. Because an aerobic exercise workout lasts for 45 to 60 minutes, the energy is predominantly supplied aerobically.

A popular term you may have heard related to anaerobic energy production is lactic acid. **Lactic acid**, or lactate, is a by-product of producing energy anaerobically. When lactic acid accumulates to high levels in the blood it causes muscular fatigue. However, the first few minutes of exercise, as well as any change of pace during the workout, would be hindered without the anaerobic energy system and its accompanying lactic acid production.

Lactic acid is not the villain of exercise it is often made out to be. With training, the body becomes better equipped to handle lactic acid. Several efficient changes occur in the body during training that result in decreased production of lactic acid and increased removal of it from the bloodstream.

Aerobic Energy Production

Group exercise classes usually last for 45 to 60 minutes. All of the movements/exercises are performed at a submaximal level of performance, meaning that you work out at an intensity below an all-out, sprinting kind of pace. Because the exercise is submaximal, the cardiorespiratory system has plenty of time to deliver the needed oxygen to the working muscles. Thus, the energy for aerobic exercise is predominantly supplied aerobically.

Aerobic exercise at varying intensity (heart rate) and duration (length of the workout) trains the energy systems as well as all the other systems. Training the aerobic energy system requires gradually increasing the amount of time spent doing an activity to give the energy system time to adapt to meeting its new demands.

Figure 5.7 *The central nervous system*

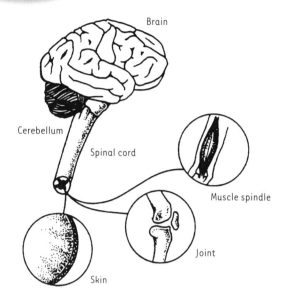

Figure 5.8 *The heart's electrical system*

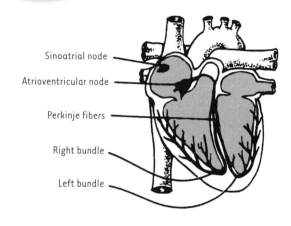

Central Nervous System

What makes the cardiorespiratory system adjust its activity rate from rest to exercise? What makes muscles contract and relax at the right time? Somehow messages must be sent throughout the body to get these systems to speed up or slow down correctly. The main switchboard that organizes these electrical messages is the central nervous system, comprised of the brain and the spinal cord (see figure 5.7). Millions of nerves of varying sizes branch off from the spinal cord and spread much like blood vessels that continually branch out from the main arteries and veins. This network of nerves throughout the body allows you to react to your environment.

Let's consider a few functions the nervous system provides for the cardiorespiratory system and the muscles at rest and during exercise. Without these little electrical signals flowing back and forth between the brain and the body systems, nothing in the body could function.

Signals to the Cardiorespiratory System

The heart has its own electrical system (see figure 5.8). The signals sent over this system are responsible for maintaining a regular heartbeat. Any interference with this electrical network results in an irregular beat, meaning that the atria and the ventricles cannot contract in normal sequence.

A clump of nerve tissue (the sinoatrial node) located in the right atrium receives signals from the brain and sets the pace for the heart to contract. Not surprisingly, this node is often referred to as the heart's pacemaker.

The atrioventricular node is located at the junction of the right atrium and the right ventricle. The atrioventricular node receives the electrical impulse from the sinoatrial node and sends it to the Purkinje fibers, which form a network that spreads the impulse throughout the ventricles. The fibers are grouped into the right and left bundles.

Electrocardiogram

An electrocardiogram (EKG) is a tool used to assess the heart's ability to transmit its electrical impulses. An electrocardiograph mechanically records the heart's electrochemical activity. When the impulse travels through the heart, electrical current generated at the surface of the heart muscle spreads into fluid surrounding the heart. A minute portion of the current flows to the surface of the body (Guyton, 1974). Electrodes properly placed on the skin around the heart (see figure 5.9) can pick up this electrical current and transmit it to a recording instrument.

Figure 5.9 depicts a normal EKG. Each segment of the line indicates a portion of the conduction of the heart's current. The curve labeled P wave is caused by the current generated as the sinoatrial node initiates an impulse through the atria. The QRS complex results from the impulse passing through the Purkinje system and the ventricles. The T wave of the line represents the recovery of the electrical changes in the ventricles. The atrial recovery is not visible on the EKG because it is masked by the strong QRS complex of the ventricles.

An EKG is often part of an exercise stress test. Because the heart is performing more work during the stress of exercise, abnormalities are more likely to show up then than during a resting EKG.

Blood Vessels

Before, during, and after exercise, the nervous system regulates the heart rate. Nerve impulses also affect the blood vessels. When necessary, such as during redis-

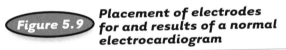

Figure 5.9 Placement of electrodes for and results of a normal electrocardiogram

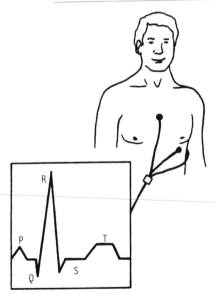

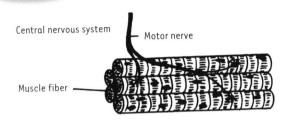

Figure 5.10 A motor unit

Central nervous system — Motor nerve

Muscle fiber

tribution of blood from the major internal organs to working limbs in preparation for exercise, the nervous system sends messages to the blood vessels supplying information to certain areas to dilate (become larger) or constrict (become smaller).

Breathing

The rate of breathing during vigorous exercise is also partially controlled by the nervous system. Messages are sent to the muscles that surround the rib cage to contract and help lift the rib cage at a faster rate.

Signals to the Muscles

Skeletal muscle fibers are united with many nerve fibers. When impulses are sent to the muscles via the central nervous system, the muscles contract, and when the impulses stop, the muscles relax. One motor nerve fiber innervates anywhere from 1 to 150 or more muscle fibers. All of the muscle fibers innervated by the motor nerve work as a unit; that is, they contract and relax at the same time. Figure 5.10 shows a single motor nerve innervating several muscle fibers.

The nervous system helps to coordinate the functioning of the body's systems at rest and during exercise. Like all other systems, it too responds to training. Its ability to send nerve impulses to the correct site, at the proper speed, and for the necessary amount of time are all enhanced through training.

Figure 5.11 *Front and back views of the human skeleton*

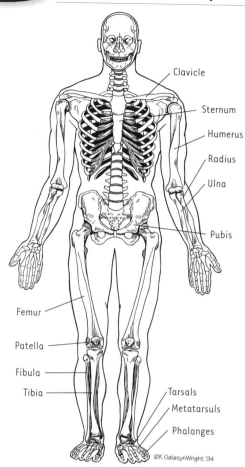

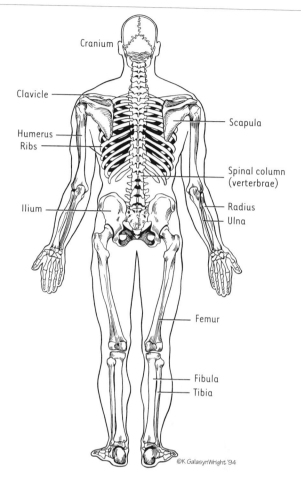

Anatomy and Biomechanics

As a YMCA Water Fitness Instructor, you need to be knowledgeable about the basics of anatomy and biomechanics. This chapter defines some key terms and presents some elementary concepts from these areas of study.

Anatomy

In this section, we will describe the different types of bones, the joints that are the linking points between bones, the positions in which the bones can move, and the muscles that move the bones.

Bones

The skeleton consists of 206 bones that provide protection for the internal organs and a leverage structure for muscles. The skeleton also allows for growth and is the largest store of calcium in the body. There are four classes of bones:

- **Long bones.** These are found in the arms and legs, and they are associated with movement.
- **Short bones.** These are found in the hands and feet. Some short bones are irregular in shape, such as the bones in the vertebral (spinal) column.
- **Flat bones.** These are found in the upper part of the skull.
- **Irregular bones.** These are found in vertebrae and the pubic area.

Figure 5.11 shows the front (anterior) and back (posterior) views of the skeleton and identifies the major bones, groups of bones, and anatomical landmarks.

Joints

A joint is the point where bones link or connect. Joints are also called *articulations*, and items associated with joints usually begin with the prefix *arthr-*, as in *arthroscope*, a device that is used to look into joint spaces of a person with *arthritis*. Joints are classified on the basis of how much movement is permitted between the bones:

- **Synarthrodial joints.** These are immovable joints or those with limited movement, such as the joints between the bones in the skull.
- **Amphiarthrodial joints.** These are joints with slight movement, as seen in the connections between vertebrae in the spinal column.
- **Diarthrotic or synovial joints.** These are joints possessing great potential for movement, as in the knee.

The diarthrotic or synovial joint is most important in physical activity. Movement occurs when the muscles move the bones through a range of motion within the limits of these joints. These joints are held together by connective tissue—*ligaments*, which cross over the joint, and *tendons*, which attach muscles to bones and also cross over joints to lend additional support. Because these joints move a great deal, the structure also provides slippery surfaces and a lubricant. The slippery surface in each movable joint is the *articular hyaline cartilage* that covers the ends of the bones. This cartilage also absorbs some of the shock of impact to reduce the chance that the bony surface will wear out. *Synovial fluid* is the lubricant secreted by the *synovial membrane* within the joint housing or capsule. In addition, *bursae*, or sacs containing synovial fluid outside the joint space, help to lubricate the movement of tendons, ligaments, and muscles over bony structures. Some of these joints (e.g., the knee) have additional cartilage in the joint space between the bones to take up some of the shock of impact. This is the type of cartilage that can be torn as a result of high-impact forces, while the smooth articular cartilage is the type that can be damaged by arthritis.

Diarthrodial (movable) joints are classified on the basis of the type of movement permitted:

- **Ball and socket joints.** These allow movement in all directions. An example is where the head of the humerus (the bone of the upper arm) fits into the shoulder.
- **Hinge joints.** These allow movement in one plane of motion. The elbow is an example.
- **Saddle joints.** These allow movement in all directions. The metacarpal-carpal joint of the thumb is an example.
- **Pivot joints.** These allow rotation around the long portion of the bone. The radioulnar joint is an example, as it allows us to rotate our wrist to make the hand face up (supinated position) or down (pronated position).
- **Gliding joints.** These allow only gliding or twisting. An example is found in the joints between the wrist bones (carpals) or the ankle bones (tarsals).

Movements

The type of movements possible at each joint is dependent on the type of joint. It is important to know the terms that describe these movements before we present a summary of the muscles involved:

- **Flexion/extension.** Flexion describes a motion that decreases the angle of a joint, and extension is a movement that increases the joint angle. If your arm is hanging straight down, flexion is the movement of your hand toward your shoulder around the elbow joint; lowering the hand back to its starting position is extension. The term hyperextension refers to the extension of a limb or part beyond the normal limit (*Stedman's*, 1976, p. 669).
- **Abduction/adduction.** Abduction describes a movement away from the center line of the body; adduction is a return to the ordinary anatomical position. Moving the leg to the side away from the body is an example of abduction.

- **Rotation.** Rotation is movement around the long axis of a bone and describes a movement either toward (inward or medial rotation) or away from (outward or lateral rotation) the center of the body. With your forearm at a 90-degree angle relative to your upper arm, and your hand in front of the body, movement of the wrist and lower arm toward the center line of the body is an example of medial rotation.

- **Pronation/supination.** If the forearm is held at a 90-degree angle relative to the upper arm, hand in front of the body with thumb up, pronation describes a movement of the forearm such that the palm turns downward, and supination is the reverse. These terms are also used to describe the manner in which the foot lands when walking or running. A person who lands with the inside or medial aspect of the foot striking first is said to be a "pronator." Many running shoes are designed to control this problem.

- **Dorsiflex/plantarflex.** These terms describe the movement of the foot from its normal position either toward the lower leg (dorsiflex) or toward the bottom of the foot (plantarflex).

- **Inversion/eversion.** Inversion is turning the bottom of the foot to the inside; eversion is turning the bottom of the foot to the outside. (Donnelly, 1990).

Muscles

Muscles are composed of muscle fibers, which are individual muscle cells. Each cell possesses the capacity to contract when stimulated by a *motor neuron*, or nerve cell. A single motor neuron may stimulate as few as 10 to more than 100 muscle fibers, and when it does, all the fibers attached to that single motor neuron fire at once. This complex of a single motor neuron and its muscle fibers is called a *motor unit*. A muscle possesses many motor units, and the tension that a muscle develops is dependent primarily on the number of motor units called into play. If more tension is needed, more motor units are recruited. When a muscle contracts, the ends of the muscle move toward the center, pulling the tendons (attached to the bones) toward each other. A variety of terms describe the different types of contractions:

- **Concentric contraction.** If the force of contraction is greater than the resistance offered, movement occurs as the bones to which the tendons are attached move toward each other. As the muscle shortens and the bones change position, however, the amount of tension needed to move the weight varies; more tension must be developed at some joint angles than at others to cause the same movement. For example, more force is required at the beginning of an exercise, such as a bicep curl, to overcome gravity than at the end of the movement.

- **Eccentric contraction.** This is a contraction in which a muscle exerts force, lengthens, and is overcome by a resistance (Study, 1991).

- **Isometric contraction.** This is also called a static contraction in that there is no movement even though the muscles are developing tension. Standing in a doorway and pushing against the door jamb is an example of this type of contraction.

- **Isokinetic contraction.** This contraction is similar to the concentric contraction, except that the speed of movement remains constant throughout the entire range of movement. To accomplish this, special "isokinetic machines" were developed to alter resistance during the movement. Closely related to these machines are those that work on the principle of variable resistance.

The major muscle groups are described in figures 5.12 through 5.17, and the action of specific muscles at each joint are listed in table 5.4. The term prime mover refers to the muscle that is primarily involved in the movement at that joint.

Muscles move the body and limbs through various planes. Normal joint ranges of motion are illustrated in figure 5.18.

Figure 5.12 **Muscles of the human body—anterior view**

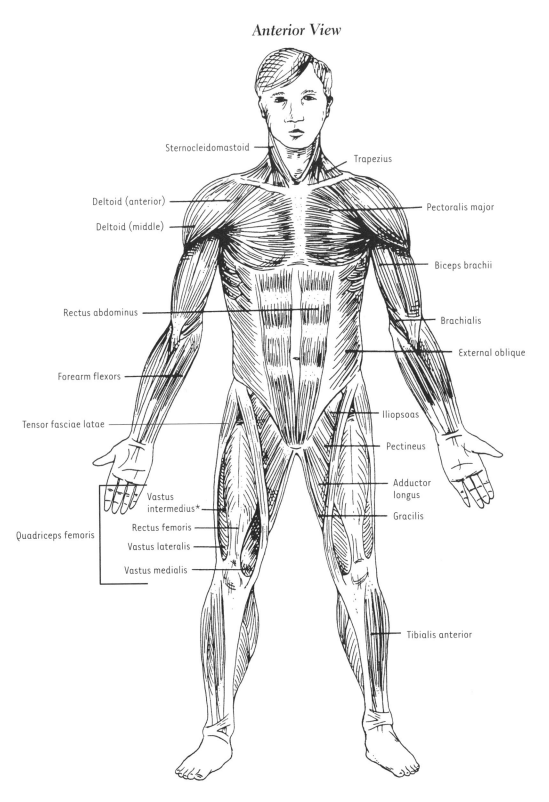

Anterior View

Sternocleidomastoid

Trapezius

Deltoid (anterior)

Pectoralis major

Deltoid (middle)

Biceps brachii

Rectus abdominus

Brachialis

External oblique

Forearm flexors

Tensor fasciae latae

Iliopsoas

Pectineus

Adductor longus

Vastus intermedius*

Gracilis

Quadriceps femoris

Rectus femoris

Vastus lateralis

Vastus medialis

Tibialis anterior

*Vastus intermedius is located under rectus femoris.

Figure 5.13 *Muscles of the human body—posterior view*

Posterior View

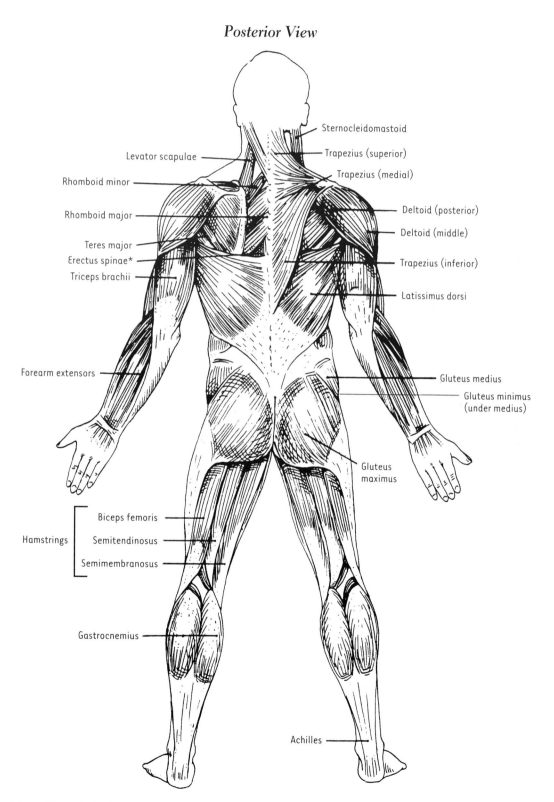

- Sternocleidomastoid
- Trapezius (superior)
- Trapezius (medial)
- Levator scapulae
- Rhomboid minor
- Rhomboid major
- Deltoid (posterior)
- Deltoid (middle)
- Teres major
- Erectus spinae*
- Triceps brachii
- Trapezius (inferior)
- Latissimus dorsi
- Forearm extensors
- Gluteus medius
- Gluteus minimus (under medius)
- Gluteus maximus
- Biceps femoris
- Semitendinosus
- Semimembranosus
- Hamstrings
- Gastrocnemius
- Achilles

*Erectus spinae is located beneath the rhomboid major.

Figure 5.14 *Muscles of the arm—anterior view*

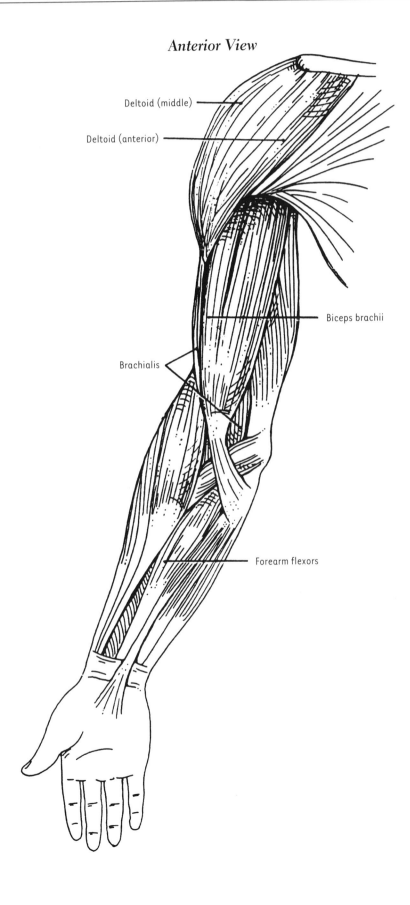

Anterior View

Deltoid (middle)

Deltoid (anterior)

Biceps brachii

Brachialis

Forearm flexors

Figure 5.15 *Muscles of the arm—posterior view*

Posterior View

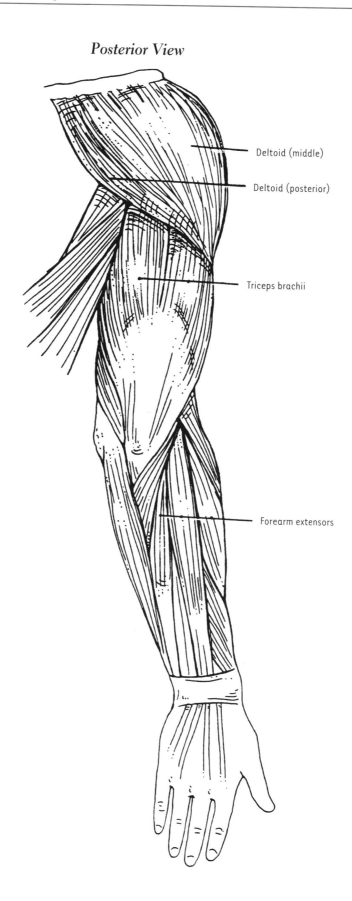

Deltoid (middle)

Deltoid (posterior)

Triceps brachii

Forearm extensors

Figure 5.16 *Muscles of the leg—anterior view*

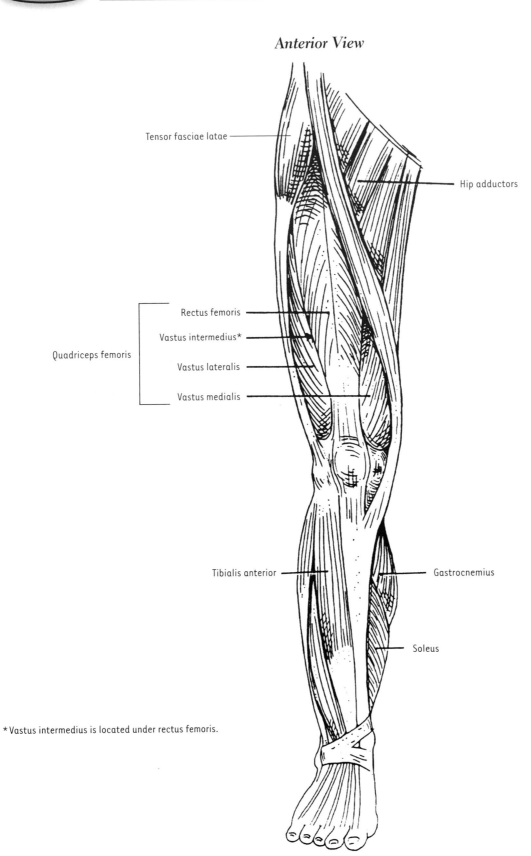

Anterior View

Tensor fasciae latae

Hip adductors

Quadriceps femoris

Rectus femoris

Vastus intermedius*

Vastus lateralis

Vastus medialis

Tibialis anterior

Gastrocnemius

Soleus

*Vastus intermedius is located under rectus femoris.

Figure 5.17 *Muscles of the leg—posterior view*

Posterior View

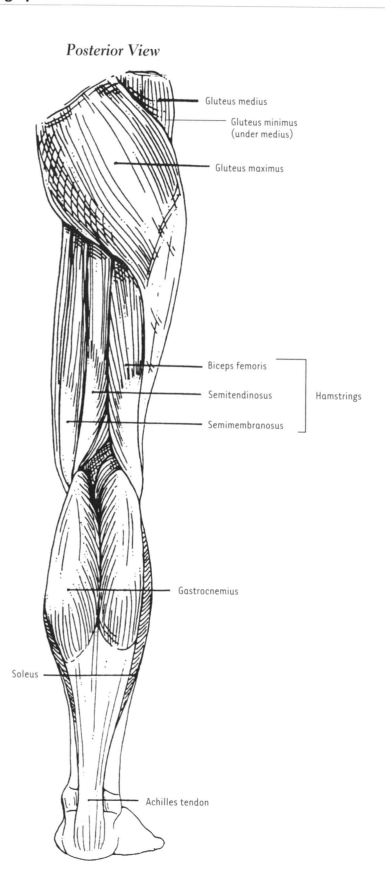

Gluteus medius

Gluteus minimus
(under medius)

Gluteus maximus

Biceps femoris

Semitendinosus

Semimembranosus

Hamstrings

Gastrocnemius

Soleus

Achilles tendon

Table 5.4 *Primary Joint Actions With Involved Muscles*

Joint	Joint action and prime movers (assisting muscles)
Scapula	**Abduction with upward rotation**—serratus anterior
	Adduction and downward rotation—rhomboid major and minor (trapezius)
	Adduction—middle fibers of trapezius, rhomboids (upper and lower fibers of trapezius)
	Elevation—levator scapulae, upper fibers of trapezius (rhomboids)
	Depression—lower fibers of trapezius, pectoralis minor
Shoulder joint	**Flexion**—anterior deltoid, coracobrachialis (deltoid middle, pectoralis major, biceps brachii)
	Extension—latissimus dorsi, teres major, posterior deltoid (long head of triceps brachii, teres minor)
	Abduction—middle deltoid, supraspinatus (serratus anterior for direct action on the scapula, anterior and posterior deltoid)
	Adduction—latissimus dorsi, teres major, pectoralis major
	Lateral rotation—infraspinatus, teres minor (posterior deltoid)
	Medial rotation—pectoralis major, subscapularis, latissimus dorsi, teres major (anterior deltoid)
	Horizontal adduction—both portions of the pectoralis major (anterior deltoid)
	Horizontal abduction—posterior deltoid (infraspinatus, teres minor)
Elbow joint	**Flexion**—biceps brachii, brachialis, brachioradialis (forearm flexors)
	Extension—triceps brachii (forearm extensors)
Radioulnar joint	**Pronation**—pronator quadratus, pronator teres (flexor carpi radialis)
	Supination—supinator, biceps brachii (brachioradialis)
Wrist joint	**Flexion**—*forearm flexors:* flexor carpi ulnaris, flexor carpi radialis (palmaris longus)
	Extension—*forearm extensors:* extensor carpi ulnaris, extensor carpi radialis longus and brevis
	Radial deviation—flexor carpi radialis, extensor carpi radialis longus and brevis (extensor pollicis)
	Ulnar deviation—flexor carpi ulnaris, extensor carpi ulnaris
Lumbosacral joint	**Forward or anterior pelvic tilt**—iliopsoas (erector spinae)
	Backward or posterior pelvic tilt—rectus abdominus, internal obliques (external oblique, gluteus maximus)

Joint	Joint action and prime movers (assisting muscles)
Spinal column (thoracic and lumbar areas)	**Flexion**—rectus abdominis (external obliques, internal obliques)
	Extension—erector spinae group
	Rotation—internal oblique, external oblique (erector spinae, latissimus dorsi)
	Lateral flexion—internal oblique, external oblique, quadratus lumborum (erector spinae)
Hip joint	**Flexion**—iliopsoas (pectineus, rectus femoris, sartorius, tensor fascia latae, adductor longus and brevis)
	Extension—gluteus maximus, biceps femoris, semitendinosus, semimembranosus
	Abduction—gluteus medius (tensor fascia latae, gluteus minimus, gluteus maximus (upper fibers)
	Adduction—adductor magnus, adductor brevis, adductor longus, gracilis pectineus
	Lateral rotation—gluteus maximus, the six deep lateral rotator muscles (sartorius, biceps femoris—long head)
	Medial rotation—gluteus minimus, tensor fascia latae (gluteus medius, semitendinosis, semimembranosis)
Knee joint	**Flexion**—biceps femoris, semimembranosus, semitendinosus (sartorius, gracilis, gastrocnemius, popliteus)
	Extension—rectus femoris, vastus medialis, vastus lateralis, vastus intermedius
Ankle joint	**Plantar flexion**—gastrocnemius, soleus (plantaris, peroneus longus, peroneus brevis, tibialis posterior, flexor digitorum longus, flexor hallucis longus)
Intertarsal joint	**Dorsi flexion and inversion**—tibialis anterior
	Inversion—tibialis posterior (flexor hallucis longus, flexor digitorum longus, gastrocnemius—medial head)
	Eversion—peroneus brevis, peroneus longus (extensor digitorum longus, peroneus tertius)

Adapted by permission from: Hislop and Montgomery, eds. (1995). *Muscle Testing: Techniques of Examination*, 6th ed., W.B. Saunders Co., Philadelphia.

Figure 5.18 *Primary Muscles and Joint Actions*

Sternocleidomastoid

Where they are:

Each side of the neck

What they do:

Each side acts independently to bend the head sideways and turn the head. They both act together to bend the head to the chest.

Joint action:

Neck rotation and lateral flexion (side bending) and rotation

Trapezius

Where it is:

This is a triangular-shaped muscle that runs from the spine to the shoulder blades.

What it does:

It draws the shoulders together and downward and generally acts as a brace for the shoulders. Weak trapezius muscles can aggravate dowager's hump and round shoulders. The trapezius takes a lot of strain if you sit hunched at a terminal or over a desk for long hours.

Joint action:

Scapular adduction, upward rotation (by upper and lower trapezius)

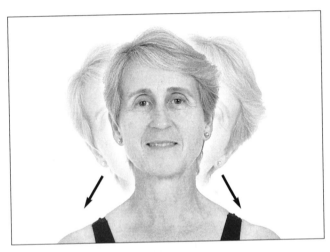

**Lateral flexion
(40–45 degrees to each side)**

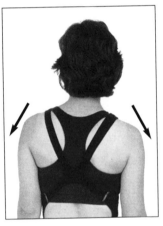

Scapular depression

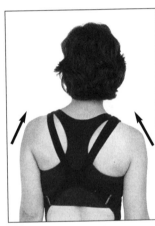

Scapular elevation

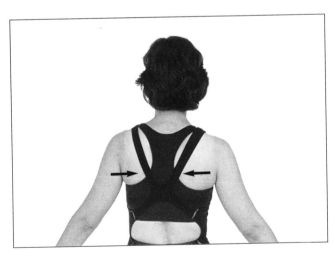

**Neck rotation
(80–90 degrees to each side)**

Scapular adduction

Deltoids

Where they are:

These muscles are over the tops of the shoulders, covering the shoulder joints like shoulder pads.

What they do:

They raise the arms up to shoulder level sideways and, in conjunction with other muscles, help rotate the arms and raise them to the front and back.

Joint action:

Shoulder flexion, shoulder abduction, shoulder horizontal abduction

Latissimus Dorsi

Where it is:

This is a broad muscle that stretches across the back into the back of the arms.

What it does:

It helps draw the arms down and back and internally rotates them. It also pulls the trunk up toward static arms (as in rope climbing).

Joint action:

Shoulder extension and adduction, medial rotation

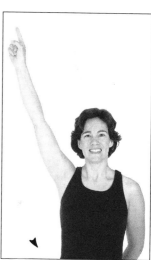

Shoulder extension (45 degrees)

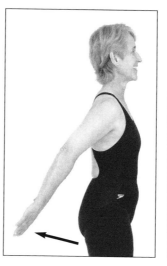

Shoulder adduction (arm swings 45 degrees across the front of the body)

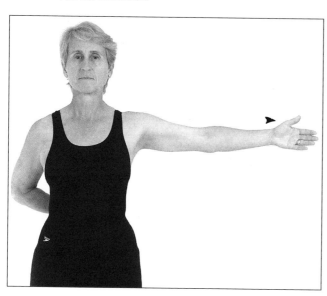

Shoulder horizontal abduction

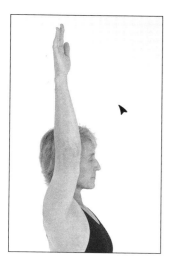

Shoulder flexion (180 degrees)

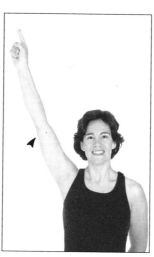

Shoulder abduction (180 degrees)

Biceps

Where they are:

These muscles are in the front of the upper arms.

What they do:

They bend the elbows.

Joint action:

Elbow flexion

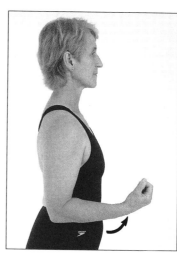

Elbow flexion (135—145 degrees

Figure 5.19 *Primary Muscles and Joint Actions*

Triceps

Where they are:

These muscles are in the back of the upper arms.

What they do:

They straighten the elbows.

Joint action:

Elbow extension

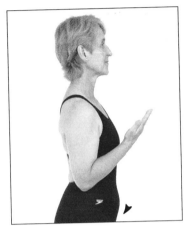

Elbow extension (extension is the return from flexion) (0–5 degrees)

Wrist flexors

Where they are:

These muscles are located on the front of the fore-arms.

What they do:

They help bend the palms of the hands toward you.

Joint action:

Wrist flexion

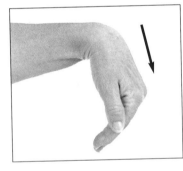

Wrist flexion (80 degrees)

Wrist Extensors

Where they are:

These muscles are in back of the forearms.

What they do:

They pull the palms of the hands away from you.

Joint action:

Wrist extension

Wrist extension (70 degrees)

Pectorals

Where they are:

These muscles are located in the upper chest.

What they do:

They draw the arms across the body and rotate the arms inward. They also help with lifting the arms above the head and lowering them back down to the sides.

Joint action:

Shoulder horizontal adduction, shoulder adduction, medial rotation

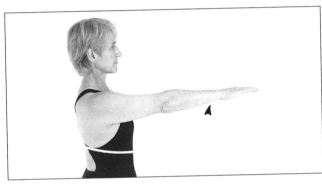

Shoulder horizontal adduction

Obliques

Where they are:

These muscles are on both sides of the front of the trunk.

What they do:

They help maintain neutral position.

Joint action:

Low back flexion, lateral flexion, and spinal rotation

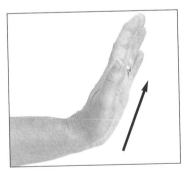
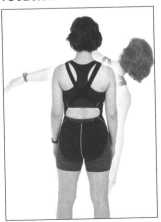
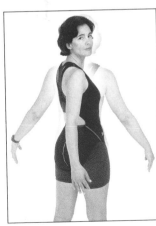

Low back lateral flexion (35 degrees left and right)

Spinal rotation (45 degrees left and right)

Rectus Abdominis

Where they are:

These muscles extend down the center of the anterior trunk to the pubic bone.

What they do:

They bend the trunk forward and help maintain neutral position.

Joint action:

Thoracic flexion, spinal or low back flexion, posterior pelvic tilt

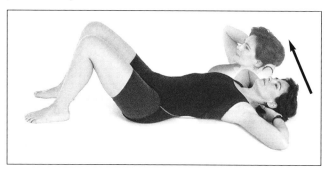

Thoracic flexion
(70 degrees)

Erector Spinae

Where they are:

They are positioned on each side of the spinal column, from neck to tailbone.

What they do:

They help the trunk to move smoothly in many planes and maintain or move the spine into an upright position. They help maintain neutral posture.

Joint action:

Low back extension, lateral flexion, and trunk rotation

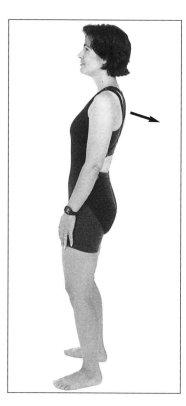

Low back extension

Gluteus Maximus

Where they are:

These muscles cover the backside of the hips (buttocks).

What they do:

They pull the legs backward and turn the legs outward. They assist in standing up from a seated position.

Joint action:

Hip extension, hip lateral rotation, posterior pelvic tilt

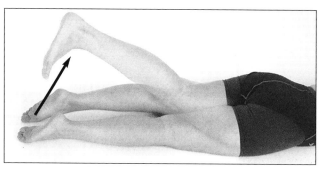

Hip extension
(10—15 degrees)

Hip Adductors

Where they are:

These muscles are on the inside of the thighs.

What they do:

They pull the legs inward.

Joint action:

Adduct the hip

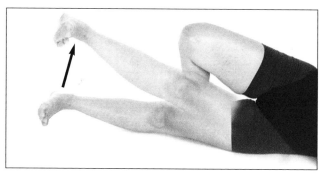

Hip adduction
(20—30 degrees)

(continued)

Figure 5.19 *Primary Muscles and Joint Actions (continued)*

Gluteus Medius (Hip Abductors)

Where they are:

These muscles sit on the upper back and side of the hips.

What they do:

They move the legs outward, away from the center of the body.

Joint action:

Hip abduction

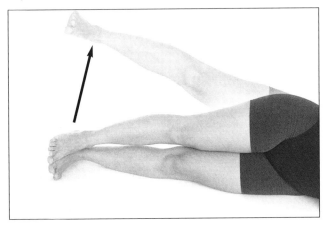

*Hip abduction
(45 degrees)*

Gluteus Minimus

Where they are:

These muscles are inside the hip area, connecting the pelvis to the femurs (thigh bones).

What they do:

They raise the legs outward to the sides and turn the legs inward. They may help lift the knees toward the chest.

Joint action:

Hip internal rotation

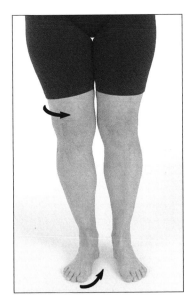

*Hip internal rotation
(35 degrees)*

Tensor Fasciae Latae (T.F.L.)

Where they are:

These muscles are on the lateral side of the thighs.

What they do:

They bring the knees toward the chest, turn the knees inward, and move the legs away from the center of the body.

Joint action:

Hip abduction from a flexed position
Internal hip rotation

Hamstrings

Where they are:

These muscles are at the back of the thighs.

What they do:

They bend the knees and help turn the lower legs inward. They extend the legs backward and help turn the legs inward.

Joint action:

Knee flexion, hip extension

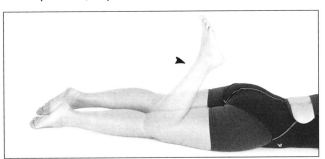

Knee flexion (120—130 degrees)

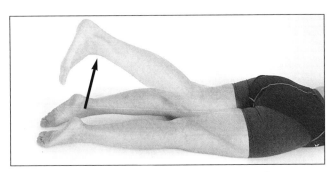

Hip extension (10—15 degrees)

Quadriceps

Where they are:

These muscles are in the front of the thighs.

What they do:

They straighten the knee.

Joint action:

Knee extension

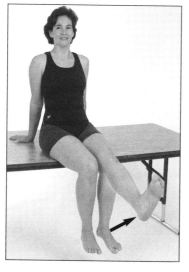

**Knee extension
(extension is the return
from flexion)
(0 degrees)**

Hip Iliopsoas (Flexors)

Where they are:

These muscles attach the lower spine to the femurs (thigh bones).

What they do:

They bring the knees to the chest.

Joint action:

Hip flexion

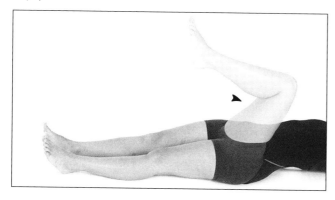

Hip flexion with knee flexion (125 degrees)

Tibialis Anterior

Where they are:

These muscles are in the front of the lower legs.

What they do:

They raise the feet up and turn the feet inward.

Joint action:

Ankle dorsiflexion and ankle inversion

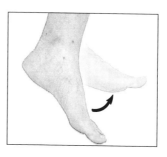

**Ankle dorsiflexion
(15—20 degrees)**

**Ankle inversion
(little toe down,
big toe up)
(5 degrees)**

Gastrocnemius

Where they are:

These muscles are in the back of the lower legs.

What they do:

They raise the heels and point the toes downward.

Joint action:

Plantar flexion of the ankle joint and assistance with flexion of the knee

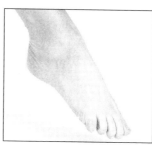

**Plantar flexion
(45—50 degrees)**

Soleus

Where they are:

These muscles are in the back of the lower legs.

What they do:

They point the toes.

Joint action:

Plantar flexion of the ankle joint

The following section presents a summary of the muscle groups involved in some of the most common physical activities (see figures 5.12 and 5.13 for labeling of muscles). We begin with walking and end with lifting heavy things.

Walking, Jogging, and Running

Walking, jogging, and running have a lot in common; they differ, however, in terms of the muscular force needed to move forward at different speeds. During walking one foot is in contact with the ground at all times, but in jogging or running there is a period of "flight" when both feet are off the ground. If a period of flight is involved, a greater amount of energy must be expended to both "take off" and "land." The primary muscle groups involved in each phase of these activities include these:

- Push-off phase—The push-off uses the concentric contraction of hip extensors.
- Bringing push-off leg forward—The concentric contraction of hip flexors initiates movement that is modified by the lateral hip rotators. The knee flexors first cause knee flexion, then, through an eccentric contraction, control the rate of knee extension prior to the foot touching down. The foot is dorsiflexed prior to landing.
- Landing—The hip extensors that initiated the push-off now contract eccentrically to slow the swing of the forward leg. When the foot touches down, the knee extensors also contract eccentrically to control the motion of the foot on the ground.

Cycling

Given that cycling is a restricted activity in that the pedals move in a fixed manner, it should be no surprise that the muscle groups involved in cycling are also somewhat limited. The hip and knee extensors develop the force to move the pedals downward, and, if toe clips are used by a cyclist skilled in their use, hip and knee flexors are involved in the return to the starting position. Without the use of toe clips, flexor activity is considerably less.

Jumping

The force needed to propel the body off the ground is generated by the knee and hip extensors as well as the plantar flexors. To absorb the forces of impact, these same muscles contract eccentrically.

Lifting and Carrying

When a person lifts an object the large, strong knee and hip extensors should be the primary muscles involved, not the muscles in the arms or along the spine. Keeping the object close to one's body reduces the stress on the back.

Biomechanical Concepts

A variety of basic principles and laws governing the movement of objects and people can, when understood, help you determine proper and improper movements.

Stability

The **center of gravity** for an average person is near the navel. The stability of an individual is greater the closer the center of gravity is to the ground and the wider the base of support. A person standing with both feet close together is less stable than when standing with feet spread apart.

Rotational Inertia

The concept of rotational inertia as applied to the body indicates the tendency of a body segment to remain at rest and not rotate around a joint. The larger the body segment and the farther the mass of the segment is from the joint (e.g., arm vs. leg), the more rotational inertia the body segment has and the greater the energy required to move that segment through a range of motion. The energy requirement can be reduced by bringing the mass of the segment closer to the joint of rotation; bringing the flexed rear leg forward during running is an application of this principle.

Torque

This is the effect produced when a muscle contraction (force) causes rotation. We will look at forearm flexion as an example, with the forearm at a 90-degree angle to the upper arm and a 10-pound weight held in the hand. The resistance is the product of the 10-pound weight and the distance from the center of the weight to the elbow joint. The muscular force needed to move that weight is dependent on the distance from the elbow that the tendon of that muscle is inserted into the bone of the forearm. The closer the biceps' insertion is located to the hand, the smaller the muscular force needed to move the resistance. In the same way, if the 10-pound weight is moved closer to the joint (to reduce the length of the lever arm), less muscular force is needed to move the resistance. This concept can be extended to the carrying of objects. The reason for carrying an object close to the body is to maintain stability and reduce the force of the back muscles needed to carry the load. If the object is held with arms outstretched, the back muscles must exert more force, which can cause back problems.

Angular Momentum

This term describes the amount of motion that takes place as a limb moves around a joint or a body rotates and is equal to the product of angular velocity and rotational inertia. The conservation of angular momentum states that once motion is initiated, angular momentum remains constant until an outside force changes it. This means that a decrease in rotational inertia during a movement results in a higher angular velocity. This is best seen when an ice skater spins around in place; as the arms are brought closer to the body to decrease rotational inertia, the velocity of rotation increases.

Bibliography

American Council on Exercise. 1993. *Aerobics instructor manual.* San Diego: American Council on Exercise.

Decker, J.I., G. Orcutt, and P. Sammann. 1989. *Y's way to fitness walking leader's guide.* Champaign, IL: Human Kinetics.

Donnelly, J.E. 1990. Living anatomy (2nd ed.). Champaign, IL: Human Kinetics.

Foster, C. 1975. Physiological requirements of aerobic dancing. *Research Quarterly* 46: 120–122.

Golding, L.A., C.R. Myers, and W.E. Sinning, eds. 1989. *Y's way to physical fitness.* 3rd ed. Champaign, IL: Human Kinetics.

Guyton, A. 1974. *Function of the human body.* 4th ed. Philadelphia: W.B. Saunders.

Hoppenfeld, S. 1976. *Physical examination of the spine and extremities.* New York: Appleton-Century-Crofts.

Kasch, F.W., and J.L. Boyer. 1968. *Adult fitness: Principles and practice.* Greeley, CO: All American Products and Publications.

Rockefeller, K.A., and E. J. Burke. 1979. Psychophysiological analysis of an aerobic dance programme for women. *British Journal of Physical Education* 13: 77–80.

Stedman's Medical Dictonary (23rd ed.). Baltimore, MD: Williams & Wilkins.

Study, M., ed. 1991. *Personal trainer manual, the resource for fitness instructors.* San Diego, CA: American Council on Exercise.

Vaccaro, P., and M. Clinton. 1981. The effects of aerobic dance conditioning on the body composition and maximal oxygen uptake of college women. *Journal of Sports Medicine and Physical Fitness* 21: 291–294.

Weber, H. 1974. The energy cost of aerobic dancing. *Fitness for Living* 8: 26–30.

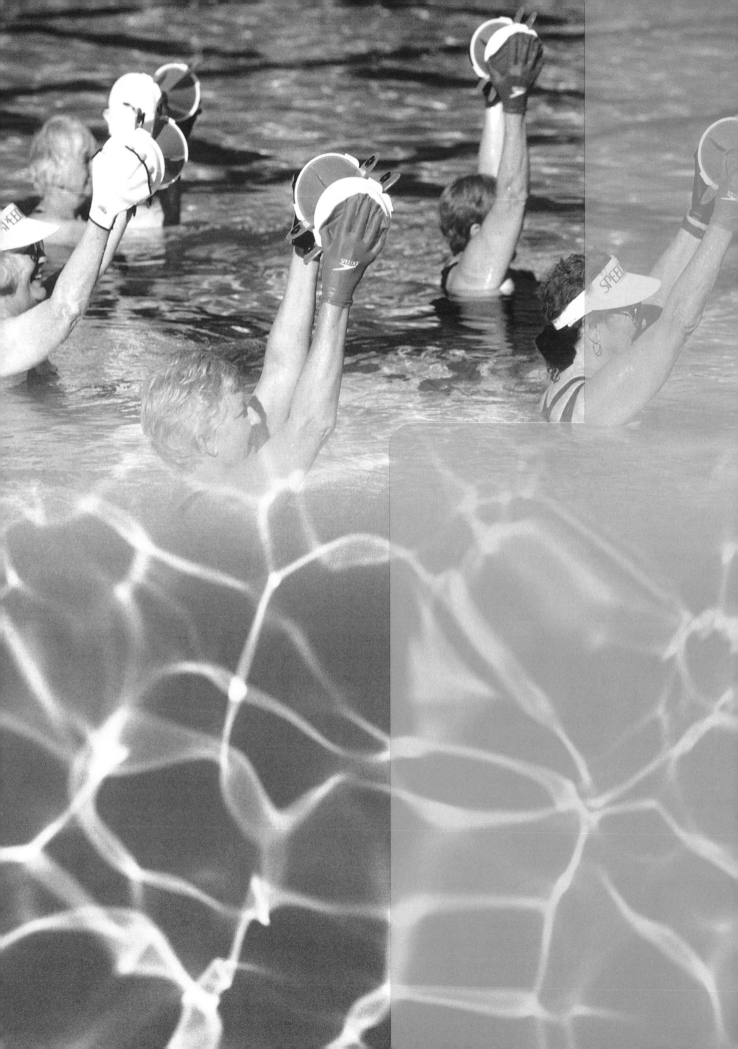

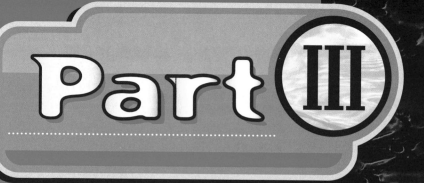

Part III

Fundamentals of Water Exercise

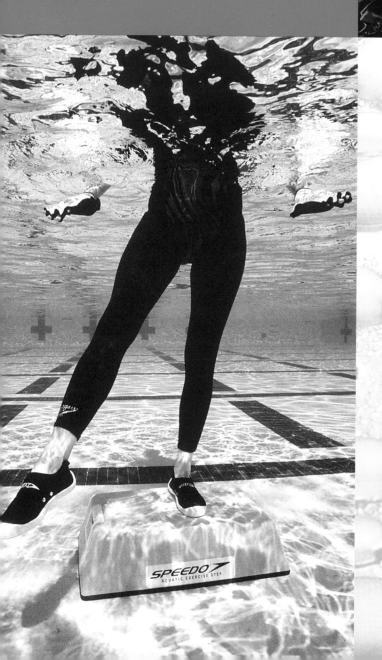

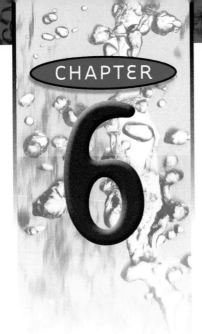

CHAPTER 6

What Research Reveals About Water Exercise

MARY E. SANDERS, CAROL KENNEDY, AND NICKI E. RIPPEE

Objectives:

- To review water exercise literature up to 1994 and its applications to water exercise training and design

- To review water exercise literature between 1994 and 1998 and its applications to water exercise training and design

I f you're unsure where water exercise fits in the total exercise picture, you're not alone. The unique environment and properties of water exercise have raised a lot of questions for fitness professionals. However, the rising popularity of water fitness, a growing body of research, and the increased experiential knowledge of water fitness experts are paving the way (or perhaps, parting the waves) for a greater understanding of water exercise in the fitness industry.

Reviewing the available research, along with the application of exercise science principles and an understanding of the properties of water, can give you a better grasp of water exercise. In addition, it can help dissolve many of the seeming contradictions of water fitness and help you determine how you can best incorporate water exercise into your fitness program options.

Water fitness is not clearly defined within fitness circles because the use of water as a training environment requires manipulating resistance and buoyancy to create work and rest, rather than manipulating gravity as we do when training on land. Unfortunately, this concept of manipulation is not always understood or applied in either research or practical settings. However, by applying exercise science and taking into account the properties of water, we can use research to answer two important questions:

- Does water exercise work?
- How do we optimize work in water to achieve fitness?

In order to ensure the most effective and safest training for your participants, it's important to understand how to apply research results to exercise design. (Research was the basis for the YMCA Water Exercise Program training methods.) This chapter reviews the literature and provides some examples of what the studies' results mean to us as water fitness instructors. It is divided into two parts: the literature up to 1994, and the literature between 1994 and 1998.

Review of Water Exercise Literature Up to 1994

In this section, we will discuss the following key questions about water fitness programming:

- Is water exercise a valid method of cardiorespiratory conditioning?
- What is the best method for monitoring intensity in the water?
- Can water exercise improve body composition?
- Can water exercise enhance muscular strength and endurance and flexibility?
- How can exercise intensity be manipulated in the water?
- How does buoyancy affect exercise?
- How important is thermal regulation?
- What are some important factors for optimal program design?

Water Exercise and Cardiorespiratory Conditioning

Investigations using single bouts of water exercise, in both **shallow** and **deep water**, indicate that training in water can improve cardiorespiratory endurance (Cassady and Nielsen, 1992; Heberlein et al., 1987; Johnson et al., 1977) because participants can achieve a training $\dot{V}O_2$ within the range recommended by the American College of Sports Medicine (ACSM).

Several deep and shallow water training adaptation studies have also reported significant improvements in cardiorespiratory fitness (Barretta, 1993; Hoeger et al., 1993; Michaud et al., 1992; Ruoti, Troup, and Berger, 1994; Sanders, 1993; Stevenson et al., 1988). But what about studies in which participants didn't reach a training threshold?

For example, Eckerson and Anderson (1992) reported an exercise $\dot{V}O_2$ below the minimum threshold even though the heart rate response was 82 percent of maximum heart rate (well within ACSM training guidelines). This study seems to indicate that water exercise is not appropriate for cardiorespiratory training. However, when the exercise protocol for this study is examined and exercise principles are applied, this "contradiction" can be explained. Let's look at the research protocol.

The exercise workout used extensive overhead arm movements above the water's surface (clapping and overhead flexion/extension of the elbows and shoulders) as well as stationary kicks, jogging, knee raises, bobbing, and jumping. The water temperature was 25 degrees to 27 degrees C (77 degrees to 81 degrees F). Working water depth was not given, but the class was conducted in the shallow end of the pool (1 meter/ 3.28 feet at the shallowest part). The participants had average body fat for their ages.

Research indicates that water temperature, body composition, and water depth would not account for the high heart rate and low $\dot{V}O_2$. However, the overhead armwork and the extensive use of the arms to create work could explain the problem. Research tells us that arm-cranking moves and armwork above the head produce a higher heart rate relative to the $\dot{V}O_2$ demands (Åstrand, Guharay and Wahren, 1968; Shephard, 1984). Resistive work with the arms produces relatively low-oxygen uptake and does not meet the criteria for aerobic training intensity (Beasley, 1989).

A closer look at research reporting achievement of a training $\dot{V}O_2$ (and a lower heart rate) reveals interesting differences in program design. Cassady and Nielsen (1992) determined that using the lower extremities produced higher work intensities. Beasley (1989) reported that travel through waist-deep water (with shoes on) elicited 87 percent of $\dot{V}O_2$max. Gleim and Nicholas (1989), Town and Bradley (1991) and Whitley and Schoene (1987) also show that travel elicits higher oxygen consumption.

Work intensities seem to vary with the skill level and motivation of the exerciser. Wilder and Brennan (1993), Ritchie and Hopkins (1991), and Ruoti, Troup, and Berger (1994) found that motivated, more highly skilled exercisers were able to achieve higher heart rates than nonskilled participants.

This research illustrates that, by making use of the water properties of turbulence and frictional resistance, work intensity can be increased by amplifying the resistance of the water acting against the body (Duffield, 1976).

APPLYING THIS RESEARCH TO YOUR PARTICIPANTS' NEEDS

- Use traveling moves that allow time and space for water to act against the body, thus increasing work intensity. We suggest a minimum of four to six feet in one direction to maximize turbulence and form drag (i.e., the shape and size of limb or body moving through the water).

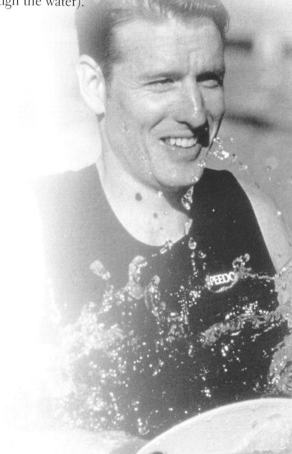

- Keep armwork below shoulder level. When the arms are sustained overhead, heart rate will overestimate the intensity of the cardiorespiratory training response.

- Because the arms and shoulders make up a small muscle group, concentrate on maximizing leg movements.

- Teach skills, and give exercise participants time to become proficient.

Monitoring Exercise Intensity in the Water

Accurately counting heart rate has proven difficult on land (Ebbeling et al., 1991); it becomes even more difficult in the dynamic environment of water. Studies such as those just mentioned show that using heart rate to measure exercise intensity in water may not be appropriate, at least if target heart rates for land exercise are applied. Heart rate as the only measure of intensity does not seem warranted for a number of reasons:

- **Heart rate and exercise design.** Using hand-held equipment increases heart rate, but this increase contributes minimally to a cardiorespiratory training effect and will not reflect adequate training intensity (McArdle, Katch and Katch, 1991).

- **Heart rate and water temperature.** Research indicates that water temperature has a decided effect on heart rate and oxygen consumption. Exercising in warm water (30 degrees to 35 degrees C/86 degrees to 95 degrees F) produces heart rates similar to land exercise (Craig and Dvorak, 1969; Evans, Cureton, and Purvis, 1978; McArdle et al., 1976). However, cycling and running in water temperatures from 18 degrees to 25 degrees C (64 degrees to 77 degrees F) produce heart rates 10 to 15 beats per minute (bpm) lower than are typical for land exercise (Craig and Dvorak, 1969; Svedenhag and Seger, 1992). So warmer water elicits higher heart rates, and cooler water elicits lower heart rates.

- **Heart rate and water depth.** What effect does water depth have on achievable heart rate? It is difficult to say from the research. There do not seem to be comparisons of deep versus shallow water work where routines were specifically designed and used for different depths. A comparison of the same water aerobics routine done in waist-deep and chest-deep (nipple-deep) water reported that the deeper water work averaged a heart rate 10 bpm lower than the shallow water work (Kennedy et al., 1989).

However, before assuming that deeper water causes lower heart rates, we must consider the properties of water. This difference in heart rate may be attributable more to the increased effect of buoyancy when a routine is taken from the more gravity-based environment of waist-deep water to the more buoyant, nipple-deep water, particularly when the exercisers are not wearing shoes.

In fact, as Kennedy et al. (1989) noted, the participants in their study exercised in bare feet and reported having trouble gaining speed during the traveling moves in deeper water. The lack of traction necessary to overcome inertia could result in lower-intensity work and account for the lower heart rates.

Researchers (Navia, 1986; Ritchie and Hopkins, 1991; Svendenhag and Seger, 1992) reported that heart rates for deep water running were lower than for treadmill running at a corresponding $\dot{V}O_2$ because of increased stroke volume. However, results of the studies by Navia (1986) and Ritchie and Hopkins (1991) suggested that the lower heart rates in water may actually correlate with an aerobic training effect that would be expected from a higher heart rate during treadmill running on land. At this point, the evidence seems insufficient to draw specific conclusions in this area. Research is needed for deep water rhythmic exercise.

The relationship among heart rate, $\dot{V}O_2$, and ratings of perceived exertion has been investigated only with deep water running. Most of these running studies show that perceived exertion tends to be higher for water running than for comparable land exercise as measured by $\dot{V}O_2$ or heart rate (Fernhall, Manfredi and Congdon, 1992; Svendenhag and Seger, 1992). However, Ritchie and Hopkins (1991) reported that perceived exertion was comparable during deep water running at a "hard" pace and during "hard" treadmill running. Again, research needs to be done specifically for rhythmic water exercise.

Even though there are many questions about monitoring exercise intensity in water, training studies using rhythmic exercises reported significant increases in cardiorespiratory endurance. These programs used a combination of perceived exertion, heart rate, and breathing rate to measure work intensity, indicating that the combination of these methods does work (Hoeger et al., 1993; Sanders, 1993). However, as

Wilder and Brennan (1993) suggested, research is needed to find an environment-specific (i.e., water-specific) means of exercise prescription.

APPLYING THIS RESEARCH TO YOUR PARTICIPANTS' NEEDS

- Heart rate is not always a valid indicator of work intensity. Heart rate can vary, depending on water temperature, skill and motivation of participants, amount of armwork, and accuracy of heart rate measurement.

- Until further research is done, you should use a combination of heart rate, perceived exertion, and breathing rate (talk test) to monitor intensity.

- Participants performing shallow water exercise should wear shoes to ensure good traction. This will potentiate work intensity.

Improving Body Composition With Water Exercise

There is a widely held opinion that water exercise is not an effective way to decrease body fat. This belief is a result of highly publicized research that reported either no fat loss or an increase in body fat with swimmers (Gwinup, 1987; Stavish, 1987). Yet other research (Maharam, 1992) has reported significant decreases in body fat with swimming. Unfortunately, not only has the public equated swim training with rhythmic water exercise, but they also seem unaware of the research showing fat loss.

Studies have shown convincingly that, for decreasing body fat, rhythmic water exercise is comparable to land-based programs. Hoeger et al. (1993) reported a 2 percent decrease in body fat as a result of participation in shallow water rhythmic exercise. This was greater than the 1.1 percent decrease experienced by subjects in a comparable low-impact land aerobics training study. Diet was not controlled in either program. Knecht (1992) conducted a 10-week shallow water exercise study that found significant improvements in body composition in comparison to nonexercising groups. Sanders (1993) conducted an eight-week combination shallow water (two sessions a week) and deep water (one session a week) rhythmic exercise program and reported significant (2.31 percent) decreases in body fat.

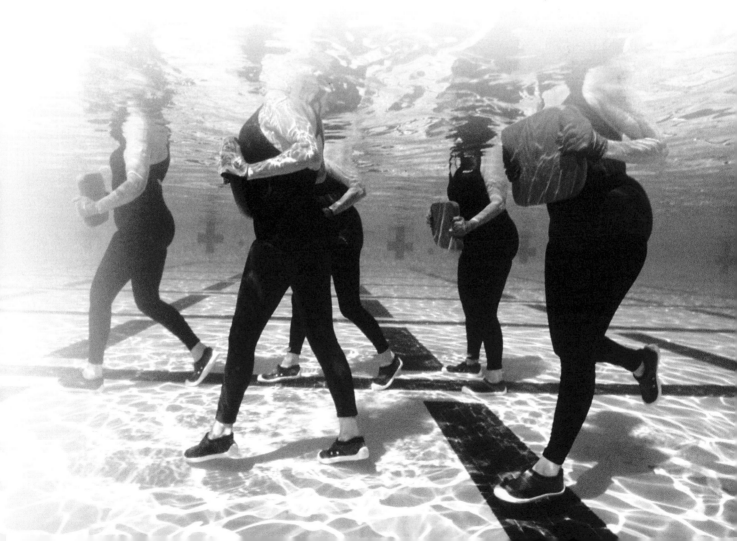

APPLYING THIS RESEARCH TO YOUR PARTICIPANTS' NEEDS

- Be aware of the evidence showing reduction in body fat resulting from participation in rhythmic water exercise. Give your participants accurate, research-based information.

Improving Muscular Strength and Flexibility With Water Exercise

Several studies have been done that demonstrate that water exercise can improve muscular strength and flexibility. Each study outlined in table 6.1 used different exercise designs and different tests to evaluate training adaptions, so only general conclusions can be drawn. The authors are not recommending these programs; each program needs to be evaluated for safety and effectiveness.

- **Muscular strength and endurance.** Each of the studies indicated significant increases in muscular strength and endurance for the areas measured. Of particular interest is the increase in abdominal strength Sanders (1993) reported, because the program did not utilize any abdominal "crunch" exercises. Improvements were attributed to the vertical, dynamic postural alignment techniques. Also of note are findings by Hoeger et al. (1993) showing that shallow water rhythmic exercise produced greater muscular strength gains than a low-impact aerobics class.

- **Flexibility.** Two studies (Barretta, 1993; Hoeger et al., 1993) reported increases in hamstring and low-back flexibility. If water exercisers simply perform land stretches in the water, they should attain flexibility gains because of the ability to overload. However, a question still remains concerning the potential for movement using the water to affect flexibility. It seems that water should work to increase range of motion, but the research produces contradictory results.

Regulating Exercise Intensity in the Water

Water, because of its viscosity, provides an accommodating resistance to work (Fawcett, 1992). To use resistance to regulate exercise intensity, a number of factors can be manipulated:

- **Speed.** Muscular work increases as faster speeds increase drag resistance to the work (Cole, Moschetti, and Eagleston, 1992). Cassady and Nielsen (1992) and Wilder, Brennan, and Schotte (1993) found that heart rate increased with speed of movement. Cassady and Nielsen (1992) also reported higher $\dot{V}O_2$ values with increased speed of lower-extremity work in water than with land exercise. However, research reinforces that we must always remember this: Unlike land exercisers, water exercisers not only move their bodies; they also have a "force" working against them. Evans, Cureton, and Purvis (1978) found that for walking and jogging in waist-deep water, approximately one-half to one-third the speed of land walking/jogging was necessary for the same level of energy expenditure because of the muscular force required to move through water. To fully utilize the resistive environment, we must change our "land" concept of speed when we put movement in the water.

- **Surface area and size of movement.** Since no one variable works alone in the interactive environment of water, other variables work with speed. Two of these are surface area and movement size. Costill (1971) found that work intensities in water were affected proportionally by the surface area placed in motion and that the velocity (speed) of the motion was determined by the level of muscular strength.

- **Turbulence and form drag.** Travel in the water creates turbulence as a result of frontal resistance, laminar flow, and drag (Duffield, 1976). This results in greater resistance to movement, thereby increasing the muscular work required. Beasley (1989), Gleim and Nicholas (1989), and Town and Bradley (1991) all found that oxygen consumption in water was highest when the subjects traveled through the water.

APPLYING THIS RESEARCH TO YOUR PARTICIPANTS' NEEDS

- To use speed for regulation of exercise intensity, exercisers need to develop appropriate levels of muscular strength and endurance.
- Larger movements at one-half to one-third of land speed are recommended to take advantage of action/reaction and inertia.
- Small, fast movements merely potentiate isometric muscle contractions and give a false illusion of work because the heart rate increases.
- Programs should include travel. For example, participants should walk in their own circles and then in the reverse direction.

Using Buoyancy

Buoyancy can assist rest or work in water. It aids limb movements toward the surface, thereby requiring less work, and resists downward movements, thereby creating more work (Fawcett, 1992). Buoyancy equipment amplifies these effects.

For example, compare a standing biceps curl using a dumbbell on land with the same exercise using a foam dumbbell in nipple-deep water. On land, this exercise works the biceps concentrically during elbow flexion and eccentrically during elbow extension. In water, the foam dumbbell minimizes work for the biceps while causing the triceps to contract eccentrically to some degree during elbow flexion (by resisting the buoyant move to the surface) and concentrically with elbow extension. The same water movement using a webbed glove (surface area resistance) will work the biceps concentrically with elbow flexion and work the triceps concentrically with elbow extension.

Therapists determine optimal exercise depth according to the amount of weight bearing a patient needs for a given injury. The exact working depth for shallow water exercise must strike a balance between creating work intensity and decreasing gravitational compression. Work in water depth above the xiphoid process (the segment of the sternum level with the nipple) should be considered deep water work, because the lungs are submerged, buoyancy increases, and cardiorespiratory response changes.

Gravitational forces are decreased up to 90 percent when the body is immersed in neck-deep water (Cole, Moschetti, and Eagleston, in press). Therefore, the deeper the water, the more difficult it is for an exerciser to control the effects of buoyancy. Individual bone density, percentage of muscle mass and body fat, and deposition of fat also affect each individual's buoyancy.

APPLYING THIS RESEARCH TO YOUR PARTICIPANTS' NEEDS

- When you analyze movements to determine what muscle group is working and how, you must consider the properties of water.
- Controlling the buoyancy effects of foam equipment in water is critical for optimum resistance benefits.
- You can maximize the resistance benefits of using a surface-area resistance device (webbed glove) by regulating speed and lever length to vary intensity.

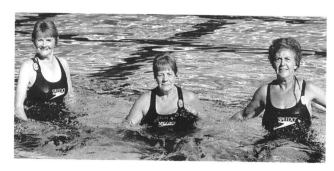

- A participant's ability to touch the bottom of the pool is not the criterion for differentiating shallow and deep water. Optimal working depth for water exercise depends on the body composition of the exerciser. A general rule of thumb is to work between the navel and nipple for shallow water.
- A program designed for deep water is necessary for water depths above the nipple.

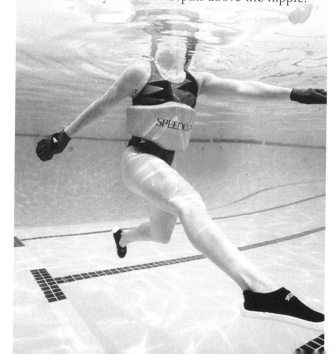

Table 6.1 Water Training Studies

Water depth and program type	Duration and frequency (weeks and days/week)	Pool water temperature	Mean age (years/range)	Intensity
Shallow water rhythmic exercise (Hoeger et al., 1993) n=20F	8 and 3	Not available	27 (15—35)	70—85% HR reserve
Shallow and deep water rhythmic exercise (Sanders, 1993) Combined groups, n=20F	8 and 3	83°F 28°C	40 (18—66)	74—84% HRmax

In the Sanders (1993) study, level of significance was preset at the p <.05. Groups 1 and 2 were found to be significantly different and were examined separately. Results are given below.

Water depth and program type	Duration and frequency (weeks and days/week)	Pool water temperature	Mean age (years/range)	Intensity
Shallow and deep water rhythmic exercise Group 1, n=10F	8 and 3	83°F 28°C	28 (18—37)	71—84% HRmax
Shallow and deep water rhythmic exercise Group 2, n=10F	8 and 3	83°F 28°C	52 (41—66)	68—80% HRmax
Shallow water rhythmic exercise** (Miss, 1988) n=6F, 6M (athletes)	9 and 3	Not available	Not available (18—25)	80% HRmax
Shallow water calisthenic exercise** (Ruoti, Troup, and Berger, 1994) n=10F, 2M)	12 and 3	86°F 30°C	65 (59—75)	80% HRmax
Rhythmic deep water exercise** (Barretta 1993) n=12F, 5M	14 and 3	Not available	29.9 (19—43)	Not available

* Significant with p <.05.

**Men and women were evaluated together. The authors assigned fitness categories according to *The Y's Way to Physical Fitness* and *Principles and Labs for Physical Fitness and Wellness.* F = Female, M = Male

From Rippee, N., and M. Sanders. 1994. Probing the depths of water fitness research. *IDEA Today* (August). Reprinted with permission by IDEA, The Health Fitness Source, (800)999-IDEA, ext. 7.

Note: This table is a review of most of the training adaptations research currently available.

RHR (BPM) (pre/post)	% fat (pre/post)	$\dot{V}O_2$max (ml/km/min) (pre/post)	Flexibility % change	Muscular strength/ endurance
77/70* (−7 bpm) (below average/ average)	26.4/24.4* (−2%) (average)	31/35.6* (+4.6 ml/kg/min) (below average/ average)	14.9/16.5 in* (health standard– high physical standard)	5—15%+ isokinetic strength
75/69* (−6 bpm) (below average/ above average)	25.41/23.1* (−2.31%) (above average/ good)	28.66/31/97* (+3.31 ml/kg/min) (below average/ average)	14.4/14.7in (health standard)	bench press (+16)* curl-ups (+17)* (below average/ above average)
79/70* (−9 bpm) (poor/average)	25.1/22.1* (−3%) (average/ above average)	32.29/36.72* (+4.43 ml/kg/min (below average/ average)	15.9/16.0 in (health standard)	bench press (+19)* curl-ups (+22)* (below average/good)
72/69* (−3 bpm) (average/above average)	25.7/24.2* (−1.5%) (above average/ good)	25.0/27.22 (+2.22 ml/kg/min) (below average/ average)	12.8/13.5 in (health standard/ high physical standard)	bench press (+12)* curl-ups (+11)* (below average/ above average)
Not available	16.7/15.42* (−1.28%)	Significant increase	Significant increase	Significant increase: muscular endurance, but not power*
72/67* (−5 bpm)	38.5/36.9 (−1.6%)	23.4/26.9* (+3.5 ml/kg/min)	Not available	Significant increase: shoulder flexion/ extension; shoulder adduction/ abduction*
Not available	26.06/24.08* (−1.98%)	33.68/35.88* (+2.2 ml/kg/min)	14.8/16.8 in*	Significant improvement: shoulder press and pull; chest press and pull; thigh flexion*

Maintaining Thermal Balance During Water Exercise

A neutral temperature exists at which the metabolic heat generated by exercise can be transferred easily to the water without costing the exerciser energy through shivering from cold water stress (Cole, Moschetti, and Eagleston, in press). Maintenance of this thermal balance is important for maximizing optimal training. Pendergast (1988) reported that exercisers who have a reduced core temperature have reduced oxygen transport, which could influence oxygen consumption capability. Avellini, Shapiro, and Pandolf (1983), Craig and Dvorak (1969), and Svendenhag and Seger (1992) also found that the vasoconstriction/dilation response to water temperatures (narrowing and dilating of the blood vessels in cooler and warmer water) is important for the central blood flow and results in cardiorespiratory adjustments.

Craig and Dvorak (1968) suggested a neutral temperature for upright, shoulder-deep water exercise that balances heat production with heat loss during various exercise intensities. They suggested a temperature of 34 degrees C (93 degrees F) for 3.1 **METs** (corresponding to the warm-up or cool-down) and 29 degrees C (84 degrees F) for 4.2 METs (corresponding to vigorous travel moves during the aerobics portion [McArdle, Katch, and Katch, 1991]). Craig and Dvorak (1968) also reported an initial drop in core temperature with immersion in water of 32 degrees C (90 degrees F) and a continued decline even with a light workload.

Research also shows amount of body fat is not always an indicator of exercisers' comfort with water temperature. Body fat proved to be a critical insulator in water colder than 25 degrees C (77 degrees F) and during immersion for three hours (Rennie, 1988). However, in a review of the literature covering thermal, metabolic, and cardiorespiratory changes in men and women during cold water stress, Graham (1988) discussed various possibilities for comfort in cool water. Fat may diminish the response to cold, but layers of muscle seem to be more critical insulators. In addition, surface area exposed to the water during exercise and body mass are related to maintenance of body temperature.

APPLYING THIS RESEARCH TO YOUR PARTICIPANTS' NEEDS

- Standing in water cooler than 32 degrees C (90 degrees F) causes dramatic cooling for exercise participants. Performing standing

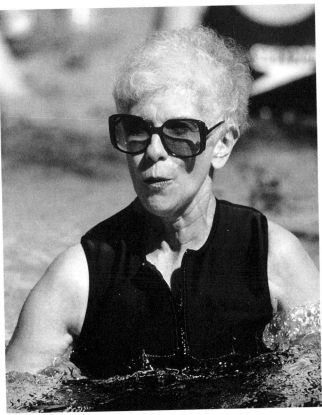

stretches has the same effect. Therefore, have participants jog while performing upper-body static stretches, and incorporate arm movements during lower-body stretches. Consider stretching only at the end of the workout or alternate stretching set with more vigorous "heat producing" sets.

- Insulation provided by additional clothing during exercise can contribute to temperature stability in very cold water. If water is cooler than the recommended neutral temperature, instructors need to encourage class participants to regulate their thermal comfort in water with extra clothing and increased work intensity.

Important Factors for Optimal Program Design

Research has documented that water exercise can improve health-related components of fitness and that these benefits are optimized when exercise design takes into account both exercise science principles and the properties of water. The unique properties of water have long been documented but must be understood in relation to water exercise, if fitness professionals are to design programs that provide an optimal training environment.

Physical therapists make use of these properties in rehabilitation (Cole, Moschetti, and Eagleston, in press; Fawcett, 1992); water exercise instructors also need to apply them, rather than merely taking land movements into the water. According to Cole, Moschetti, and Eagleston (1992), "the properties of water provide the greatest advantages for aquatic programs."

Though they are not directly addressed by this research, the following suggestions for program design seem to be supported:

- Exercise speed and number of repetitions must be individualized by each exerciser. The effects of buoyancy, body composition, deposition of fat, and limb length are such critical factors in regulating work intensity and are so different for each exerciser that not everyone in class can work at the same pace. Instructors need to teach participants to take personal responsibility for regulating work intensity according to their needs, rather than letting the beat of the music set the pace.

- Water is a forgiving environment, but it does not give us a license to use exercises that pose a potential risk for injury. Several training studies reviewed are still using exercises with a high potential for causing neck, shoulder, and back pain. (For example, performing continual calisthenic exercises while hanging backward on the pool wall may be contraindicated for the shoulders.) Instructors must choose movements responsibly and evaluate exercises for safety as well as water-specific benefits.

- Research and the properties of water make it clear we cannot simply drop land exercise into water and assume it will work the same way it does on land. For example, the training technique of **plyometrics** may be valid for creating work in water, but because of the effect of buoyancy, the movements will not be "plyometric" or elicit the same training response as they would on land. Plyometrics utilizes body mass and gravity to provide the rapid eccentric lengthening the technique requires. Buoyancy prevents the "all-important rapid prestretch" (McArdle, Katch, and Katch, 1991) from occurring.

We must keep in mind exercise science principles and the unique qualities of water when we design water exercise programs, evaluating movements with regard to the effects water has on the body.

Review of Water Exercise Literature From 1994 to 1998

Since 1994, we have seen many new research studies on water fitness. There seems to be a continuing interest by researchers in learning more about this activity and why it produces so many wonderful results for people. We have a great deal of anecdotal evidence on how water exercise improves people's health. We hear testimonials from our participants on how they have less back pain, enjoy their sport activities more, have more energy to play with their grandkids, and so on. We are just now beginning to understand why this is happening and how we can make our water fitness sessions more safe and effective for our participants.

This second section reviews more recent studies reported from 1994 to 1998. To help fitness professionals translate this current research, we give examples of applications of the studies' results. Using a combination of published studies and experience, we attempt to answer the following often-asked questions:

1. Why reduce the speed of movement in the water? How does this affect intensity?
2. What types of class formats are effective for water fitness sessions, and how can we help our participants improve?
3. Can water exercise help with weight management? Can it help prevent bone loss?
4. Can water exercise maintain or improve functional performance on land?

Speed of Movement

Frangolias and Rhodes (1995) compared metabolic responses to both land treadmill and deep water running in 13 runners who had previously trained in deep water for at least six months. The results showed that when deep water runners and treadmill runners were working at the same VO_2max and perceived exertion their stride frequency was 39 percent slower in the water. This study supports prior research that suggests we reduce the speed of movement from land to water by one-third to one-half. If we try to keep the same cadence in the water as on land we may end up learning what Wilder, Brennan, and Schotte (1993) discovered. The Wilder study looked at heart rate and cadence during deep water exercise and concluded that cadence was an effective quantitative measure for exercise prescription. However, in reviewing the study, we found that many of their 20 subjects dropped out

Motivation is important for the noncompetitive participant to gain benefits from water fitness activities.

of the study at different times. This suggests that if we use the same cadence for all participants we will not be meeting their needs and varied fitness levels.

Brown et al. (1997a) measured physiologic responses of men and women at treadmill-matched walking/running cadences and found that physiologic responses during deep water running were significantly greater when compared with land treadmill running at matched running cadences. Water runners cued to work at the same running cadence as on land produced higher submaximal responses, indicating that when speed was matched (land and water), the energy cost necessary to do the work was higher. In another study by Brown et al. (1997b), it was noted that during pilot work for the study, at a given cadence, when the lower-body range of motion was varied by the investigators, smaller ranges lowered exertion responses, indicating that speed of movement and working range of motion were related with regard to intensity. As runners slowed down their water movement, they also made their workout easier.

Two other studies examined energy expenditure during treadmill running on the land and in the water. Napoletan and Hicks (1995) made comparisons in energy expenditure between walking on a land treadmill and on a treadmill in the water at two different depths (mid-thigh and xiphoid level). The study suggested that walking at a speed of 2 miles per hour at both water levels required greater energy expenditure than land treadmill walking at the same speed. When subjects ran at 3.5 miles per hour at xiphoid depth, the energy expenditure was not significantly different than land running at the same speed. It was assumed that this difference was due to buoyancy's effect to "float" the body during the flight phase of the running gait. However, when running at 3.5 miles per hour in thigh-deep water, where the flight phase is eliminated, subjects achieved their highest energy expenditure and perceived the exercise as the most difficult when compared to land or chest depth at the same speed. Since most water exercise sessions are held in water that is at least waist deep, the variable times for individual body types to work through the flight phase are different. Additionally, if participants

are traveling without a treadmill, it could be assumed that at 3.5 miles per hour, energy expenditure in water would be greater. Generally, matching land speed requires more energy expenditure and varies with water depth and land prescriptions. In addition, land-based movement combinations should be adjusted to water speed. Byma, Craig, and Wilmore (1996) and Hered, Darby, and Yaekle (1997) found similar results. All studies concluded that water walking/running felt harder and required more energy than the same movement performed on land.

During a water step test, Wieczorek et al. (1996) found that stepping up and down at a cadence of 90 bpm elicited a heart rate response of only 39.4 percent of max heart rate. Seefeldt et al. (1997) studied 22 college-age females participating in an 11-week aquastep class. The subjects were pre- and post-tested for changes in $\dot{V}O_2$, body composition, flexibility, and treadmill time. The moves used were basic steps, v-steps, knee lifts, repeater steps, and some water-specific moves at a tempo between 80 and 120 beats per minute. Results indicated that there were no significant differences between pre- and posttesting for any of the parameters measured. Thus we cannot assume that taking a "land-based" activity and putting it into the water will be beneficial. We need to make sure we are creating "water-specific" moves all of the time and not just part of the time.

In another study, Evans and Cureton (1998) looked at bench height and different movements on the step while working at a cadence of 116 bpm and measuring $\dot{V}O_2$. They found that the water basic step (land move performed in the pool) elicited a lower $\dot{V}O_2$ response at all bench heights. The water jax (jumping jack with bench straddled) elicited the highest $\dot{V}O_2$ response and was higher than the land basic step. This study shows that a land step class taken directly into the pool at a set speed may not provide adequate overload for cardiorespiratory training. By using water-specific movement, however, the set cadence was adequate for training. These studies remind us of the need to be sure to create water-specific movement patterns all of the time in order to maximize the health benefits to our participants.

Finally, when subjects were asked to set their own pace, investigators found motivation to be a key element in self-directed cadence speeds. Gehring, Keller, and Brehm (1997) asked noncompetitive runners and competitive runners to replicate land training intensity during deep water running. Noncompetitive runners failed to replicate land training pace. However, competitive runners were able to achieve training intensities similar to land training by running. Hoeger, Varner, and Fahleson (1995) performed a similar test with water aerobics and found the same results using noncompetitive female subjects. Motivation is important for the noncompetitive participant to gain benefits from water fitness activities. We wonder if music tempo should be our only form of motivation, as it is with land-based group exercise classes, or whether we should be thinking about other forms of motivating participants. For example, we can educate them about muscle movement, the purpose of the exercises, and how training can be optimized through proper technique.

APPLYING THIS RESEARCH TO YOUR PARTICIPANTS' NEEDS

Land-based cadences may elicit higher energy expenditure depending on water depth, the size of the movement, muscular strength/endurance, body composition, and the motivation of the participant to work at a speed sufficient enough to make a difference. Instructor-set cadences may over- or underexert individuals depending on water depth, skills, and movement. How can we optimize the use of speed or cadence to create safe and effective training? Here's some suggestions:

- Allow participants to progressively increase the intensity of the moves by beginning slowly, emphasizing a full **range of motion**, and then gradually increasing speed without compromising range of motion, until they find the resistance level that is appropriate for them.

- **Intensity** can be regulated by slowing down or speeding up, depending on the strength and skill level of the participants as well as the type of motivation provided by the instructor. Motivate participants to increase their intensity by giving them cues such as "Push water out of your way" and by encouraging them to work at their own level.

- The "float or flight" phase of every movement, where the participant is suspended above the pool floor, varies in shallow water. Body composition differences and water depth will dictate individual time to land on the pool bottom and continue landing on a beat. Allow participants to choose a stride or movement frequency that allows time for these differences.

- Reduce the initial speed of movement by one-third to one-half of land speed before increasing the speed of the movement. If the pace is set by the music tempo, coach the participants to adjust the size of the movement based on their individual needs.

- Generally, walking and running at a given speed require more energy in water than on land, and the energy costs vary with water depth. Consequently, adjust speed when transferring land-based movements to water.

- During water exercise, the arms move through water's resistance to provide balance. For participants unaccustomed to working their arm muscles, moving at fixed speeds fatigues these muscles, minimizing their effectiveness as stabilizers for the remainder of the workout. Coordinate arm and leg patterns to balance work and rest, adjusting armwork to maximize cardiorespiratory training by the legs when targeting that objective.

- Do not assume that land-based step moves elicit the same cardiorespiratory response in the water as they do on land. Whether you are creating moves for a personal training session or a group class, design water-specific moves to maximize participant's results.

- Athletes or participants training to improve sports performance need to consider proper mechanics during resisted work in the water. Adjust speed to vary training intensities without compromising body mechanics. When speed variations no longer provide training overload, add equipment, so speed can again be applied for overload at a higher base load.

Interval Training and Progressive Resistance Overload

Wilber et al. (1996) studied 16 land-only trained male runners by comparing physiological responses during submaximal deep water running and land treadmill running at the same $\dot{V}O_2$. There was a 31 percent difference in blood lactate levels between the two types of activities, with the water eliciting the higher response. Lactate, or lactic acid, is a waste product of anaerobic energy production known to cause localized muscle fatigue (Study, 1991). It was concluded that the natural resistance of the water and the constant use of the arms create more of an anaerobic response, causing the higher lactate level response to exercise, especially in nonwater trained participants. Michaud et al. (1995b) also studied land-only trained male runners and found similar increases in blood lactate levels. It was suggested that interval-type workouts with short periods of rest be performed rather than continuous runs due to this rise in blood lactate levels. In another study by Michaud et al. (1995a), 10 healthy sedentary subjects participated in an eight-week progressive interval-style deep water running program. Land and water $\dot{V}O_2$max tests were performed before and after the training. Results indicated that the deep water running produced gains in $\dot{V}O_2$max of 10.6 percent for treadmill running and 20.1 percent for deep water running. Thus, interval-style training does, in fact, enhance function on land.

Frangolias, Rhodes, and Tauton (1996) believe that many of the studies on water running performed in the early 1990s used subjects unfamiliar with water running and therefore concluded that water training was not as effective as land training for maintaining and/or improving land $\dot{V}O_2$. They believe that if the activity is performed with poor technique there will be minimal transfer of cross-training benefits. Frangolias and Rhodes (1995) also did a study comparing metabolic responses for both treadmill and deep water running in 13 land- and water-trained runners. They found lower $\dot{V}O_2$max with similar peak blood lactate levels and lower stride frequency values when comparing land and water exercise. They felt that the active musculature and muscle recruitment patterns differ in water exercise due to the high viscosity friction of water and the nonweight-bearing nature of deep water running. In other words, the water is much like a giant resistance machine. As we muscularly adapt to the resistance of the water, we need to increase speed and surface area to challenge and improve our participants.

Arthur Weltman (1995) recently published a monograph on the blood lactate response to exercise. He believes the blood lactate response to exercise may be a more accurate estimate of endurance performance than $\dot{V}O_2$max because $\dot{V}O_2$max is limited by central circulation, and blood lactate responses to exercise appear to be limited by skeletal muscle at the cellular level. It is possible the reason that we are seeing increased lactate response during deep water exercise in land-trained but not water-trained participants is because the land-trained participants are not accustomed to overloading the muscles, especially the smaller muscles of the arms, on a continual basis. Training in the water involves strength/endurance training for skeletal muscles due to the constant resistance of the water. It would appear that a combination of deep water exercise and land training would be beneficial to performance, as it has the potential to increase $\dot{V}O_2$max and decrease blood lactate levels in general for both land and water performance.

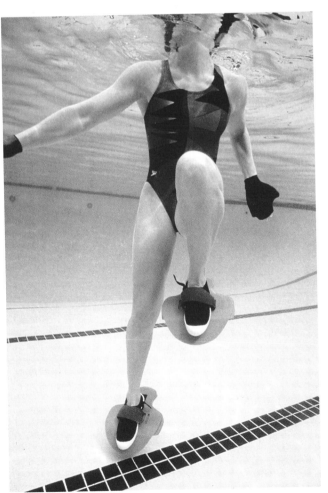

Quinn, Sedory, and Fisher (1994) studied seven women in a 14-week training study. The first 10 weeks subjects were land trained. After land training, they trained only in the water for four weeks. The subjects' VO_2 increased with the land training and then practically decreased back to pretesting levels after the water exercise training. The authors suggested that to improve results they might have tried interval training as opposed to the steady-state training selected in this study. Robert, Jones, and Bobo (1996) found similar results when comparing the physiological response of exercising in the water and on the land. It was thought that the participants were not motivated to work as hard in water as they did on land. One of the reasons the participants did not show results could be because they had not developed strength to move forcefully enough through the water to increase their overall energy expenditure. We see many land-trained participants come into water exercise and say they are not getting their heart rates up but that it is a tough workout from a perceived exertion standpoint. If we look at the water as a giant resistance arena then this makes sense. One must possess the strength to increase from a cardiorespiratory standpoint. Just as runners do **fartlek training** on the track (interval training in which the exerciser bases interval length on how he or she feels), water exercisers need to do interval training for optimum effectiveness of training.

APPLYING THIS RESEARCH TO YOUR PARTICIPANTS' NEEDS

When you look at further research on water exercise, check if the subjects have been "water trained." If they have not been, then you can expect to see that their cardiorespiratory fitness will be lower in the water. To truly get the benefits from water exercise, here are some tips to consider:

- Be aware that many land-trained participants don't feel cardiorespiratory overload during water exercise. This may be because they are not yet strong enough to overload their cardiorespiratory systems, even though their muscles are challenged.

- Incorporate interval-style segments instead of all steady-state work, especially for participants who have not trained extensively in the water. Interval training can enhance exercisers' ability to remove blood lactate and reduce discomfort.

- During the rest period of the interval work, encourage participants to move through a full range of motion, practice the move to check biomechanics, and then power the move during the interval segment. Vary segments using 10-, 15-, 20-, 25-, or even 30-second work/rest intervals. Not only is this effective but it also motivates participants by using different muscle types, providing a variety of movements, changing the pace, and anticipating rest. Use motivating music during the work and soft music during the rest.

- Keep in mind that untrained water participants may have an increased lactate response during deep water exercise because they are not accustomed to using their arms during a workout or to overloading their muscles on a continual basis.

- When participants have been in the program for a long period of time, have them use equipment to create an overload, so they can build more strength and endurance in the water. This is called the principle of adaptation. Once participants adapt to the water's resistance, progressively overloading to enhance gains will be important. Have strong participants gradually increase the intensity, then use equipment to increase surface area.

- Assume participants are at different levels within a water fitness session. Encourage the use of different sizes of equipment to individualize the overload. If all participants had the same equipment, it would be like taking them all into the weight room and putting them on the same level of resistance. We know that people's abilities are different, so we need to individualize, so that most of them maintain or improve their fitness levels.

- Due to water's constant resistance, workouts in the pool involve strength and endurance training for specific skeletal muscles. Remember that cross training on land and in the water can help balance any risk to untrained participants, can vary the physiological challenges to the body, and can make effective training more time efficient.

Water Exercise and Weight Management

Weight control is a primary motivator for many people to exercise. Although water exercise is increasing in popularity, due to its many unique properties and benefits, many exercisers ask the question, "Will water exercise help me meet my weight management goals?"

A number of research studies have indicated that rhythmic, upright exercise in the water can increase energy expenditure. In theory, if water exercise increases energy expenditure as do other physical activities on land, the additional energy output should lead to the control of weight and body fat. But several research studies have questioned whether water exercise is in fact effective for weight loss.

The Gwinup Study

Extensive media coverage of one study (Gwinup, 1987) was paramount in forming the public's perspective on water exercise. Gwinup designed a training study in which he compared the effects of swimming (not upright water exercise), stationary cycling, and walking on overweight women. Subjects exercised for one hour daily for approximately six months with no diet manipulation. Body fat was not estimated; however, one skinfold was taken at the triceps site at both the beginning and end of the study as an indicator of body fat change.

Results indicated that the body weight of the women who walked or cycled decreased 10 to 12 percent, while the body weight of the swimmers showed a nonsignificant increase. The skinfold measurement also decreased for the walkers and cyclists, but did not change for the swimmers. Gwinup concluded that while swimming was enjoyable and promoted fitness, it was not effective for weight or fat loss.

The media's enthusiastic coverage of Gwinup's findings was unfortunate because the study had some design flaws:

- The exercise sessions were not monitored; therefore, exercise intensity and adherence may have varied greatly among the exercise groups. Fitness was assessed not with a VO_2max test but by measuring resting pulse rates. Therefore, fitness gains could not be assessed or compared among the groups. The bottom line is that the actual energy expenditure over the six-month period undoubtedly varied among the walkers, cyclists, and swimmers.

- One skinfold measurement is not an appropriate indicator of body composition. Since the subjects' body composition was never actually estimated, there was no way to measure either body fat or lean mass changes that may have occurred as a result of the exercise interventions. It is possible that the work performed against the resistance of the water could have caused the swimmers to gain weight due to an increase in muscle mass.

- Finally, the subjects' diets were not manipulated or measured. Since diet is a major component of weight loss, the lack of control of this factor is a major design flaw in the study. Gwinup proposed that the swimmers actually increased their food intake to compensate for the energy lost through the increased activity. He further speculated that this increased food intake was to maintain subcutaneous body fat levels to provide insulation against the cool pool water (74 to 78 degrees F). He presumed that activity in the cold water stimulated the appetite mechanism to increase calorie consumption. Since diet was not controlled or measured, it is virtually impossible to attribute any weight or body fat changes solely to the exercise intervention.

The three major design flaws of this study preclude drawing any concrete conclusions from it regarding the efficiency of swimming as an exercise method to induce weight loss. Based on the data of Gwinup's study, it cannot be concluded either that swimming does or does not induce the loss of body weight or fat. Furthermore, the conclusions drawn from this swimming study should not be applied to upright water exercise, which is a different modality.

Weighing the Evidence

It is unfortunate that Gwinup's study received such coverage from the media in the 1980s; it is even more unfortunate that the flawed study has received endorsements from the popular press (Bailey, 1994). In 1997, Oprah Winfrey's personal trainer quoted this study on Oprah's popular TV show and spurred even more inaccurate perceptions about the effects of water training. Fortunately, a few training studies on the topic of body composition and upright water exercise have since become available in peer-reviewed journals. Let's examine some of these studies.

Hoeger et al. (1993) conducted a study that used an eight-week shallow water rhythmic exercise intervention. Subjects exercised three times a week at 70 to 85 percent of heart rate reserve for 20 minutes per session. Exercisers used long-lever resistance movements and no buoyancy or resistance equipment. Using skinfold measurements, the authors found a significant 2 percent decrease in body fat.

Abraham, Szczerba, and Jackson (1994) used an 11-week, three-day-a-week water aerobics program to assess changes in VO_2max, body weight, and percent body fat. Class length was 50 minutes, and the average training heart rate was 79 percent of maximum heart rate. Results showed that while body weight and VO_2max did not show significant changes after training (although VO_2 did improve by 5.6 percent), percent body fat showed a significant decrease of 1.4 percent. Two three-day dietary analyses provided an indication of dietary habits. The analyses determined no differences in total caloric intake between the experimental and control groups. The researchers concluded that this type of water exercise program provided health and fitness benefits for relatively inactive college women.

Conflicting evidence indicates that upright water exercise does not reduce body fat levels. Ruoti, Troup, and Berger (1994) conducted a 12-week training study with elderly subjects. The training protocol consisted of 40 minutes of traditional shallow water exercise movements at approximately 80 percent of maximum heart rate. Body fat percentage was estimated from body density determined by hydrostatic weighing. Members of the exercise group significantly improved their VO_2max, resting heart rate, and work capacity in the water, but failed to significantly decrease their percentage of body fat.

In another study by Campbell et al. (1990), subjects exercised at moderate intensity (60 to 80 percent of maximum heart rate) three days a week for 12 weeks. Each session lasted 20 minutes. The subjects consisted of normal-weight adults, overweight adults, and overweight teens. Skinfolds indicated a nonsignificant increase in percent body fat in the overweight adults and a nonsignificant decrease in the percent fat of the normal-weight adults. Overweight teens had a significant decrease (1.5 percent) in body fat. No dietary analysis was used in this study, a potentially significant flaw in the study's design.

Why are there so many different answers to the weight, body fat, and water exercise question? To comprehend the seemingly conflicting study results, you must understand the difficulties with research on weight or body composition. Since humans are not laboratory rats, nearly all research must take place while the subjects are interacting with their environment. Controlling physical activity and dietary intake is extremely difficult under these circumstances. Unfortunately, these two factors can have major implications for the changes in a subject's weight and body composition. The best studies attempt to have subjects maintain their normal activity levels so that the additional caloric costs are due solely to the exercise intervention. In addition, since studies rarely control dietary intake, some form of assessment must be used to determine if there is a significant difference in dietary intake between the control and exercise groups. If there is a significant difference, there is an unmeasurable bias on the impact of the exercise intervention.

Other factors for research include the following:

- **Metabolic demand.** To produce a change in body composition or weight, the metabolism steady state has to be changed through alterations in energy expenditure or energy intake. It is possible that some of the exercise interventions used in upright water exercise research were simply not strenuous enough to produce the required caloric deficit. A study conducted by Lieber, Lieber, and Adams (1989) may support this theory. Although this study did not use upright water exercise, the results did show that 11.5 weeks of swim training at 75 percent of treadmill VO_2max for 60 minutes, three days per week, significantly reduced body fat (2.4 percent) in sedentary young men. This reduction in body fat was not significantly different from the reduction (1.8 percent) experienced by subjects who performed a comparable amount of run training on land.

- **Body composition methodology.** The best studies of body composition are conducted by research laboratories and require extensive equipment and training. Study data are only as good as the assessment instruments or techniques used. Also, the method of body composition assessment must be appropriate for the population being studied.

• **Statistics/design.** When the number of subjects who complete a study decreases, the statistical power of the study decreases. Researchers are less able to detect any differences between treatment conditions. A reduction in statistical power also means that the ability of the experiment to provide an adequate test of the research hypotheses is decreased. One of the best ways to increase statistical power is to increase the number of subjects assigned to each experimental group.

APPLYING THIS RESEARCH TO YOUR PARTICIPANTS' NEEDS

• Tell your students the truth: The jury deciding the efficiency of upright water exercise for modifying body weight and composition is still out. In theory, since water exercise increases energy expenditure, it should promote weight loss and body composition alterations as long as the energy deficit is sufficient to disrupt the exerciser's metabolic balance. Also, since water provides resistance, water exercise training may result in positive strength gains and increases in muscle mass. The addition of muscle mass could increase the resting metabolic rate, and that increase, over time, could potentially result in weight and body fat changes.

• Reinforce the basics: Weight management and body composition status are based on energy intake and energy expenditure. The control of this status involves a combination of psychological and physiological factors, and the control mechanisms are not easily understood.

• According to Gaesser (1996), we should throw out weight as our main focus and concentrate instead on metabolic fitness first. Many people who are within the normal weight range are not healthy. In his opinion, health should not be measured by size alone, but also by metabolic parameters such as cholesterol, blood pressure, and blood glucose levels. The idea is to encourage people to shape up "without necessarily changing shape." This type of program may encourage people to begin getting healthy by focusing on the positive results "inside," without the fear of failing to appear "thin" on the outside. Yo-yo dieting, weight fluctuations, and dieting without exercise may be the reason for weight gain and other health-related problems. Gaesser suggests that some body fat in certain locations may be beneficial to protect against certain diseases and cancers. Insurance and drug companies, along with the fashion industry, have all endorsed thinness, and unfortunately, Gaesser believes it is "fitness professionals who have done more than any other group to make lean synonymous with health, and fat with unhealthy" (p. 31). As fitness professionals, we need to provide responsive feedback so our participants can achieve both healthy and realistic objectives for health.

Water Exercise and Prevention of Bone Loss

While body fat is foremost in the minds of many exercisers, bone is an important component of body composition. Researchers in Japan investigated the effects of water exercise on bone loss in healthy Japanese postmenopausal women (Tsukahara et al., 1994). Cross-sectionally, the bone density of the veteran water exercisers (water exercise participants for an average of 35.2 months) was significantly greater than that of beginning water exercisers or sedentary controls. Longitudinally, bone mineral density decreased 0.92 percent a year for the nonexercising controls, where it increased 1.55 percent a year for the veterans and 2.16 percent per year for the newcomers. The authors concluded that consistently participating in water exercise may be an important avenue for preventing bone loss.

Functional Exercise

Athletes who need to seek effective and safe cross-training alternatives may be interested in water exercise if it can supplement their training programs for land-based performance. Bushman et al. (1997) examined the effects of four weeks of deep water run training on land running performance in competitive athletes. Their results indicate that deep water run training did provide sufficient stimulus to maintain land running performance. Participants were able to run the same 5K time on a land treadmill after training only in the water for four weeks. Eyestone et al. (1993) performed a similar study using a two-mile run pre- and posttest and found similar results. Wilber et al. (1996) found that deep water running by land-trained runners may offer an effective training alternative to land-based running for the maintenance of aerobic performance for up to six weeks. Morrow, Jensen, and Peace (1996) also found that deep water run training was as effective as

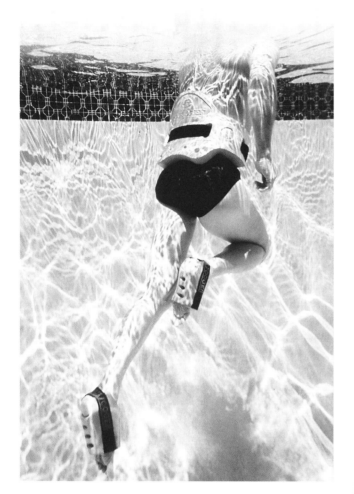

from a sitting position, balancing, and climbing stairs. These gains led to a more active, confident, and healthy lifestyle with greater independence for most of the subjects.

Another study by Simmons and Hansen (1996) measured the effectiveness of water exercise on postural mobility in the well elderly. Four groups of older adults (average age 80 years) trained either on the land or in the water. Results showed that the water exercisers who performed activity in the pool increased their functional reach almost every week, the land exercisers increased only during the first week, and the people who sat in the water and socialized and land sitters who played cards did not increase at all. Water exercisers demonstrated the greatest gains in functional activity. This implies that the type of activity and the environment seemed to affect postural skill outcome. Australian studies by Landgridge and Phillips (1988) and Smit and Harrison (1991) evaluated therapeutic aquatic exercise programs for patients with chronic back pain. Results showed that most participants had less back pain after completing the exercise programs. Improvement in quality of life for ADL were also reported by almost all subjects.

land-based running for the improvement of land treadmill VO$_2$ and a 2.4K run.

Athletes are not the only ones to benefit from water training. Improved quality of living may also be attributed to training. A recent study (Gold, 1998) involving 10,000 women between the ages of 40 and 55 found that 20 percent have trouble with simple functional physical tasks of daily living. These tasks are as basic as walking one block, climbing a flight of stairs, carrying groceries, bathing, and dressing. A current challenge for fitness professionals is to design exercises that simulate **activities of daily living (ADL)** on land. Sanders, Constantino, and Rippee (1997) performed a water exercise training study targeted to minimize the effects of aging and to improve land function for older women. Specificity of training was applied to exercise designs that strengthened and stretched muscle groups typically weak and tight from poor habits of daily living. Additionally, training progressions used coordinated land movement patterns, including movement errors and recovery skills. After 16 weeks, the subjects improved significantly in both muscular endurance and ADL tasks, such as standing

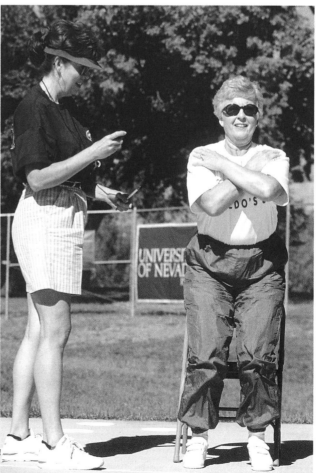

Two other studies investigated functional outcomes of exercises endorsed by the Arthritis Foundation Certification Program. In a study conducted by Templeton, Booth, and O'Kelly (1996), participants with rheumatic diseases (average age 62.5) participated in eight weeks of aquatic therapy. Results demonstrated a significant gain in active joint motion and improvement in 18 ADL. Investigators assumed that the decreased pain and difficulty in performing tasks contributed significantly to increases in functional status and range of motion. These encouraging results were supported by a study conducted by Suomi and Lindaur (1997), who measured the effects of hip and shoulder strengthening and range-of-motion exercises in 17 women suffering from arthritis involving the hip joints. Results indicated significant increases in isometric strength (10–17 percent) and range of motion for the affected hip joint of the exercise group. It was interesting to note that there were no significant gains for the unaffected shoulder joints in the exercise group. The program appears to have been effective in increasing strength and range of motion for the arthritic joints, but the intensity may not have been great enough to induce changes in joints unaffected by the condition.

APPLYING THIS RESEARCH TO YOUR PARTICIPANTS' NEEDS

Encourage athletes and nonathletes to cross train in water to increase the volume of their training without increasing the risk of injury, if they need variety or a reduction in the amount of land training performed due to injury. Also, encourage them to take a break from the land and train by substituting water-based training for a period of about four to six weeks. Listed below are other suggestions:

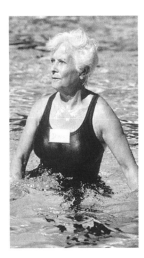

- Include water exercises that are specifically designed to target ADL within your water program, especially when working with older adults. For example, squats performed in shallow water or on the step may improve participants' ability to stand from a sitting position on land.

- People with special medical or chronic conditions can be taught water exercise skills in the safety of water to help maintain their ability to perform daily tasks and/or to improve an injury or condition. Always make sure to work with medical providers to ensure you respond to the specific needs of your participants.

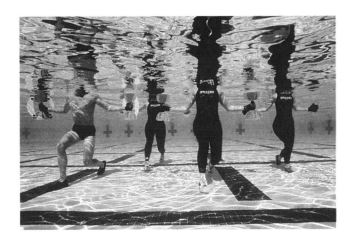

- Functionally targeted, individually paced water exercise progressions were shown to increase muscular strength and endurance for lower and upper body. Individualize the overload, using speed, surface area, and equipment to optimize resistance work. Select equipment that has various overload options. For example, webbed gloves allow you to increase the surface area progressively by first making a fist with the hand, then opening the hand, and finally opening the fingers. This piece of equipment also provides better progressive overload in many functional planes of movement.

For more information on functional exercise, see chapter 13.

Conclusion

As researchers continue to ask questions, water fitness will continue to evolve. These questions should be followed by quantification and results that can be applied to exercise and program design to ensure safe and effective training. The challenge for us as fitness professionals is to continually evaluate our programs in response to the growing body of literature and be open to change, while keeping pace with the most accurate information available.

When you look for new information from the research literature, make sure your sources are peer-reviewed journals in exercise science, rather than popular magazines. Articles in peer-reviewed journals should explain what questions the study was attempting to answer, summarize any biases or factors to be taken into account when reviewing the study's results, describe what the results mean, and mention further research that needs to be done.

Bibliography

Abraham, A., J.E. Szczerba, and M.L. Jackson. 1994. The effects of an eleven-week aqua aerobic program on relatively inactive college age women. *Medicine and Science in Sports and Exercise* 26(5): S103.

American College of Sports Medicine. 1990. The recommended quantity and quality of exercise for developing and maintaining cardiorespiratory and muscular fitness in healthy adults. *Medicine and Science in Sports and Exercise* 22(2): 265–274.

American Council on Exercise. 1993. *Aerobics instructor manual*. San Diego, CA: ACE.

Åstrand, I., A. Guharay, and J. Wahren. 1968. Circulatory responses to arm exercise with different arm positions. *Journal of Applied Physiology* 25: 528–532.

Avellini, B., Y. Shapiro, and K. Pandolf. 1983. Cardiorespiratory physical training in water and on land. *European Journal of Applied Physiology and Occupational Physiology* 53: 255–263.

Bailey, C. 1994. *Smart exercise* (ch. 6). New York: Houghton Mifflin.

Barretta, R. 1993. Physiological training adaptations to a 14 week deep water exercise program. Unpublished dissertation, University of New Mexico, Albuquerque.

Beasley, B. 1989. Prescription pointers on aquatic exercise. *Sports Medicine Digest* 11(1).

Brennan, D.K., T.J. Michaud, R.P. Wilder, and N.W. Sherman. 1992. Gains in aquarunning peak oxygen consumption after eight weeks of aquarun training. *Medicine and Science in Sports and Exercise* 24(5): S23.

Brown, S., L. Chitwood, K. Beason, and D. McLemore. 1997a. Deep water running physiologic responses: Gender differences at treadmill-matched walking/running cadences. *Journal of Strength and Conditioning Research*, 11(2): 107–114.

Brown, S., L. Chitwood, J. Alvarez, K. Beason, and D. McLemore. 1997b. Predicting oxygen consumption during deep water running: Gender differences. *Journal of Strength and Conditioning Research* 11(3): 188–193.

Bushman, B., M. Flynn, F. Andres, C. Lambert, M. Taylor, and W. Braun. 1997. Effect of 4 weeks of deep water run training on running performance. *Medicine and Science in Sports and Exercise* 29(5): 694–699.

Byma, H.K., J.N. Craig, and J.H. Wilmore. 1996. A comparison of the effects of underwater treadmill walking on oxygen consumption, heart rate and cardiac output. *Journal of Aquatic Physical Therapy* (November): 4–11.

Campbell, K.D. et al. 1990. Effect of water exercise on body composition in overweight females. Presentation at American Alliance for Health, Physical Education, Recreation and Dance, Annual Convention, New Orleans, LA.

Cassady, S.L., and D.H. Nielsen. 1992. Cardiorespiratory responses of healthy subjects to calisthenics performed on land versus in water. *Physical Therapy* 72(7): 62/532–68/538.

Cole, A., M. Moschetti, and R.E. Eagleston. (in press). Lumbar spine aquatic rehabilitation in *A sports medicine approach, handbook of pain management*, ed. A. Cole, 2nd ed. Baltimore: Williams and Wilkins.

Cole, A., M. Moschetti, and R. Eagleston, 1992. Getting backs in the swim. *Rehabilitation Management* (August/September): 62–70.

Corbin, C.B., and R. Lindsey. 1994. *Concepts of physical fitness*. 8th ed. Madison, WI: Brown and Benchmark.

Costill, D.L. 1971. Energy requirements during exercise in the water. *Journal of Sports Medicine* 11: 87–92.

Costill, D., P.J. Cahill, and D. Eddy. 1967. Metabolic responses to submaximal exercise in three water temperatures. *Journal of Applied Physiology* 22: 628–632.

Craig, A.B. Jr, and M. Dvorak. 1969. Comparison of exercise in air and in water of different temperatures. *Medicine and Science in Sports and Exercise* 1(3): 124–130.

Craig, A.B. Jr., and M. Dvorak. 1968. Thermal regulation of man during water immersion. *Journal of Applied Physiology* 25: 23–35.

Duffield, M.H. 1976. *Exercise in water.* Baltimore: Williams and Wilkins.

Ebbeling, C.B., C.J. Ebbeling, A. Ward, and J. Rippe. 1991. *Comparison between palpated heart rates and the heart rates observed using the polar favor heart rate monitor during aerobics exercise class.* Exercise Physiology and Nutrition Laboratory, University of Massachusetts Medical School (unpublished study).

Eckerson, J., and T. Anderson. 1992. Physiological response to water aerobics. *Journal of Sports Medicine and Physical Fitness* 32(3): 255–261.

Evans, B.W., K.J. Cureton, and J.W. Purvis. 1978. Metabolic and circulatory responses to walking and jogging in water. *Research Quarterly* 49: 442–449.

Evans, E., and K.J. Cureton. 1998. Metabolic, circulatory and perceptual responses to bench stepping in water. *Journal of Strength and Conditioning Research* (Summer).

Eyestone, E., G. Fellingham, J. George, and G. Fisher. 1993. Effect of water running and cycling on maximum oxygen consumption and 2-mile run performance. *American Journal of Sports Medicine* 21(1): 41–44.

Fawcett, C.W. 1992. Principles of aquatic rehab: A new look at hydrotherapy. *Sports Medicine* 7(2): 6–9.

Fernhall, B., T. Manfredi, and K. Congdon. 1992. Prescribing water-based exercise from treadmill and arm ergometry in cardiac patients. *Medicine and Science in Sports and Exercise* 24(1): 139–143.

Frangolias, D., and E. Rhodes. 1995. Maximal and ventilatory threshold responses to treadmill and water immersion running. *Medicine and Science in Sports and Exercise* 27(7) 1007–1013.

Frangolias, D., E. Rhodes, and J. Tauton. 1996. The effect of familiarity with deep water running on maximal oxygen consumption. *Journal of Strength and Conditioning* 10(4): 215–219.

Gaesser, G. 1996. *Big fat lies, the truth about your weight and your health.* New York: Fawcett Columbine.

Gehring, M., B. Keller, and B. Brehm. 1997. Water running with and without a flotation vest in competitive and recreational runners. *Medicine and Science in Sports and Exercise* 29(10): 1374–1378.

Gleim, G.W., and J.A. Nicholas. 1989. Metabolic costs and heart rate responses to treadmill walking in water a different depths and temperatures. *American Journal of Sports Medicine* 248(5), March-April.

Gold, E. 1998. Interview by author. University of California, Medical School, Davis, The study of women across the nation (SWAN).

Graham, T.E. 1988. Thermal, metabolic and cardiovascular changes in men and women during cold stress. *Medicine and Science in Sports and Exercise,* 20(5): S185–S191.

Gwinup, G. 1987. Weight loss without dietary restriction: Efficacy of different forms of aerobic exercise. *American Journal of Sports Medicine* 15(3): 275–279.

Heberlein, T., H. Perez, J. Wygand, and K. Connor. 1987. The metabolic cost of high impact aerobics and hydro-aerobic exercise in middle-aged females. *Medicine and Science in Sports and Exercise* 19(2): Supplement S89, #531.

Hered, S.L., L.A. Darby, and B.C. Yaekle. 1997. Comparison of physiological responses to comparable land and water exercises. *Medicine and Science in Sports and Exercise* 29(5): Abstract #923.

Hoeger, W., T. Gibson, J. Moore, and D. Hopkins. 1993. A comparison of selected training responses to water aerobics and low-impact aerobic dance. *National Aquatics Journal* (Winter): 13–16.

Hoeger, W., J. Varner, and G. Fahleson. 1995. Physiologic responses to self-paced water aerobics and treadmill running. *Medicine and Science in Sports and Exercise* 27(5): Abstract 83.

Hoeger, W., T. Gibson, J. Moore, and D. Hopkins. 1993. A comparison of selected training responses to water aerobics and low impact aerobic dance. *National Aquatics Journal* (Winter): 13–16.

Hoeger, W.K., D.R. Hopkins, D.J. Barber, and T. Gibson. 1992. Comparison of maximal VO_2, HR and RPE between treadmill running and water aerobics. *Medicine and Science in Sports and Exercise* 24(5): S96.

Johnson, B.K., J. Adamcyzk, S.G. Stromme, and K.D. Tennoe. 1977. Comparison of oxygen uptake and heart rate during exercise on land and in water. *Physical Therapy* 57(3): 273–278.

Kennedy, C., V. Foster, M. Harris, and J. Stokler. 1989. *The influence of music tempo and water depth on heart rate response to aqua aerobics.* Paper presented at IDEA Foundation International Symposium on the Medical and Scientific Aspects of Aerobic Dance, October, San Diego, CA.

Knecht, S. 1992. Physical and psychological changes accompanying a 10 week aquatic exercise program. *AKWA Letter* 5(5): 6.

Landgridge, J., and D. Phillips. 1988. Group hydrotherapy exercises for chronic back pain sufferers. *Physiotherapy* 74(6): 269–273.

Lieber, D.C., R.L. Lieber, W.C. Adams. 1989. Effects of run training and swim training at similar absolute intensities on treadmill VO_2max. *Medicine and Science in Sports and Exercise* 21(6): 655-661.

Maharam, L. 1992. Swim yourself thin. *Fitness Swimmer* (June): 50–51.

McArdle, W.D., J.R. Magel, G.R. Lesmes, and G.S. Pechar. 1976. Metabolic and cardiovascular adjustment to work in air and water at 18, 25 and 33°C. *Journal of Applied Physiology* 40: 85–90.

McArdle, W.D., F.I. Katch, and V.L. Katch. 1991. *Exercise physiology, energy, nutrition, and human performance.* 3rd. ed. Philadelphia: Lea and Febiger.

Michaud, T.J., D.K. Brennan, R.P. Wilder, and N.W. Sherman. 1992. Aquarun training and changes in treadmill running, maximal oxygen consumption. *Medicine and Science in Sports and Exercise* 24(5): S23.

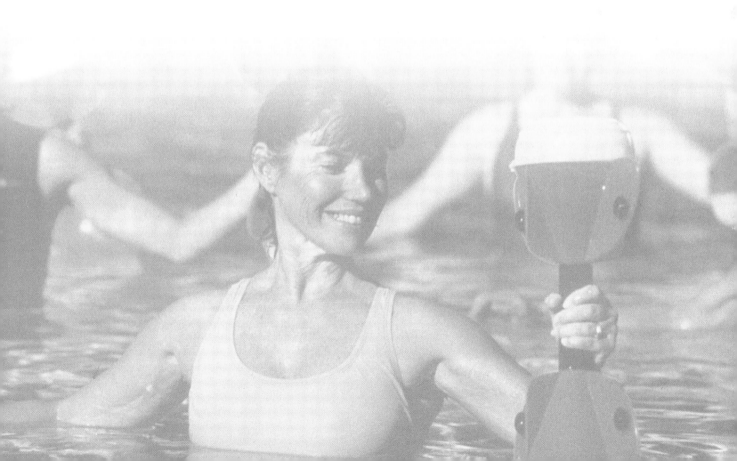

Michaud, T.J., D.K. Brennan, R. Wilder, and N. W. Sherman. 1995a. Aquarunning and gains in cardiorespiratory fitness. *Journal of Strength & Conditioning Research* 9(2): 78–84.

Michaud, T. J., J. Rodriguez-Zayas, F. F. Andres, M. G. Flynn, and C. Lambert. 1995b. Comparative exercise responses of deep water and treadmill running. *Journal of Strength and Conditioning* 9(2): 104–109.

Miss, M. 1988. Comparison between the effects of a nine week exercise program on land or in the water on selected components of physical fitness. Unpublished thesis for master of science degree, University of Illinois at Chicago, Chicago, IL.

Morrow, M.J., R.L. Jensen, and C.R. Peace. 1996. Physiological adaptations to deep water and land based running training programs. *Medicine and Science in Sports and Exercise* 28(5): Abstract 1252.

Napoletan, J.C., and R.W. Hicks. 1995. The metabolic effects of underwater treadmill exercise at two departments. *APTR* 3(2): 9–14..

Navia, A.M. 1986. Comparison of energy expenditure between treadmill running and water running. Thesis, University of Alabama, Birmingham.

Pendergast, D.R. 1988. *Medicine and Science in Sports and Exercise.* Supplement. 20(5): S170–175.

Quinn, T., D. Sedory, and B. Fisher. 1994. Physiological effects of deep water running following a land-based training program. *Research Quarterly for Exercise and Sport* 65(4): 386–389.

Rennie, D.W. 1988. Tissue heat transfer in water: Lessons from the Korean divers. *Medicine and Science in Sports and Exercise* 20(5): S177–S183.

Ritchie, S., and W. Hopkins. 1991. The intensity of deep water running. *International Journal of Sports Medicine* 12: 27–29.

Robert, J.J., L. Jones, and M. Bobo. 1996. The physiological response of exercising in the water and on the land with and without the X1000 Walk'n Tone Exercise Belt. *Research Quarterly for Exercise and Sport* 67: 310–315.

Ruoti, G., J. Troup, and R. Berger. 1994. The effects of nonswimming water exercises on older adults. *Journal of Sport and Physical Therapy* 19(3), March, 140–145.

Sanders, M.E. 1993. Selected physiological training adaptations during a water fitness program called Wave Aerobics. Thesis, University of Nevada, Reno, Microform Publications, University of Oregon, Eugene.

Sanders, M., N. Constantino, and N. Rippee. 1997. A comparison of results of functional water training on field and laboratory measures in older women. *Medicine and Science in Sports and Exercise* 29(5), Abstract 630.

Seefeldt, L., A. Abraham, D. Waterfield, and J. Cavanaugh. 1997. The effects of an eleven week aqua step exercise program on maximum oxygen consumption, body composition and flexibility in college age women. *AKWA Letter* 10(4): 10.

Shephard, R. 1984. Tests of maximal oxygen uptake: A critical review. *Sports Medicine* 7: 77–80.

Simmons, V., and P. Hansen. 1996. Effectiveness of water exercise on postural mobility in the well elderly: An experimental study on balance enhancement. *Journal of Gerontology: Medical Sciences* 51A(5): M233–M238.

Smit, T., and R. Harrison. 1991. Hydrotherapy and chronic lower back pain: A pilot study. *Australian Journal of Physiotherapy* 37(4): 229–234.

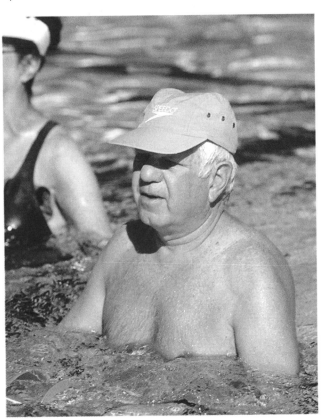

Stavish, J.M. 1987. Walk-jog versus swim training: Effects on body composition and aerobic capacity. Unpublished thesis, San Diego State University, San Diego, CA.

Stevenson, J., S. Tacia, J. Thompson, and C. Crane. 1988. A comparison of land and water exercise programs for older individuals. *Medicine and Science in Sports and Exercise* 20:S537.

Study, M., ed. 1991. *Personal trainer manual, the resource for fitness instructors.* San Diego, CA: American Council on Exercise.

Suomi, R., and S. Lindaur. 1997. Effectiveness of Arthritis Foundation program on strength and range of motion in women with arthritis. *Journal of Aging and Physical Activity* 5: 341–351.

Svedenhag, J., and J. Seger. 1992. Running on land and in water: Comparative exercise physiology. *Medicine and Science in Sports and Exercise* 24:1155–1160.

Templeton, M.S., D.L. Booth, and W.D. O'Kelly. 1996. Effects of aquatic therapy on joint flexibility and functional ability in subjects with rheumatic disease. *Journal of Orthopedic and Sports Physical Therapy* 23(6): 376–381.

Thomas, D.Q., and K.A. Long. 1994. Generalizability of deepwater exerciser blood pressure. *Research Quarterly for Exercise and Sport* 65S (March): A30.

Town, G.P., and S.S. Bradley. 1991. Maximal metabolic responses of deep and shallow water running in trained runners. *Medicine and Science in Sports and Exercise* 23(2): 238–241.

Tsukahara, N., A. Toda, J. Goto, and I Ezawa. 1994. Cross-sectional and longitudinal studies on the effects of water exercise in controlling bone loss in Japanese postmenopausal women. *Journal of Nutrition and Science Vitaminology* 40(1): 37–47.

Vikery, S.R., K.J. Cureton, and J.L. Langstaff. 1983. Heart rate and energy expenditure during aqua dynamics. *Physician and Sports Medicine* 11: 67–72.

Weltman, A. 1995. *The blood lactate response to exercise* (Monograph #4). Champaign, IL: Human Kinetics.

Whitley, J.D., and L.L. Schoene. 1987. Comparison of heart rate responses; water walking versus treadmill walking. *Physical Therapy* 67: 1501–1504.

Wilber, R., R. Moffatt, B. Scott, D. Lee, and N. Cucuzzo. 1996. Influence of water run training on the maintenance of aerobic performance. *Medicine and Science in Sports and Exercise* 28(8): 1056–1062.

Wilder, R.P., and D.K. Brennan. 1993. Physiological responses to deep water running in athletes. *Sports Medicine* 16(6): 374–380.

Wilder, R., D. Brennan, and D. Schotte. 1993. A standard measure for exercise prescription for aqua running. *American Journal of Sports Medicine* 21(1): 45–48.

Wieczorek, M., D. DeMore, M. Tucker, P. Shea, M. Brokes, C. Kauffman, A. Marchese, K. Row, R. Babb, and P. J. Sorg. 1996. Comparison of heart rate, blood pressure and rate of perceived exertion on land versus water with aerobic stepping. *The Journal of Aquatic Physical Therapy* 4(5): 4–10.

Physical Laws and Properties of Water

MARY E. SANDERS AND MARY CURRY

Objectives:

- To examine the physical environment of water, comparing land to water.

- To identify how the physical laws and properties of water act against the body during immersion and movement through the water.

- To apply the properties to water exercise and class design.

Participants can achieve fitness throughout their lives by working out at a challenging pace, safely, in the water. Research has shown that when the intensity of exercise in water equals the intensity of exercise on land and the exercises have been chosen to target the same specific training objectives (cardiorespiratory, muscular endurance, etc.), training results are equivalent. Thus, instructors who match the **properties of water** with appropriate training guidelines for cardiorespiratory endurance, muscular conditioning, flexibility, and body fat loss can achieve results in those areas (Barretta, 1993; Hered, Darby, and Yaekle, 1997; Hoeger et al., 1993; Ruoti, Troup, and Berger, 1994; Sanders, 1993).

A few training studies of shallow water training programs have targeted land-based functional activities of daily living (ADL) skills. The results of these studies suggest that people in such shallow water training programs improved both the quantity and quality of their land activities (Sanders and Maloney-Hills, 1998; Simmons and Hansen, 1996; Templeton, Booth, and O'Kelly, 1996). The net result is that participants have stronger, leaner, and healthier bodies that allow them to achieve or maintain a happier, fully active lifestyle.

Conditions for exercise in water differ from those for exercise on land. Instructors must understand these differences before they can design safe and effective exercises. In this chapter we cover the major differences in eight areas:

- Buoyancy
- Hydrostatic pressure
- Gravity versus buoyancy
- Speed, power, and force
- Inertia
- Resistance
- Leverage
- Action and reaction

For each of these, we describe the following:

1. The physical laws that pertain to water
2. How those laws affect the body during submerged exercises
3. How both the physical laws and the physiological responses of the body in water apply to effective exercise and class design

Buoyancy

Archimedes' principle describes *buoyancy* as the upward thrust exerted on an immersed object at rest as a force equal to the weight of fluid that is displaced. The force of the buoyancy will vary depending on water depth; the amount of body surface area immersed in the water; and body weight, height, bone density, and composition.

The arms and legs have a different degree of buoyancy depending on body composition and lever

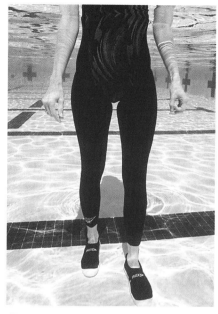
1 Shallow depth

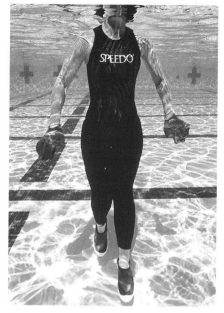
2 Transitional depth

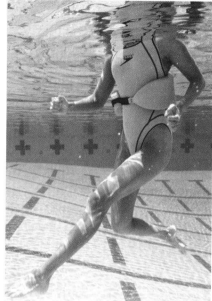
3 Deep water depth

length. For example, lifting an arm overhead and out of the water decreases the buoyancy of the body.

Gravitational forces decrease as a body goes deeper into the water:

- At waist depth (with lungs not submerged), gravity decreases by 50 percent; the feet are used as a base of support.
- When the water is above the nipple (the lungs are submerged), gravity decreases by 85 percent; feet are still a base of support but less stable.
- When the water is neck deep, gravity decreases by 90 percent. If the person is not wearing buoyancy equipment, the feet are still a base of support but less stable. If the person is wearing buoyancy equipment and is suspended in the water, the feet are not a base of support.

People may find it difficult to balance in the water because of the effects of buoyancy pushing upward. Achieving balance and stability when the lungs are submerged is more difficult because the body must balance the **center of buoyancy** at the lungs with the center of gravity at the hips.

EXERCISE DESIGN CONSIDERATIONS

- Teach balance skills such as **sculling** and coordinated arm/leg patterns.
- Provide participants with webbed gloves to wear on their hands. These increase surface area, which helps them balance.

- Don't determine the optimal shallow water depth for exercise by the participants' ability to touch the bottom of the pool (Kennedy et al., 1989). Instead, consider participants' body composition, their stability and control of movement, and their ability to move quickly through the water by propelling themselves with their feet.
- Vary the force of the buoyancy by changing depths. In the shallow water, mimic deep water exercises, in which the feet do not touch the bottom, by having participants lift their feet off the bottom and work suspended in the water.

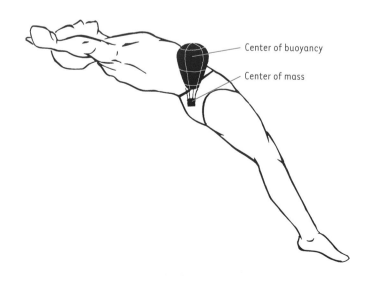

Center of buoyancy

Center of mass

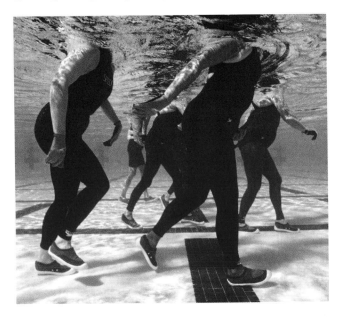

- Perform a cross-country ski movement with legs and arms working in unison, then perform the movement with legs and arms in opposition.

- Jog in shallow water (water line between the navel and nipple), and gradually move into deeper water. Feel the difference that depth makes on the force of buoyancy, control of movements, and speed of movements.

- Perform a scissors movement in shallow water, first in a "rebound position" (pushing forcefully off the pool floor) and then in a "suspended position" (with feet raised off the floor, mimicking deep water). Feel how the impact and buoyancy changes. How do the arms and legs need to work together for balance and stability?

- Address differences in buoyancy at various water depths and for different individuals. Design exercises for each depth that take into account the amount of buoyancy acting on the body. Frequently cue participants to correct their posture, as buoyancy may take them out of good alignment.

TECHNICAL DRILLS FOR THE POOL

- First jog in shallow water with your hands out of the water, then with arms hanging straight down at your sides (no movement), and finally with arms performing a figure-eight scull in the water. Which of these three upper-body positions provided the most stability or support for the movement?

Hydrostatic Pressure

Hydrostatic pressure is defined as the thrust of the molecules of a fluid on the entire surface area of an immersed body. Hydrostatic pressure against the body increases with depth. It affects the body in the following ways:

- When the lungs are submerged, the increased hydrostatic pressure makes breathing more difficult. Breathing and inflating the lungs against the pressure help participants maximize lung volume and adjust to the feeling of pressure against the chest.

- The increase of pressure aids venous circulation and contributes to the reduction of edema, especially in the lower body. In a vertical position, the greatest pressure is at the feet.

- Systolic blood pressure may increase initially upon immersion as a response to hydrostatic pressure on the body. In deep water exercise, heart rate decreases as stroke volume increases.

EXERCISE DESIGN CONSIDERATIONS

- Cue your participants to breathe, fully inflating the lungs against the pressure. Watch that they don't hold their breath.

- Teach your participants that their bodies will normally rise on inhalation and descend with exhalation.

- Allow participants with high blood pressure to adjust to deep water gradually, starting in shallow water and exiting in shallow water.

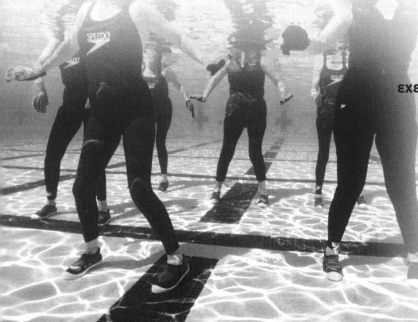

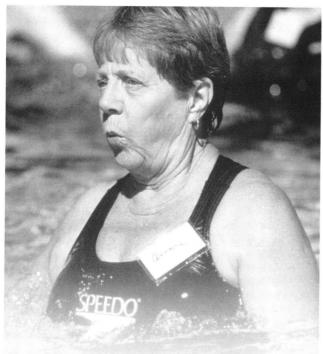

- Using heart rates to estimate exercise intensity in water may not be appropriate, as research shows that water depth (increased hydrostatic pressure), temperature, amount of armwork used, and the use of handheld equipment all affect heart rates. Instead, use a combination of perceived exertion (RPE) and the talk test to monitor intensity.

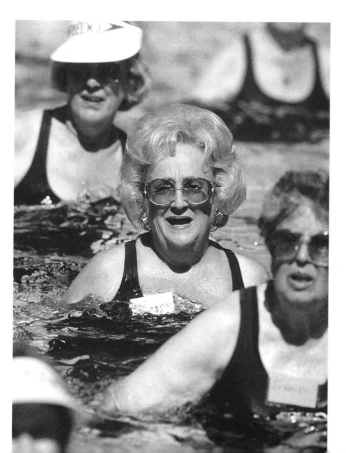

TECHNICAL DRILLS FOR THE POOL

- In shallow water, submerge your lungs and shoulders, scull, and straddle your legs. Inhale and feel your feet rise off the pool floor; exhale and feel your body descend.
- Wearing buoyancy equipment in deep water, legs hanging vertically and arms outstretched horizontally, practice breathing and inflating your lungs. Feel your body rise on inhalation and descend on exhalation.

Gravity versus Buoyancy

On land, gravity is the primary force acting against the body. Work is created by lifting upward against gravity.

In water, buoyancy is the primary acting force. Intensity increases as arms and legs move downward against buoyancy.

Buoyancy assists upward movements and provides some resistance to downward movements (Fawcett, 1992). With buoyancy-assisted movements, the arms and legs involved float to the surface. The degree of assistance depends on individual body composition. With buoyancy-resisted movements, the parts of the body involved push down against the water, creating work. The amount of work depends on the surface area involved, the lever length, and body composition.

Consider the differences between which muscles are assisted or resisted on land and in the water:

Table 7.1 **Comparison of Muscle Land Work (Standing Upright) vs Water Exercise**

Land Exercise

Assisted	Resisted
Triceps	Biceps
Abdominals	Erector spinae
Adductors	Abductors
Latissimus dorsi	Deltoids

Water Exercise

Assisted	Resisted
Abductors	Adductors
Deltoids	Latissimus dorsi
Biceps	Triceps

Adapted from Kennedy and Sanders, 1995.

Here's an example of how to use this difference: The biceps are considered strong muscle groups on land. They can be assisted in water, while the weaker triceps can resist buoyancy for a natural overload.

EXERCISE DESIGN CONSIDERATIONS

- Design exercises that work in opposition to buoyancy to add resistance or that work in the same direction as buoyancy to assist movements. For example, have participants push a kickboard down partially below the water as they walk to work the midback muscles. Determine how buoyancy's force creates work or rest; examine the mechanics of the movement; and manipulate range of motion, speed, and surface area against buoyancy's force.

- Use a step or platform to increase the effect of gravity and reduce buoyancy by decreasing water depth.

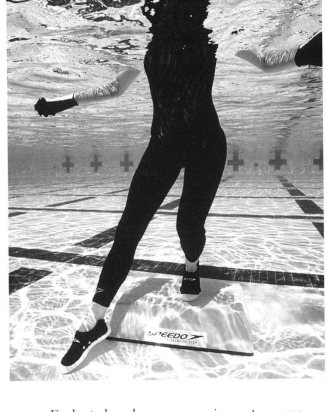

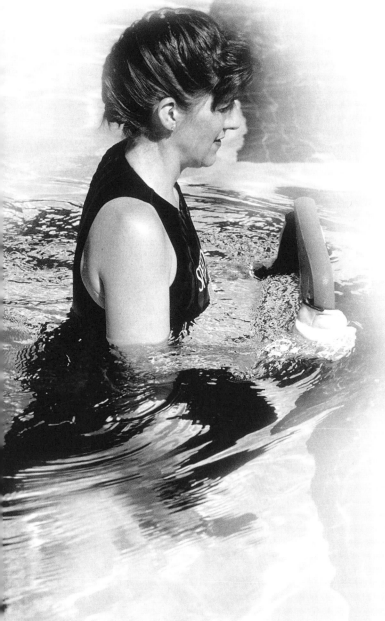

- Evaluate how buoyancy equipment can provide assistive or resistive effects. Example: If a buoyant barbell is held during elbow flexion, it assists the biceps while the triceps contract eccentrically toward the surface and resist the buoyant force. Extending the elbow to move the buoyant barbell requires the triceps to contract concentrically.

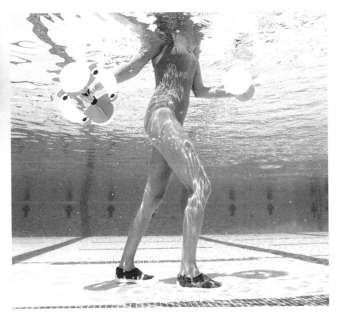

TECHNICAL DRILLS FOR THE POOL

- Test the effects of buoyancy-assisted movements by placing your hands at your sides in water. Notice how your arms have a tendency to float to the surface.
- Perform a biceps curl (elbow flexion and extension) in chest-deep water and then a kick in front (hip flexion and extension). Determine what part of each movement is assisted by buoyancy and what part is resisted.

 Video References:

The Introduction to the Speedo Aquatic Fitness System. 1994. Session 1, Buoyancy.

Specificity of Training and Deep Water Program. 1995. Introduction.

Speed, Power, and Force

Speed is a direct measure of the rate of covering distance or rate of motion of a moving object (Brancazio, 1984). The speed of performing an exercise in water is different than on land, because movement of the body in water involves overcoming the additional force of the water working against it. Faster movement through the water results in greater drag and resistance, which increases the muscular work required for movement (Shanebrook and Jaszczak, 1976).

Power is the rate of doing work, the amount of work done divided by the time required to do it (power = work done/time). Power is the result of exerting more force during a movement.

A force is any action that can cause an object to accelerate (Brancazio, 1984). The larger the force pushing against the water, the greater the acceleration and the resulting speed. The body will accelerate in the direction of the force acting on it. Therefore, as participants exert more force (without changing any other variables), the result is an increase in resistance and exercise intensity.

Water has some specific effects on participants' ability to move with speed, power, and force:

- The lack of traction, an inability to overcome inertia, and the floating effects of buoyancy can prevent participants from attaining the speeds necessary to produce optimal resistance against the body.
- Greater muscular work is required to maintain faster speed against the increased forces of resistance than with comparable movement on land.

- Heart rates increase with the speed of movement through water.
- Lower-body movements performed in water result in higher oxygen uptake $\dot{V}O_2$ than similar exercises performed on land.
- Research shows that only one-half to one-third the speed achieved during land walking and jogging is necessary for the same level of energy expenditure for walking and jogging in waist-deep water.
- Buoyancy can affect speed and force. Too much buoyancy can make it difficult to stabilize and to apply sufficient force through the water.

EXERCISE DESIGN CONSIDERATIONS

- Increase the speed, power, or force of a movement without compromising range of motion to increase the intensity of the movement. Allow participants to adjust the speed of movement at any time during the workout.
- Use equipment to affect exercise intensity by altering the speed, power, and force of the movement. For example, participants who wear water shoes will have better traction, allowing them to push more forcefully through the water with greater speed, increasing resistance and exercise intensity.
- Use exercises that train for power to train participants for ADL, such as going up and down stairs or walking with greater speed. This type of training in your exercise design would include using the working position of "rebound" (pushing forcefully off the pool floor) during both traveling and stationary movements or mimicking the "bounding" movements of stair climbing.

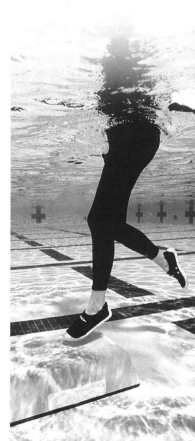

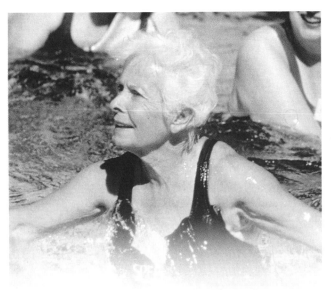

- Teach participants to regulate speed, range of motion, and surface area on their own. Working on the beat of the music may compromise one or more components, resulting in undertraining or overtraining some participants (Rippee and Sanders, 1994). Allow participants to find their own internal "beat" and range of motion—class *should* look a little chaotic!

- Make sure your participants are working in the proper water depth so they can balance and apply force through water to maximize the results of the exercises. This is especially important for exercises that travel through the water.

TECHNICAL DRILLS FOR THE POOL

- Working at navel depth, jog forward with hands clasped behind your back. (Water shoes will help with traction.) Change your force through the water. Does your speed change? Does the intensity change as you speed up or slow down?

- Working in the shallowest water possible, match a movement to the beat of the music. While maintaining the beat, move to deeper water and note any changes in the size or control of the movement.

- Partner up in navel-depth water. Turn on the music and, facing your partner, perform jumping jacks, staying on the beat for one minute. Then choose a different beat that is faster or slower and work on that beat for one minute. Check your intensity. Can you stay with your partner and the beat the entire minute? Monitor your intensity; does it match the training objective?

- Wearing gloves, slice your hands through the water while performing a rotator cuff movement. Maintaining the same size movement and surface area of the hands, increase the speed of the movement. Feel the increased resistance to the movement.

 Video Reference:

The Introduction to the Speedo Aquatic Fitness System. 1994. Session 1, Speed, Power & Force.

Inertia

According to Newton, *inertia* is the tendency of a body to remain in a state of rest or of uniform motion in a straight line until acted on by a force to change that state. Once the body has overcome the inertia of still water to begin movement, currents are created that can be used for resistance. These can assist movements in the same direction or resist movements in the opposite direction.

A change in direction creates opposing currents. Repeatedly moving back and forth quickly in the same area challenges balance, stability, and control as the body moves against the force of the currents.

The currents are the greatest for participants working in the center or back of a group traveling in the same direction. These strong currents will carry them along.

EXERCISE DESIGN CONSIDERATIONS

- Allow participants time during changes of direction to overcome the currents slowly, while maintaining balance and good body alignment. When participants travel as a group, cue them to stop traveling and stabilize (jog in place and scull) before changing the direction of travel. This allows the current to subside prior to changing direction.

- Be aware of the placement of participants in the class. Traveling in the center or back of the

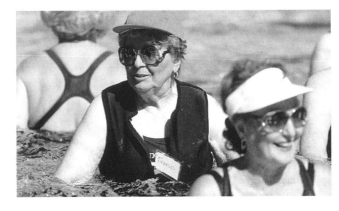

group may be less work than leading, due to the strong currents. Put the stronger participants on the outside of the group, but be watchful of the weaker ones, who may be carried along and even knocked off their feet!

- Provide balance exercises by traveling and then stopping, using the currents created by a body, limb, or hand moving through the water to challenge balance. Performing these exercises can improve core or trunk (abdominals, obliques, and erector spinae) strength by creating currents, then stopping the body so the stabilizers have to work against the water's movement.

- Use the water's current to create work or rest within your exercise design. When a traveling pattern is repeated back and forth quickly, the intensity of the work increases as the number of repetitions and speed rises.

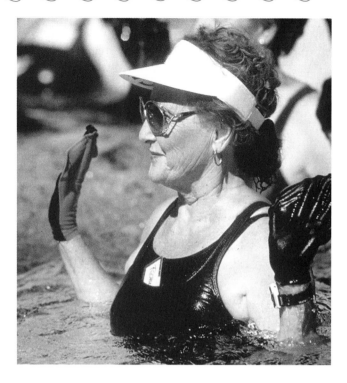

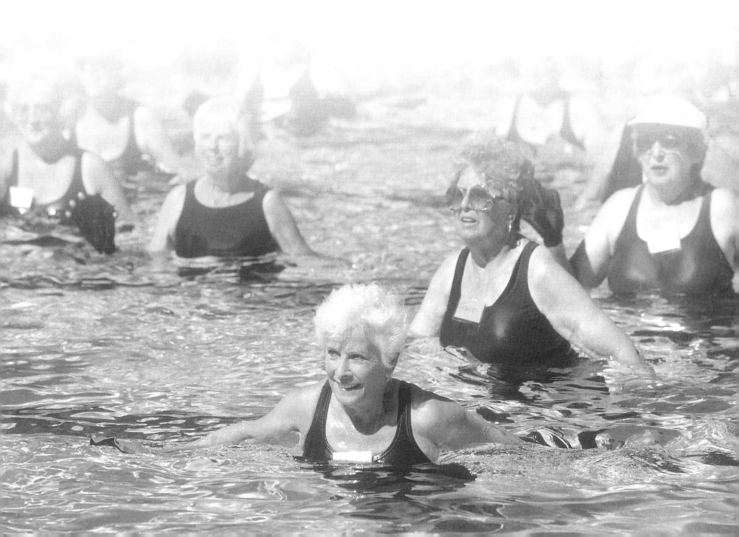

TECHNICAL DRILLS FOR THE POOL

- At a shallow depth, walk or jog in a variety of directions and styles (zigzag, scoot using giant steps, walk backward), then count to three and freeze. Stabilize yourself against the pushing and pulling current. Increase the challenge by standing on one leg or bringing your arms out of the water when you freeze.

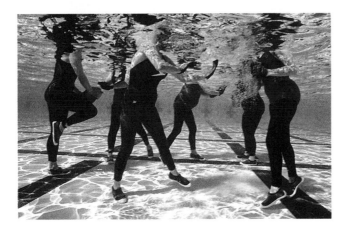

- Choose a partner. One of you performs stationary sculling for stability as the other one runs in a circle pushing water toward the partner (both directions) to create turbulence around you both. Make the drill harder, first by standing on one leg, then by bringing the arms out of the water. Feel the core stabilizers engage and help provide stability against the turbulence. Then change roles with your partner and do it again.

- Jog back and forth, changing directions without allowing the current to subside. Increase the speed at which you repeat the pattern. Feel it become harder and harder to continue to push against the current. What training objective could you target by performing this drill?

- Walk in a circle, moving in the same direction. Feel the current carry you along. Reverse the direction and move into the current. Feel the difference.

- Walk in single or double lines in a snakelike pattern. Feel the directional changes of the current challenge your balance and create work as you power through the water.

 Video Reference:

Introduction to the Waterfit Aquatic Fitness System, Shallow Water. 1994. Session 1, Inertia.

Resistance

Water provides resistance because of its viscosity. *Viscosity* is the tension between molecules of water. Think of it as the "thickness" of a liquid. When the body is submerged, resistance can be manipulated in any plane, pattern of movement, or body position. Resistance can be influenced by one or more of these variables as a body moves through water: form drag, turbulence, eddy currents, speed, leverage, action/reaction, and inertia. Small changes in these resistance variables can have marked effects on exercise intensity.

Form drag relates to the surface area and the shape of the object moving through the water. Drag acts to resist motion. It increases as an object's surface area increases, and the intensity of work required to move the object through water also increases. Reducing the surface area and streamlining will decrease drag. Limbs, the position of the body, or equipment can be dragged through the water to change the body's shape, thus changing the work intensity.

Turbulence is moving, choppy water with multidirectional force. It is created by objects moving through the water. Faster speeds and objects that are not streamlined create greater turbulence.

Eddy currents are created as the body moves through the water. As you move forward, the water flows from an area of higher pressure in front of the body to an area of reduced pressure behind the body.

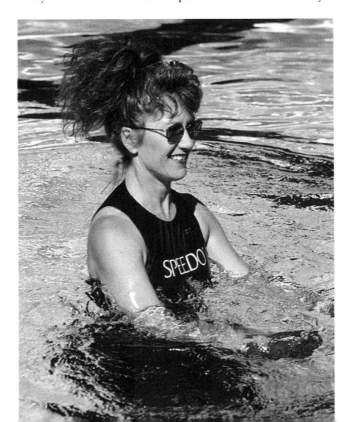

These currents create drag on the body, thus increasing resistance to movement.

Speed, leverage, action/reaction, and inertia are other variables that influence resistance. Refer to other sections of this chapter.

The results of many training studies have shown that the resistance of water provides enough intensity to significantly improve muscular strength and endurance, especially for the upper body. The resistance of movement performed at an average speed in water is estimated to be about 12 to15 times that of air, based on water being about 800 times more dense than air (di Prampero, 1986). Lower-body movements performed in water result in higher oxygen uptake VO_2 than similar exercises performed on land.

Research shows oxygen consumption to be highest when individuals travel through water at their optimal working depth at maximum speed (Town and Bradley, 1991). Lack of traction, inability to overcome inertia, and the floating effects of buoyancy may prevent participants from obtaining the speeds necessary to produce the form drag in front of the body, drag, and turbulence required for optimal resistance against the body.

EXERCISE DESIGN CONSIDERATIONS

- Design exercises using speed, water currents, and form drag to gradually increase the exercise intensity.

- Think of the pool as a giant resistance machine, in which muscular endurance can be targeted "on demand" with the initiation of movement.

- Use "travel sets" in the workout at sufficient speeds to reach cardiorespiratory training objectives during the workout. Cue the use of proper upper-body skills to assist with leg movement through water.

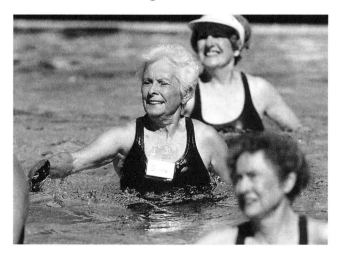

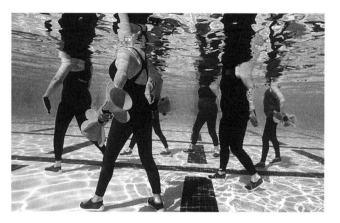

- Use equipment to vary the water flow and change the resistance to movement through the water. Equipment can change the intensity of the work by making movements more or less streamlined. In this way, you can regulate intensity to help participants achieve muscular training adaptations.

TECHNICAL DRILLS FOR THE POOL

- With elbows at the waist, pull your hands up toward your face. Vary the size and speed of the movement each time in order to observe the turbulent water on the surface. As you pull harder, moving more water, the turbulence appears to increase at the surface.

- Choose a partner and jog one behind the other. The person behind should step outside into the wake turbulence created by the leader traveling forward, then close behind the leader into the "eddy space" and get pulled along. Repeat this exercise across the width of the pool. Try various formations and pool patterns to increase this effect on the body.

- Jog forward, hands clasped behind your back. Try to maintain the same speed while you move your elbows out; then slice the water with your hands; then open your arms out and drag your fully opened hands while wearing webbed gloves. Now, jog backward and reverse the sequence, slowly decreasing the resistance and streamlining your body. Feel the changes in intensity. Blend this drill with a "Traveling Set" during your workout and change the movement to increase form drag and intensity!

 Video Reference:

Introduction to the Waterfit Aquatic Fitness System, Shallow Water. 1994. Session 1, Resistance.

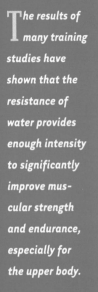

The results of many training studies have shown that the resistance of water provides enough intensity to significantly improve muscular strength and endurance, especially for the upper body.

Leverage

The lever length of limbs (arms and legs) affects the shape of the body moving through the water and the center of balance of the body:

- The longer the lever, such as an extended rather than a flexed arm, the greater the surface area and drag force through the water, and thus the greater the resistance to movement. Specific muscle groups may be recruited and overloaded as the lever length changes.

- As the lever length increases—the arms or legs work extended—the center of balance moves away from the center of the body, requiring greater stabilization by the trunk muscles to maintain balance. As the lever length decreases, the center of balance moves closer to the working joint and to the center of the body. This reduces the work intensity for the trunk stabilizers.

EXERCISE DESIGN CONSIDERATIONS

- Try modifying surface area (change lever length) and speed to provide appropriate resistance for changes in exercise intensity.

- Cue participants to change from a short lever to a longer lever slowly to protect the joints and to establish proper stabilization prior to increasing resistance.

- As a movement is enlarged by increasing the lever length, participants should coordinate synergistic arm or leg movements to balance the movement. For example, participants should kick side to side with coordinated extended arms.

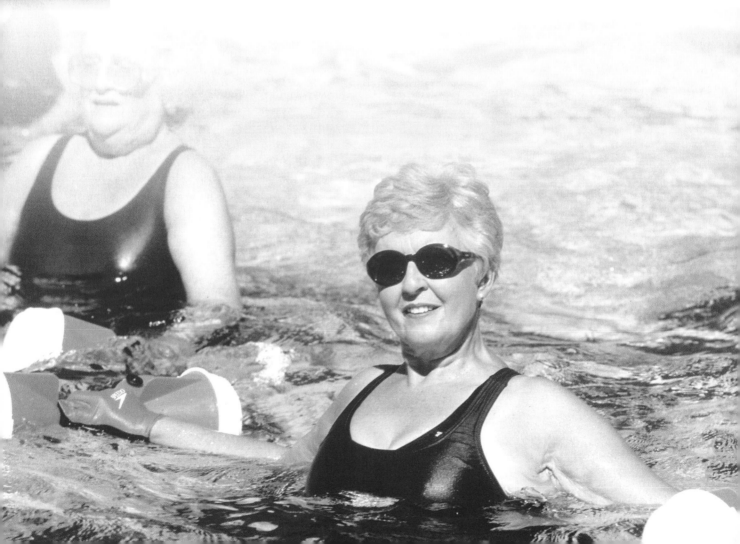

TECHNICAL DRILLS FOR THE POOL

- Walk forward with a bent knee (march). Stop and stabilize, then walk forward with straight legs, pulling them down heel first as you move forward. Feel the increased resistance with the increase of the lever length.

- Try one or more of the following "Short to Long" drills:

  ➤ Stationary jog, sculling for balance and stability, then extend the lever by kicking in front.

  ➤ Rock side to side, arms pressing out at the sides. Then extend the lever to a kick side to side, extending the arms long and working in opposition.

  ➤ Rock forward and back, sculling at the sides. Then enlarge the move and extend the front leg, enlarging the scull for balance.

  ➤ Take a neutral stance and pretend to play the piano with arms bent (short lever movement from the elbows). Then extend the arms (long lever movement from the shoulders) and continue playing. Watch for proper alignment in the extended position. Don't lean forward!

 Video Reference:

Introduction to the Waterfit Aquatic Fitness System, Shallow Water. 1994. Session 1, Leverage.

Action/Reaction

Newton's third law states that for every action there is an equal and opposite reaction. In the water, the harder you press against the water, the harder it pushes back against your body, creating variations in intensity for training. This law can be used to increase or decrease resistance, assist or resist travel, and oppose movement and create work. Long levers produce the greatest action/reaction response.

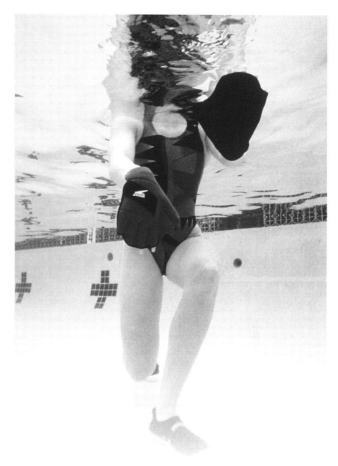

EXERCISE DESIGN CONSIDERATIONS

- Determine the direction of assistance and use that information in your exercise design to either assist or resist travel. For example, as the arms are pulled backward, the body is pushed forward, and travel is assisted forward. To resist travel when the arms pull backward, use an exercise that opposes forward movement such as jumping or kicking backward. The result is increased intensity.

- The size of a movement is as important as speed in regulating intensity. Small, quick movements may impede travel, while larger movements performed with sufficient speed can assist travel.

- To increase the efficiency of travel through the water, use large movements that push the water in the opposite direction.

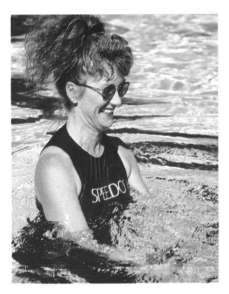
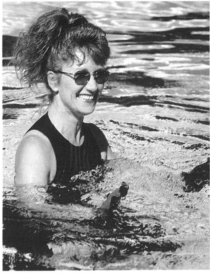
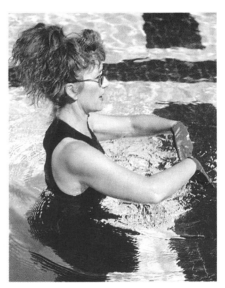

TECHNICAL DRILLS FOR THE POOL

- Try the following sculling drill wearing webbed gloves:
  - ➤ Scull with a flat hand, jogging in a stationary position. This emphasizes balance and stability.
  - ➤ Then scull with the fingers up, pushing the water forward. This assists traveling backward. If you then scull with the fingers pointed down, pushing the water backward, it will assist travel forward.
  - ➤ Next try sculling with the fingers pointed down, pushing the water backward, and travel backward. You should feel resistance. If you then scull with the fingers up, pushing the water forward, and travel forward, you also should feel resistance.
  - ➤ Finally, try a suspended jog and use a flat hand scull for lift.
- Wearing buoyancy equipment, kick short, fast kicks in front of your body. Now lengthen the leg levers—kick from the hip—and watch how the reaction to the move increases. Add your arms by rowing back to front. Feel how they assist travel.
- In a neutral working position with chest submerged, row your arms from front to back while tucking your knees to your chest. Feel the assistance to travel. Repeat by rowing back to front through the water. Now row front to back while you tuck jump backward; feel the resistance to travel and the intensity change.

 Video Reference:

Introduction to the Waterfit Aquatic Fitness System, Shallow Water. 1994. Session 1, Action/Reaction.

Bibliography

American College of Sports Medicine. 1990. Position stand: The recommended quantity and quality of exercise for developing and maintaining cardiorespiratory and muscular fitness in healthy adults. *Medicine and Science in Sports and Exercise* 22(2): 265–274.

American Council on Exercise. 1991. Personal trainer manual, the resource for fitness instructors. San Diego, CA: American Council on Exercise (formerly IDEA Foundation).

American Red Cross. 1992. *Swimming & diving.* St. Louis: Mosby Lifeline, Mosby-Year Book.

Barretta, R. 1993. Physiological training adaptations to a 14 week deep water exercise program. Unpublished dissertation, University of New Mexico, Albuquerque.

Beasley, B.L. 1989. Prescription pointers, aquatic exercise. *Sports Medicine Digest* 11(1).

Brancazio, P.J. 1984. *Sport science, physical laws & optimal performance.* New York: Simon & Schuster.

Cassady, S.L., and D.H. Nielsen 1992. Cardiorespiratory responses of healthy subjects to calisthenics performed on land versus in water. *Physical Therapy* 72(7): 62/532–68/538.

DiPrampero, P.E. 1986. The energy cost of human locomotion on land and in the water. *International Journal of Sports Medicine* 7: 55–72.

Fawcett, C.W. 1992. Principles of aquatic rehab: A new look at hydrotherapy. *Sports Medicine Update* 7(2): 6–9.

Gleim, G.W., and J.A. Nicholas. 1989. Metabolic costs and heart rate responses to treadmill walking in water at different depths and temperatures. *American Journal of Sports Medicine*, March–April, 17(2): 248–252.

Hered, S.L., L.A. Darby, and B.C. Yaekle. 1997. Comparison of physiological responses to comparable and water exercises. *Medicine and Science in Sports and Exercise Abstract* 24(5): 523.

Hoeger, W., T. Gibson, J. Moore, and D. Hopkins. 1993. A comparison of selected training responses to water aerobics and low impact aerobic dance. *National Aquatics Journal* (Winter) 13–16.

Kennedy, C., V. Foster, M. Harris, and J. Sockler. 1989. The influence of music tempo and water depth on heart rate response to aqua aerobics. Paper presented at the IDEA Foundation International Symposium on the Medical and Scientific Aspects of Aerobic Dance, October, San Diego, CA.

Kennedy, C., and M. Sanders. 1995. Strength training gets wet. *IDEA Today* (May).

Lamb, D.R., C.V. Gisolfi, and E. Nadel. 1995. Perspectives in exercise science and sports medicine. *Exercise in Older Adults* 8.

Miles, D., and P. Buchanan. 1991. *The Aquamotion water fitness manual.* J. MacDonald, 1048 "C" Palmetto Way, Carpinteria, CA 93013.

Moschetti, M. 1990. *Aquaphysics made simple.* Aptos, CA: AquaTechnics.

Rippee, N., and M. Sanders. 1994. Probing the depths of water fitness. *IDEA Today*, August.

Ruoti, G., J. Troup, and R. Berger. 1994. The effects of nonswimming water exercises on older adults.

Journal of Sport and Physical Therapy 19(3).

Sanders, M.E. 1990. The big chill is no thrill. *AKWA Letter* 4(3), (September): 1–13.

Sanders, M.E. 1992. *The Introduction to the Speedo Aquatic Fitness Program or The Art & Science of Wave Aerobics.* Educational video.

Sanders, M.E. 1993. Selected physiological training adaptations during a water fitness program called Wave Aerobics. Thesis, University of Nevada, Reno, Microform Publications, University of Oregon, Eugene.

Sanders, M., and C. Maloney-Hills. 1998. Aquatic exercise for better living on land. *ACSM's Health & Fitness Journal* 2(3): 16–23.

Schenkman, M. 1989. Interrelationship of neurological and mechanical factors in balance control. Balance Proceedings of the APTA Forum, Nashville, Tennessee, June 13–15.

Shanebrook, J. and R. Jaszczak. 1976. Aerodynamic drag analysis of runners. *Medicine and Science in Sports and Exercise* 8: 43–45.

Simmons, V., and P. Hansen. 1996. Effectiveness of water exercise on postural mobility in the well elderly: An experimental study on balance enhancement. *Journal of Gerontology: Medical Sciences* 51A(5): M233–M238.

Templeton, M.S, D.L. Booth, and W.D. O'Kelly. 1996. Effects of aquatic therapy on joint flexibility and functional ability in subjects with rheumatic disease. *Journal of Orthopedic and Sports Physical Therapy* 23(6): 376–381.

Town, G.P., and S.S. Bradley. 1991. Maximal metabolic responses of deep and shallow water running in trained runners. *Medicine and Science in Sports and Exercise* 23(2): 238–241.

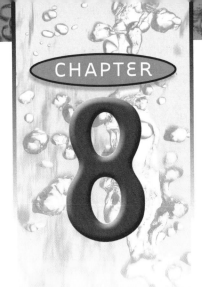
Fundamental Skills and Exercise Design

MARY E. SANDERS AND MARY CURRY

Objectives:

For three depths of water:

◎ Define fundamental skills used for balance, safety, and comfort.

◎ Define the characteristics of each depth, the basic moves, and appropriate equipment.

◎ Use the S.W.E.A.T. formula to adjust basic moves to water properties in order to create new exercises, regulate exercise intensity, and assist with balance.

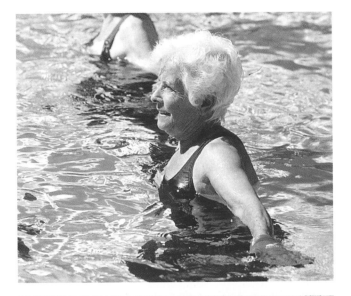

In this chapter we'll describe fundamental water exercise skills and discuss how to design water-specific exercises for three depths of water: shallow, deep, and the depth in between called transitional. Before we go into the specifics of exercise design for the water depths, though, we'll start with some general information that's applicable to all three depths.

All Depths

Here is where we'll discuss those fundamental skills that you'll need to teach participants regardless of water depth. We'll also look at equipment and a formula for exercise design—the **S.W.E.A.T.** formula—that is applicable to all depths.

Fundamental Skills

Skills that all water-fitness class participants need to know include sculling, how to recover to a stand from a horizontal position, proper body alignment, and thermoregulation (keeping the body warm). You also need to teach participants how to monitor their own exercise intensity.

Sculling

Sculling is a skill used to increase propulsion through the water and assist balance by providing lift. The figure-eight motion of sculling, especially when participants wear webbed gloves (made of soft Lycra or stiffer neoprene-type fabric), can be used to assist with good neutral posture, to resist or assist travel and direction changes, and to increase intensity for the upper body.

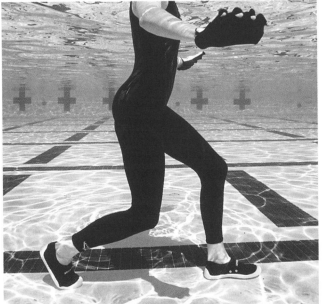

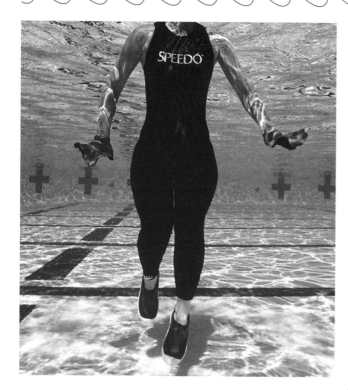

Guide participants to move their hands with palms facing downward and a little to the side. Have them practice making a figure-eight motion with both hands at their hips, then at the surface, pretending to smooth sand. Ask them to feel the resistance of water on the palms of their hands as they "lean" slightly on the supportive surface or "table top."

Buoyancy pushing upward against the surface area of the hand or the webbed glove provides a base of support for the body. It helps participants stabilize when they are pushed or pulled off center. As the participants push downward, the upward force of buoyancy (action/reaction) helps them to stand more erect.

 Video Reference:

Introduction to the Waterfit Aquatic Fitness System, Shallow Water. 1994. Session 2. Fundamental Skills, Sculling

Recovery to a Stand

Teach recovery to a stand in case participants lose their footing. The least desirable position for fearful participants is on their back or front in a horizontal position; they will feel less afraid if they know how to bring the body back to a more comfortable vertical position. Recovery is a particularly important skill to have when using flotation devices (especially on the ankles), since balance is more difficult and a fall to the prone position (face-down) can create an uncomfortable and undesirable hyperextension of the back.

Observing participants as they practice recovering also allows you to check their comfort level in the water. In order to perform this skill, participants must move from a horizontal to a vertical position in the water. If a participant is afraid to lie on his or her back or front, it suggests that this participant may be afraid of water and might panic if balance is lost.

Teach participants to protect their backs by starting face down in the prone position, turning the head to the side (the body follows the head), rolling over to the face-up supine position, and recovering according to the instructions illustrated in the video.

Recovery can be a difficult skill for people who have a lot of body fat or large breasts and underdeveloped abdominal strength. You may need to screen participants to identify those who cannot perform this skill. In shallow or transitional depths, they may be able to participate when a buddy system is in place, but they must be able to perform the skill in order to participate in deep water classes.

 Video Reference:

Introduction to the Waterfit Aquatic Fitness System, Shallow Water. 1994. Session 2. Fundamental Skills, Recovery to a Stand.

Proper Body Alignment

Before beginning a movement, participants should center their bodies, with the ears, shoulders, hips, and heels lined up. This is called the **ready position** (or **athletic stance**), a balanced stance from which many movements originate. A contraindicated exercise is any movement performed without good body mechanics.

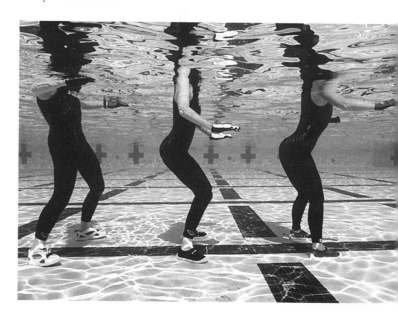

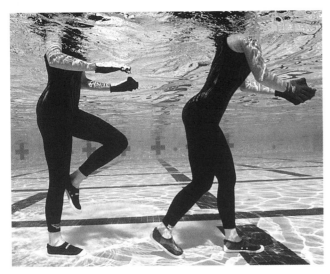

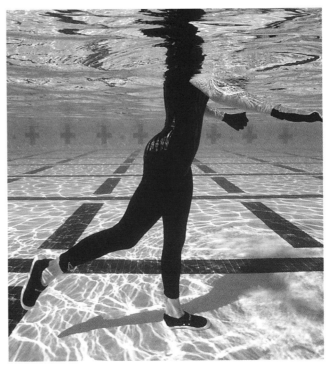

Monitor participants and correct them or change the moves as necessary to maintain proper body alignment (perform the cha-cha-cha). Here are some tips you can give them to stay in alignment:

- Hold the chin in neutral position; do not extend it. When the chin is forward from neutral, the lower back is stressed. Present a stable lumbar spine against resistance when moving backward by tightening the abdominals. Keep the chin in for the power back movement; push with the hips, engaging larger back muscles; and move with good posture.

- When the leg is extended to the back, check that ears, shoulders, and hips are lined up.
- For rebound movements, land through the foot—first toes, then the ball of the foot, then the heel to the flexed knee (like running uphill).
- Press the heels to the floor regularly.
- When jogging, bring the knees forward in front of the shoulders. Lean slightly forward to avoid hyperextending the back.
- In deep water, maintain balance by keeping the knees slightly flexed and forward, ahead of the shoulders.

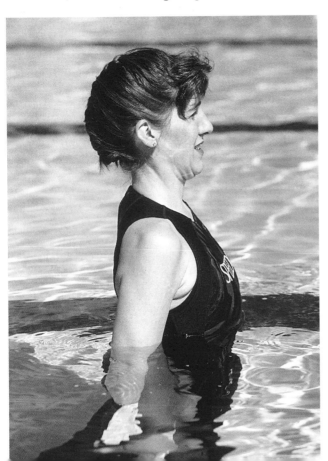

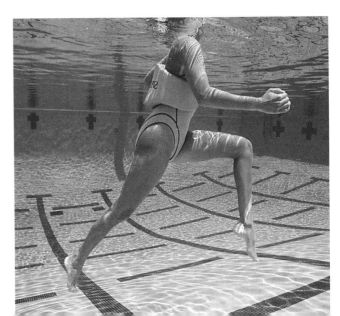

- Adjust the body to cool water temperatures by immersing the armpits, the front of the neck, and the sides of the chest. This may help reduce shoulder shrug and tension. Move to keep warm and relaxed.

If participants cannot maintain proper body position and control movements, then move them to shallower water (which will reduce the effects of buoyancy so they can gain control). Have them move more slowly with force and control or change the exercise. It takes good abdominal strength to maintain good posture during exercise. It may take participants some time to develop that basic strength.

 Video Reference:

Introduction to the Waterfit Aquatic Fitness System, Shallow Water. 1994. Session 2. Fundamental Skills

Thermoregulation

Do your participants bolt quickly to the locker room after class to warm up? Do they leave early, drop out, or complain about being cold? Although many variables can affect participants' temperature perception, including air, wind, water, and facility types, you can keep your participants comfortable by proper cueing and exercise design. To do this, though, both you and your participants need to understand thermoregulation in the water.

Normal body temperature is approximately 98.6 degrees F (37 degrees C), and body temperatures can vary throughout the day. Additionally, women's body temperatures vary with menstrual cycles, pregnancy, and menopause. The human body can maintain a constant body temperature even with environmental variations through physiological responses such as shivering or voluntary actions such as moving or putting on additional clothing.

The body can lose heat in four ways:

1. *Convection* occurs when the body comes in contact with air or water that has a lower temperature. While in contact with the body, the air or water is warmed, then carried away by streaming (movement).

2. *Conduction* is the transfer of heat energy away from the body by substances with which it is in direct contact. Conduction can occur in any medium—solid, liquid, or gas. Water's heat conductivity is 240 times greater than air (Hayward, 1990).

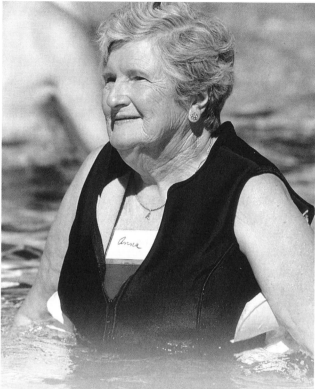

3. *Evaporation* is heat lost through the evaporation of water from the skin, such as perspiration. Evaporation accounts for about two-thirds of the normal resting heat loss from the skin and respiratory tract (Thorton, 1990).

4. *Radiation* is the direct emission of heat energy to and from mostly solid objects. The body gains great heat from sources such as the sun and fire.

Bodies also respond to being immersed in cold water in various ways. Because the skin cools, the peripheral blood vessels constrict. This causes an increase in the heart rate that may, in turn, cause an increase in blood pressure. Such a response can be a problem for participants with heart problems. Take health histories to identify such participants, and urge them to work with their physicians and to immerse themselves gradually.

When blood vessels in the skin and skeletal muscles constrict strongly, they create an outer shell that protects the body's core against further heat loss. This cooling of muscles and nerves results in slower, weaker, and poorly conditioned movements. To combat this, encourage participants to immerse themselves slowly. Follow this with relaxed, large muscle group movements that produce and conserve heat. Watch participants for shrugged shoulders and pinched faces, signs of tension and cold.

The areas of highest heat loss on the body are along the sides of the chest, the front of the neck at the carotid artery, the groin area, and the armpits (the warmest areas prior to immersion). Suggest to participants that they splash pool water on these warm spots prior to full body immersion. To conserve warmth, encourage them to wear more clothing, such as surfer undershirts that cover the neck, armpits, shoulders, and chest; tights; unitards; or "Chill Vests." If you're outside and it's windy, position participants with their backs to the wind to decrease the effects of wind chill heat loss from the face and neck. If you are facing the wind, make sure you protect yourself.

Other risk factors that can contribute to cooling are fatigue, hunger, dehydration, improper nutrition, immersion time and depth, medications, use of tobacco or caffeine (which are vasoconstrictors), and the use of alcohol (which is a vasodilator). Suggest that participants limit their intake of caffeinated beverages. Encourage participants to drink water and eat a high carbohydrate diet, which slows skin cooling (Strauss, 1985). For those who always feel cold, suggest that they check whether they are getting enough iron in their diet. Some conclusions drawn from research indicate that iron-deficient women experience cold sooner and are less tolerant of lower temperatures (Kirn, 1988).

Large individuals with a high percentage of body fat usually cool more slowly than small individuals with a low percentage of body fat. However, large individuals who lack the muscular conditioning that allows them to move at a high enough intensity through the water may actually cool more quickly than less-fat people.

Keep in mind that a person's amount of body fat may not be the only critical factor for body comfort. Delhagen (1987) found that well-conditioned runners discharged more heat than the normal person and were at greater risk for hypothermia when exposed to cool temperatures.

Finally, Collins (1989) found that men were three times more sensitive to cold when the skin was already cold. So, it's best to start warm and stay warm.

A Workout That Keeps Participants Warm

Design your program to keep participants warm and comfortable throughout the entire workout:

- Work out in the sunny area of the outdoor pool, if possible. If indoors, close the doors and windows to reduce wind chill. Wind chill markedly increases heat loss by radiation, convection, and evaporation (ACSM, 1986).

- Remind participants to layer on vests and leggings to reduce heat loss and stay warm.

- If you can, format the class to alternate less active work involving smaller muscle groups such as the biceps/triceps with more vigorous sets involving large muscles such as the quadriceps/hamstrings.

- Be organized so there is no waiting to begin, and use workout music with exercise transitions cued by a quick fade in/out of the music with no breaks.

- Although the muscle groups used and major work areas may change, keep the entire body in motion. Combine simultaneous upper- and lower-body movements to keep participants moving continuously at a low intensity. For example, perform upper-body resistance sets while jogging lightly.

- Cue participants to increase the speed, size, and force of movements to maintain a higher workload, which produces more heat.

- Cue your participants to keep their "heaters" going by moving their legs when they begin to chill. Be sure to design exercises that encourage legwork and, if necessary, add a "heater" set to the workout on demand to keep participants warm.

- Check for comfort during class by asking the participants "Are you warm?" (Don't even use the word "cold"!)

- If participants become too cool during deep water workouts and the air temperature is greater than the water temperature, move them to shallower water to reduce the amount of body surface directly exposed to the water, thus decreasing heat loss. Participants may also be able to move with greater force, power, and intensity in the shallower water, thus improving heat production.

- End the workout with a light, buoyant "warm"-down incorporating large, easy movements that will keep participants warm for the trek to the locker room and beyond. Encourage participants to go directly to the showers to chat if the air temperature is cool.

Recommended Water Temperatures

A general rule of thumb is to keep the air temperature approximately 3 degrees higher than the water temperature. Air temperatures higher than 3 degrees F above water temperature will cause program participants to perceive the water as being cold. However, the intensity of the training (based on the level of aerobic activity and the amount of heat generated from cardiorespiratory-targeted training) and the health and fitness of your participants must also be considered.

Recommended water temperatures for the comfort of your water exercise participants when considering exercise intensity are as follows:

- Competitive athletic training conducted at a high intensity (above 4.2 METs): 80–83 degrees F (26–28 degrees C)

- Fitness classes (at 4.2 METs, vigorous aerobics): 83–86 degrees F (29–30 degrees C), an approximate neutral temperature where most people can balance heat production with heat loss (Cole and Andres, 1987; Craig and Dvorak, 1968)

- Functional water fitness classes targeting activities of daily living: 83–86 degrees F (29–30 degrees C) for moderate intensity (below 4.2 METs) and stop-and-go activities (Sanders and Maloney-Hills, 1998)

- Arthritis classes: 83–88 degrees F (28–31 degrees C), depending on training intensity, with 86 degrees F (30 degrees C) being the most comfortable for a wide variety of exercises performed at low to moderate intensity (YMCA, 1997)

Monitoring Exercise Intensity

As was described in chapter 5 (see "Heart Rate"), exercise intensity for water fitness classes can be measured using heart rate, RPE, or the talk test. Teach your participants whichever methods you choose to use. Encourage them to work at an intensity that provides enough overload for work, but does not make them uncomfortable. (It's impossible for you to know what level is appropriate for each participant.) If they experience any pain or limitations in range of motion, they should modify the move or replace it with a similar move. Teach them the 4 S's to lower intensity:

> *Slow* down the move.
>
> Make the movement *Smaller*.
>
> *Stabilize*—check that the move is coordinated and stable or scull and lightly jog as you adjust your stabilizers for control.
>
> *Substitute* a similar move that feels more comfortable. For example, if jogging bothers their knees, they can march instead or can move to deeper water to reduce the amount of weight on the knees.

Review the 4 S's frequently and check that everyone understands how to use them. By teaching participants this simple skill, they can take control of their own workouts, systematically modifying them to lower intensity for personal comfort and safety.

 Video Reference:

The Golden Waves Program, Functional Water Training for Health. 1998. Section 3. Cardio Set, Interval Training.

To conserve warmth, encourage them to wear more clothing, such as surfer undershirts that cover the neck, armpits, shoulders, and chest; tights; unitards; or "Chill Vests."

Basic Equipment for Safety and Exercise Performance

The following basic equipment comfortably and safely enhances the effectiveness of exercises for your participants:

- **Webbed gloves.** Webbed gloves increase the surface area of the hands so participants can "lean" on them for effective support and balance, especially during big leg movements. This extra surface area acts as a "table top," assisting participants with upper-body posture as the lower body works through the resistance of the water. Additionally, the surface of the gloves enhances the action/reaction effect, so participants can more effectively use their hands to help change direction or adjust body positions. Finally, they provide on-demand variable resistance for upper-body muscular conditioning when participants change hand positions as follows:

    Level 1: Slicing hands (lowest intensity)

    Level 2: Fisting hands

    Level 3. Cupping hands

    Level 4: Webbing hands open (highest intensity)

Gloves are made in soft or stiffer fabrics so participants can choose the level of support or resistance they want.

- **Water shoes.** Participants should wear shoes for safe footing from the locker room to the pool. During class, shoes effectively provide good traction for faster travel through the water and cushion the foot for comfort. Worn in deep water, shoes can add extra drag resistance. During step work, participants should be required to wear water shoes that provide good toe protection, cushioning, and support.

- **Fitness apparel.** Water exercise is not swimming or sunbathing. Apparel should be comfortable and allow freedom of movement. Women can wear fitness suits that provide extra support or jog bras under suits. Additionally, participants can wear tights to decrease heat loss, increase the visibility of the legs so instructors can provide feedback, and make participants feel comfortable as they walk from the locker room into the pool.

 Video Reference:

Introduction to the Waterfit Aquatic Fitness System, Shallow Water. 1994. Section 4. Monitoring Exercise Intensity.

Shallow Water

Shallow water is defined as water that is navel to nipple depth measured with the individual standing on the bottom of the pool. In this section we'll examine how to design water-specific exercises in shallow water.

Basic Moves

The basic moves for shallow water are as follows:

1. Walking
2. Jogging
3. Kicking
4. Rocking
5. Jumping
6. Scissors

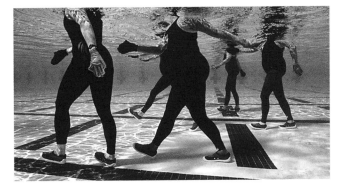

Walking

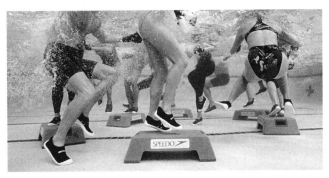

Jogging

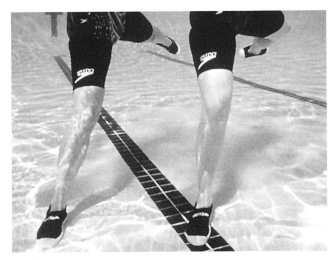

Rocking

They have their origin in dance moves. Every movement on land can be tracked to a variation of one of these basic moves. Each basic move can be varied slightly to create progressions of exercise intensity and to change the impact on the body. Instead of developing complicated choreography, use simple variations on the same basic movement to create new moves that balance muscle use, adjust intensity for cardiorespiratory or muscular endurance, and allow you to respond to participants' needs on the spot. Instead of memorizing steps, you'll be able to create thousands of movements based on simple variations of basic movements, giving you the freedom to grow your own workouts.

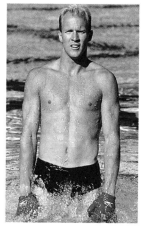

Jumping

Designing Exercises for Shallow Water

Each basic move can be manipulated by using the **S.W.E.A.T.** formula, taking into account the properties of water to create new moves, to change intensity, and to ensure muscle balance. This simple acronym helps you remember ways to vary a move to create a new one. Each letter stands for a specific use of water properties and has a specific training goal.

In the rebound position, partici[...] fully off the bottom of the pool ve[...] the effects of gravity, speed, form [...] lence, and impact. Intensity can b[...] flexing more deeply on landing, which increases the distance traveled upward. Using more power increases the speed and intensity.

In the neutral position, participants lower their bodies into the water. Buoyancy is enhanced and the levers now move through the water, with more horizontal movement possible. The effect of gravity is decreased and hydrostatic pressure is increased. Some vertical moves will be shorter due to the limited distance between the surface and the bottom; however, with the assistance of buoyancy, long lever horizontal moves are more effective. As more of the lever is submerged in a resistive environment, intensity can be increased through leverage, form drag, action/reaction, and speed.

In the suspended position, participants lift their feet off the bottom. Impact is eliminated and the properties of water movement are enhanced. Buoyancy, speed, inertia, resistance, leverage, and action/reaction are more important, especially as participants balance in this state. Symmetrical lever moves, along with sculling and trunk stabilization, are important while participants work mostly through the horizontal plane (while still maintaining vertical trunk orientation).

In the extended position, participants stand tall and work in a normal posture.

S. = *Change Surface area and Speed.*
These two variations alter intensity by changing resistance. Increased lever speed increases resistance, and decreased lever speed decreases resistance. Changing the shape of the body moving through the water (adding or removing surface area) affects form and wave drag and eddy and frontal resistance.

W. = *Use the Working positions of rebound, neutral, suspended, and extended.*
Working position is the most critical factor in designing workouts and movements. By changing the working positions, we can increase or eliminate the effects of gravity on the body. We can mimic the buoyant state with suspension. Each time the position is changed, the intensity is affected as different properties of water come into play.

E. = *Enlarge a movement, using the property of buoyancy to support the lever.* Extending to a fuller range of motion increases form drag, surface area, and intensity and encourages movement around the joint for greater flexibility.

A. = *Work Around the body or joint to achieve muscle balance.* Changing the planes of movement around the entire body or even around a single joint encourages participants to work through the resistance of water. It also encourages new neurological firing, increasing the number of muscle fibers recruited to perform a move. This enhancement can lead to improvements in muscular strength and endurance.

T. = *Traveling or propelling the body through the water has been shown to create the highest intensity possible.* All of the properties and forces of water apply here and create work against the body. Travel is one of the best ways to create high-intensity work.

By applying the **S.W.E.A.T.** formula to the six basic moves, you can utilize the properties of water; affect exercise intensity; and provide progression, muscle balance, and exercise variation. Entire workout sets can be developed by applying **S.W.E.A.T.** to a single move.

Regulating Intensity Using the S.W.E.A.T. Formula in Shallow Water

Let's examine how many different moves can be created by applying the **S.W.E.A.T.** formula "tools" to one basic move, scissors (moving arms and legs as if cross-country skiing). We'll identify the intensity changes that result from each tool as it's applied.

> ### S. = Change Surface area and Speed.
> To vary surface area:
>
> - *Change the position of the hands from slicing to palms flat, pushing and pulling the water.*
> - *Change the legs by rotating the toes out.*
>
> To vary speed:
>
> - *Increase or decrease speed to change resistance level.*

Both surface area and speed variations affect intensity. Slower, smaller moves are easier, while larger moves performed at greater speeds are harder. Allow participants to adjust speed and surface area for their own fitness.

> ### W. = Vary Working positions.
> To vary working positions:
>
> - *Perform the move in rebound, maximally flexing and extending.*
> - *Slow down and change to neutral position. Lower the body to allow buoyancy to support it and extend the legs to a fuller range of motion forward and back.*

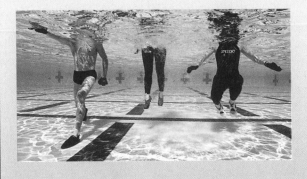

> - *Slow the move again and change to suspended. Use the arms to help create lift, work with the feet completely off the bottom, and enlarge the scissors to a comfortable range of motion. Moving this way there is no impact.*
> - *Slow the move and change to extended position.*

Rebounding creates more impact and challenges lower-body muscular strength and endurance while allowing overloading of the cardiorespiratory system. The neutral position decreases impact, but increases participants' ability to extend to fuller ranges of motion. When the move is performed in this large range at sufficient speed, cardiorespiratory training can occur. The suspended position may challenge both range of motion and muscular endurance and permit cardiorespiratory work, depending on participants' body composition. Leaner participants need to work harder to keep their heads above water, while participants with high body fat may be assisted by buoyancy and not have to work hard at all.

All the working positions can challenge cardiorespiratory endurance, depending on the speed of the scissors, and they can provide an effective system for changing impact.

> ### E. = Enlarge the movement.
> To enlarge the movement:
>
> - *Begin with a small scissors, then ask participants to gradually enlarge the range of motion, making it as big as they feel comfortable performing. Then change the size, making it smaller; then change again.*
> - *To increase the challenge for cardiorespiratory and muscular endurance, ask participants to try to maintain the same speed as they enlarge the scissors move. Enlarging the move while slowing down the speed can be used to target range-of-motion training.*
>
> ### A. = Work Around the body or a particular joint.
> To work around the body:
>
> - *Scissors front and back.*
> - *Change the working plane to the side, working a jax (a jumping jack).*
> - *Change to the diagonal plane.*

As the planes of movements change, new muscle groups are engaged or the same muscles are assisted by different muscle groups. This provides "fresh" muscles to the working body so cardiorespiratory training can continue without local muscle fatigue.

> **T. = Travel.**
> To travel:
> - *Move forward.*
> - *Move backward.*
> - *Move sideways.*
> - *Move diagonally.*

Both cardiorespiratory and muscular endurance intensity can be increased by traveling through water. The speed of travel dictates resistance levels against the body.

S.W.E.A.T. *Shallow Water Combinations*

We've just created 15 different movements and changed intensity while applying the tools of **S.W.E.A.T.** to the basic scissors move. What else can we create?

Let's try combining the elements of **S.W.E.A.T.** to develop more movement and intensity variations:

- Change the Surface area and Speed of the hands (speed up and wear webbed gloves), then the legs (turn the toes out).
- Change the Working position from rebound to suspended and Speed up!
- Change to a diagonal plane and Travel forward, then backward, slow down, and move to the suspended position.

The combinations are limitless. Allow participants at least six repetitions before changing each element, and be sure to cue to slow down before changing working positions or planes around the body. Check participants' body alignment, then gradually make the change.

 Video Reference:
Introduction to the Waterfit Aquatic Fitness System, Shallow Water. 1994. Session 5, The Basic Moves and SWEAT.

Deep Water

Deep water is a depth measured on the individual "standing" in a vertical position when the lungs are submerged, usually about armpit depth or deeper. At this depth, the feet may be touching the bottom lightly or not at all.

The Difference Between Shallow and Deep Water

In deep water, some fluid dynamics are exaggerated. For example, an action causes a more pronounced reaction, as there is no center of gravity to stabilize the body. In deep water, the body works in an open kinematics environment; no contact is made with the ground during a movement sequence.

Resistance in deep water increases exponentially with force, just as it does in shallow water; however, it may be more difficult to achieve the same speed in deep water as in shallow water, as there is no stable center of gravity from which to push off. In shallow water, speed is one of the primary intensity regulators, but comparable speeds may be more difficult to achieve in deep water.

Buoyancy is enhanced as the lungs become submerged. Deep water exercisers need to balance between the center of buoyancy (at the lungs) and the center of gravitational balance (at the heavy pelvic girdle). The degree of buoyancy and the ability to balance between these two points vary from individual to individual and depend on body composition and fat distribution (where the most fat is located on the body). Exercise design must address these differences in balance, especially when buoyancy equipment is used. Equipment that is too buoyant can make it difficult for participants to balance and push with force through the water. The effects of buoyancy and action/reaction may move the body randomly around

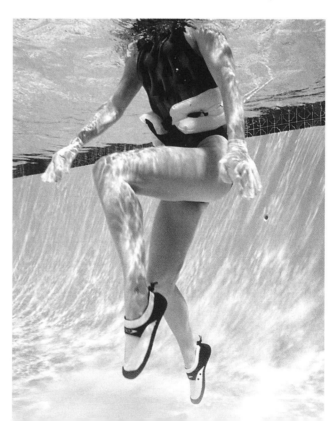

in the water. Too little buoyancy may create a "survival" workout, in which participants use the same movements over and over again during the session to simply stay afloat. Finding a balance is essential to creating a safe and effective workout.

Leverage and range of motion may be enhanced in deep water, as participants are encouraged to "stand tall" and reach for the bottom. Without the limitation of the pool bottom, and with the support of buoyancy gear such as a flotation belt, a greater variety of movements is possible.

Hydrostatic pressure increases with depth. This may make breathing feel more difficult and may give participants the sensation of working at a higher intensity than they actually are achieving. Exercisers should be trained to breathe from the diaphragm to achieve peak cardiorespiratory conditioning and will need to adjust to the sensation of pressure against the lungs as they inhale. "Top breathing" or shallow breathing may not lead to maximal VO_2 improvements.

The viscosity of deep water is the same as shallow water at any given temperature. However, the volume surrounding a submerged body is greater and feels heavier. Participants may not perform movements as

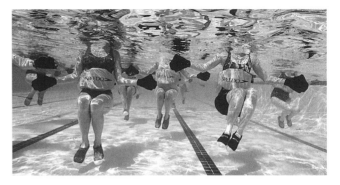

quickly in deep water, and you may need to slow down transitions so participants can adjust their balance.

Speed and acceleration may be limited by the increase in resistance and the exaggerated action/reaction effect of movement through the water as the entire body is submerged with no base of support using the feet. Buoyancy is exaggerated and is more difficult to overcome in order to gain sufficient speed to achieve appropriate intensity. Using equipment can provide additional surface area and drag that enhance intensity without having to rely on the speed of small surfaces such as hands and feet to create work. Equipment can make a move less streamlined, create turbulence, and increase intensity at a lower speed.

Fundamental Skills

Some of the shallow water skills can be used in deep water. Sculling is especially important to maintain balance and postural stabilization, to assist travel, and to change from vertical to horizontal. Other skills are modified for the bottomless environment; for example, recovery to a stand is modified by teaching participants to simply "hang" vertically with the head out of the water, instead of standing.

Before you begin instruction, you should screen your participants to see what water skills they already possess. Begin by talking to participants and observing them in the water. Find out if they have a fear of water (hydrophobia) and if they can swim. See if they are able to get from the middle of the pool to the edge without assistance. Those who have difficulty doing this may wear a flotation belt or vest that is firmly attached to the body. Handheld devices such as noodles or foam dumbbells are not adequate for safety in deep water.

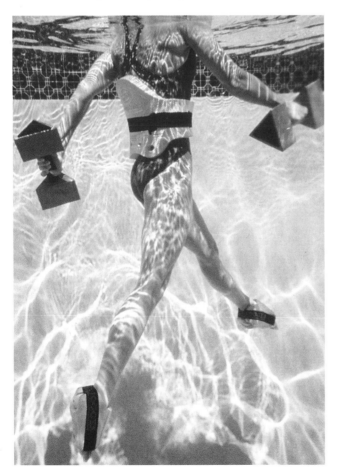

To work out in deep water, participants must be able to recover from a horizontal position to a vertical one in the water. They also should be able to stay in a simple resting position, such as a back float.

Another skill that participants need to know is treading water. It builds participants' confidence to know how to keep their heads above water when they are vertical. Treading can be performed with or without a firmly attached buoyancy device, but only swimmers should be allowed to tread without a buoyancy device.

Having participants know how to change direction during traveling moves is important for class management. Participants wear webbed gloves and use sculling motions that are coordinated with lower-body moves to move left, right, diagonally, forward, and backward effectively.

For safety, you, as an instructor, should know the following:

- Early-warning signs and signs of distress in swimmers
- Basic rescue assists with equipment
- The facility's emergency action plan
- How to correctly assist an ill or injured person from the water
- How to administer rescue breathing in and out of the water

 Video Reference:

Specificity of Training and Deep Water Program. 1995. Sessions 2 and 4.

Deep Water Equipment for Safety

Two types of equipment can help your participants work out in deep water safely: webbed gloves and buoyancy equipment. Webbed gloves assist participants with stabilization, travel, and lift. Buoyancy equipment provides support so participants can exercise suspended in the water. This gives participants freedom of movement and an ability to maximize range of motion that may not be possible on land. It also provides stabilization, balance, and lift. Without added buoyancy, participants would work the same muscle groups to fatigue by simply struggling to stay afloat. Some people may have sufficient body fat to perform the entire workout without gear; however, it may be difficult for them to relax and recover during the workout. These people may benefit most from a flotation belt that allows them to customize the amount of buoyancy.

Refer to chapter 12 for equipment choices, evaluation, and applications.

 Video Reference:

Specificity of Training and Deep Water Program. 1995. Sessions 2 and 4.

Deep Water Orientation and Proper Body Alignment

When participants move from shallow water into deep, they must make a number of adjustments. They must learn to balance movement and become accustomed to the buoyancy, the bottomless environment, and the hydrostatic pressure that affects the entire trunk. Teach them the **A.B.Y.S.S.S.** skills in the following order to help them achieve a smooth transition and prepare for exercise:

> **A. = Adjust the buoyancy for good body alignment.**

Have participants "hang" with their legs extended. Check to see if any of the flotation belts or devices need to be turned, tightened, or inflated or deflated so participants can comfortably maintain vertical position with water depth at the shoulders. As participants' lungs are submerged and their feet no longer are touching the bottom, their centers of balance will be more around the chest. Participants need to learn how to find proper alignment in the deep water, which also helps improve posture on land.

> **B. = Breathe against hydrostatic pressure.**

When a body is surrounded with water, hydrostatic pressure pushes in equally at any given depth. If the lungs are submerged, this new pressure can make breathing seem more difficult. In deep water, participants sometimes think they are working harder than they actually are because they have to inflate their lungs against the surrounding pressure.

Have participants face each other and practice breathing full breaths, watching each other rise and fall with each ventilation and exhalation. It takes about six breaths for a person to become accustomed to the new pressure and effectively breathe fully.

> **Y. = Yield to the bottomless environment.**

To help participants adjust to the bottomless environment and a new range of motion downward, have them practice jogging. Cue them to extend fully downward and feel the greater freedom.

> **S. = Scull for balance and locomotion.**

113

...ractice sculling in a number of posi-
...urface, submerged to the hips, at the sides,
...n front of the body. Have them practice propeller
sculls to travel forward, sideways, and backward.

S. = Synergize or coordinate arms and legs.

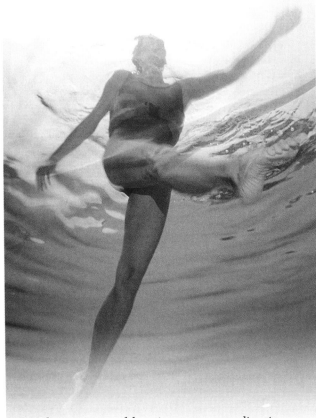

By working arms and legs in proper coordination, participants can successfully balance suspended moves. Have them practice a scissors move with the same arm and leg forward and feel how off balance it is. Then have them work with arms and legs in opposition (just like walking) and feel how better balanced they are. During the exercises, they can modify moves with this skill to help with balance.

S. = Practice Safety skills.

Without being able to touch the bottom, changing positions from horizontal to vertical and back is more challenging. Have participants practice this skill. Keep in mind it will be performed differently depending on the type and placement of buoyancy equipment being used.

 Video Reference:

Specificity of Training and Deep Water Program. 1995. Sessions 2 and 4.

Designing Exercises for Deep Water

The basic moves in deep water are slightly different based on working in the suspended position all the time. In deep water, the basic moves of jogging and bicycling are very similar. Let's examine the basic deep water moves:

Jogging (legs work from the hip using an up/down motion)

Bicycling (legs work from the hip: up, around, and down)

Kicking (legs work from the hip: forward and backward)

Scissors

Tilting

You can again use the **S.W.E.A.T.** formula to design movements, but since the environment is different from shallow water, the formula is slightly different. Let's examine how the five deep water basic moves are manipulated.

S. = Change Surface area and Speed.

Increasing Surface area and Speed increases intensity. In deep water, participants must work harder to stabilize the body before increasing Surface area (by adding more force) or Speed.

W. = Vary Working positions.

In relation to the surface of the water, the body can work vertically, in a vertical tilt (about 45 degrees), or horizontally. Another variation is seated (90-degree flexion at the hips).

Arms can be worked submerged at the hips, at the waist, and at the surface. To add weight downward, making the body "heavy" to increase lower-body work, arms can be lifted slightly above the surface and gradually moved to fully overhead.

Note: *Participants with high blood pressure should limit or avoid arm overhead movements.*

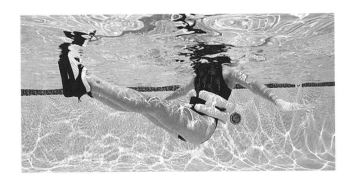

Legs can be used to perform "Power Pops," vertical propulsion work using powerful leg moves to lift the body upward and slow the body down (catching) before descending underwater. This is great cardiorespiratory training. Note that the Working positions and the skill required to perform them change with the type of buoyancy equipment used. Water noodles and buoyancy dumbbells require different skills (non-swimmers should not use this equipment as the sole support for the body).

E. = Enlarge the movement, especially downward.

Encourage using the maximal range of motion. Check that participants can stabilize the body and control the effects of buoyancy upward, which could push the limbs beyond functional range of motion.

A. = Work Around the body and joints.

Before changing the plane of movement, be sure participants' bodies are stabilized in ready position. Check body alignment frequently. Changing planes away from the center of balance requires constant trunk adjustments to effectively stabilize the body.

T. = Travel.

Travel can increase intensity in deep water also. Use webbed hands to assist movement; change directions; and focus on using the legs only, arms only, and a combination of arms and legs. Arms may need to work harder for efficient movement, so be sure to stretch or rest the upper body as needed.

Regulating Intensity Using the S.W.E.A.T. Formula in Deep Water

Let's examine how many different moves can be created by applying the S.W.E.A.T. formula "tools" to one basic move in deep water, the bicycle. We'll identify the intensity changes that result from each tool as it's applied.

S. = Change Surface area and Speed.

To vary surface area:

- *Change the position of the feet by working toes up, down, in, or out.*

To vary speed:

- *Increase or decrease speed to change resistance levels.*

Vary the intensity with both Surface area and Speed for cardiorespiratory and muscular endurance training.

W. = Vary Working positions.

For body position, tilt the bicycle to the side, forward, and back while maintaining a stationary position.

For arm position, vertical bicycle lifting one arm at a time until both arms are overhead.

For "Power Pops," bicycle upward, lifting the body above the surface as far as possible.

The body position requires trunk strength and control, and the arms must be coordinated to maintain a stationary position. The arm position progressively adds weight downward, making participants work harder to stay level, with the head above the surface. "Power Pops" are effective cardiorespiratory training, especially for people with low body fat.

E. = Enlarge the movement.

To enlarge the movement:

- *Cue participants to "jump over the barrel" or "ride a big bike" while maintaining speed.*

Intensity increases as the size of the movement is enlarged and speed is maintained.

A. = Work Around the body.

To work around the body:

- *Bicycle with knees out, then change to bicycling with knees at a diagonal.*

New muscles are engaged to maintain cardiorespiratory training intensity.

T. = Travel.

To travel:

- *Bike forward, backward, sideways, and around in a circle (both directions).*
- *Vertical bike up to horizontal.*
- *Bike up and down from vertical to horizontal on a diagonal.*

Both cardiorespiratory and muscular endurance can be targeted by pushing the body "purposefully" through the water.

We've just created 27 moves from the bicycle basic move and changed intensity many times.

 Video Reference:

Specificity of Training and Deep Water Program.
1995. Sessions 2 and 4.

S.W.E.A.T. *Deep Water Combinations*

Let's sample a few combinations to create more movements:

- Speed up bicycling with toes up, travel forward, and tilt forward.
- Change to a stationary bicycle, one arm submerged, one arm overhead. Circle around in place… then reverse direction.
- Change to knees opened out to the sides, vertical tilt back, travel backward, speed up, and bicycle to vertical.

 Video Reference:

Specificity of Training and Deep Water Program.
1995. Sessions 2 and 4.

Transitional Water

Transitional water is defined as a depth that is nipple to neck depth, where the lungs are submerged and the feet can touch the bottom.

Differences Among Shallow, Deep, and Transitional Water

Transitional depth needs to be addressed differently than either shallow or deep; however, it shares some of the same characteristics of both. As the feet can still touch the bottom, it is similar to shallow water, but as the lungs are submerged as in deep water, the greater effect of buoyancy makes developing speed by walking or running on the bottom more difficult and less effective for cardiorespiratory training. To optimize resistance in this depth, the basic moves from both shallow and deep water can be modified so participants can gradually increase intensity. Consider these two ways to work this depth most effectively:

- Modify shallow water moves for the new depth and additional buoyancy.
- Have participants wear flotation belts and combine both shallow water and deep water modified movements.

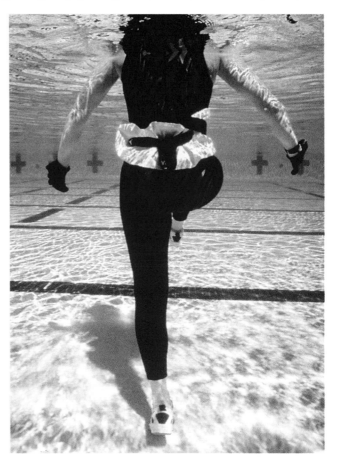

Sculling

Modify sculling to help create lift by having participants work the hands down lower near the hips. This supports the body in a tall stance so the head does not submerge during some of the moves.

You also may need to cue participants to scoop with their hands to help pull the hips under the shoulders for good posture. For example, during a kick to the rear, scooping the hands in front, submerged to the waist, prevents the hips from floating up and help keep the feet grounded for balance.

Designing Exercises for Transitional Water

In this section, we'll design water-specific exercises for transitional depth, using basic moves from both shallow and deep water.

Basic Moves From Shallow Water

These are the shallow water moves that can be modified for use in the transitional depth (no buoyancy equipment used):

Walking

Jogging

Kicking

Rocking

Jumping

Scissors

For *walking*, movement speed is slower due to buoyancy. Hands should work near the waist with a breaststroke action, thumbs up, to get enough speed to propel the body forward. In this depth, the work is primarily performed by the arms. Because buoyancy is so great, the feet do not provide effective traction.

For *jogging*, sculling is done near the hips to increase lift. To maximize intensity, alternate jogging to travel with jogging with vertical propulsion (jump and jog suspended), landing tall.

For *kicking*, sculling is done near the hips. Scooping pulls the hips down for balance during a kick to the rear. Check participants' kick heights to prevent them from going beyond a safe range of motion. Encourage them to land tall.

For *rocking*, instead of having participants lean forward and back away from the body center, have them rock by standing tall and working from the trunk so they can land tall and optimize the range of motion.

For *jumping*, have participants use the scoop motion with the hands on landing to bring the legs quickly back down to the bottom. They should land tall after jumping.

For *scissors*, have participants start tall and center, use a flat scull, and jump to a scissors, suspended. Have them land tall in the center and repeat the jump scissors leading with the other leg.

The **S.W.E.A.T.** formula as used in shallow water can be applied the same way in transitional depth by using these modified basic moves. For example, when thinking about **T.** for Travel, modify basic moves by using vertical propulsion moves (jumping or rebounding) instead of traveling moves, since traveling moves primarily work the arms and may not optimize cardiorespiratory work.

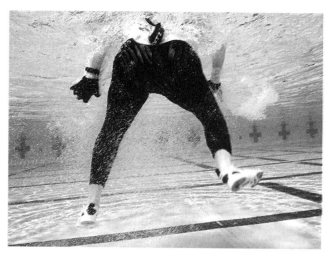

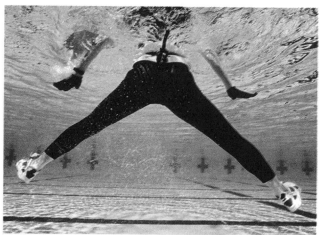

Basic Moves From Deep Water

These are the deep water moves that can be modified for use in the transitional depth (using a flotation belt):

Jog

Bike

Kick

Tilt

Scissors

When participants wear flotation belts, all the moves can be performed the same way, except that you need to cue participants to minimize downward extension.

The **S.W.E.A.T.** formula can be applied the same way as in deep water, and **A.B.Y.S.S.S.** can be modified to check alignment and orient participants to the equipment and the suspended position.

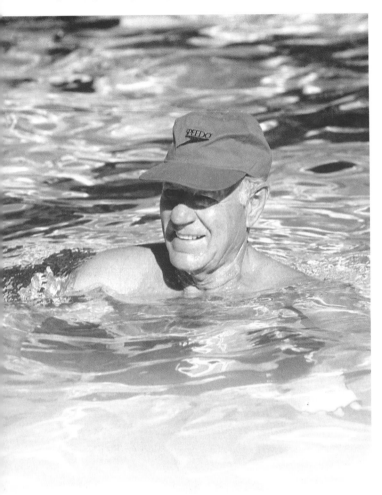

Combining Moves From Shallow and Deep Water to Optimize Transitional Work

By combining the moves from both shallow and deep water depths and modifying them for the transitional depth, you can create a new program. Have participants wear flotation belts during the entire workout. A good choice is an inflatable belt so participants can decide how much buoyancy they'll use. Blend modified shallow moves with deep water suspended moves to create a fun and effective program. Wearing belts allows participants to stay suspended for a long time, and modifying shallow moves makes it possible to work wearing a flotation belt during the entire workout. Participants can rebound off the bottom and change to being suspended without missing a beat. It's truly the best of both worlds!

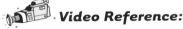 **Video Reference:**

Specificity of Training and Deep Water Program. 1995. Session 2.

Bibliography

Abraham, A., J.E. Szczerba, and M.L. Jackson. 1994. The effects of an eleven-week aqua aerobic program on relatively inactive college age women. *Medicine and Science in Sports and Exercise* 26(5): S103.

American College of Sports Medicine. 1992. *ACSM fitness book.* 2nd ed. Champaign, IL: Human Kinetics.

American College of Sports Medicine. 1990. The recommended quantity and quality of exercise for developing and maintaining cardiorespiratory and muscular fitness in healthy adults. *Medicine and Science in Sports and Exercise* 22: 265–274.

American College of Sports Medicine. 1986. *Resource manual for guidelines for exercise testing and prescription.* (3rd ed.). Philadelphia: Lea & Febiger.

American National Red Cross. 1983. *Lifeguard Training Manual,* St. Louis: Mosby-Yearbook.

Archer, S. 1998. Water exercise liability. *IDEA Health & Fitness Source* 16(2): 71–77.

Bailey, C. 1994. *Smart exercise,* ch. 6. New York: Houghton Mifflin.

Beasley, B.L. 1989. Prescription pointers, aquatic exercise. *Sports Medicine Digest* 11(1): 1–3.

Burns, N., ed. 1990. Unusual environments and human behavior. *Physiological & Psychological Problems of Man in Space* 13: 321-334.

Campbell, K.D. et al. 1990. Effect of water exercise on body composition in overweight females. Presentation at American Alliance for Health, Physical Education, Recreation and Dance, Annual Convention, New Orleans, LA.

Cole, A., Moschetti, M., Eagleston, R.E. (in press). Lumbar spine aquatic rehabilitation. In *A Sports Medicine Approach, Handbook of Pain Management,* ed. A. Cole, 2nd ed. Baltimore: Williams & Wilkins.

Cole, L.K., and F. Andres. 1987. Physiological and perceptual responses to running in the water (Research abstracts session). Aquatic Symposium, NSPI, 3. (Contact Laura K. Cole, University of Toledo, Exercise Physiology Lab, Toledo, OH 43606.)

Collins, R.L., ed. 1989. *AOPA's handbook for pilots.* Frederick, MD: AOPA.

Craig, A.B. Jr., and M. Dvorak. 1968. Thermal regulation of man during water immersion. *Journal of Applied Physiology* 25: 23-35.

Delhagen, K. 1987. Cold water survival. *Runner's World* (May).

Evans, B., K. Cureton, and J. Purvis. 1978. Metabolic and circulatory responses to walking and jogging in water. *Research Quarterly* 49: 442–449.

Fawcett, C. 1992. Principles of aquatic rehab: A new look at hydrotherapy. *Sports Medicine* 7(2): 6–9.

Gwinup, G. 1987. Weight loss without dietary restriction: Efficacy of different forms of aerobic exercise. *American Journal of Sports Medicine* 15(3): 275–279.

Hayward, J.S. 1990. Hypothermia, frostbite and other cold injuries, immersion hypothermia. *Physician and Sportsmedicine* (January): 66–73.

Hoeger, W., T. Gibson, J. Moore, and D. Hopkins. 1993. A comparison of selected training responses to water aerobics and low-impact aerobic dance. *National Aquatics Journal* (Winter): 13–16.

JAMA, The Journal of the American Medical Association. 1989.

Hypothermia Prevention (Morbidity & Mortality Report) (January 27): 513.

Kerasote, T. 1989. Summer's greatest danger. *Sports Afield* (July).

Kirn, T. 1988. Do low levels of iron affect body's ability to regulate temperature, experience cold? *Journal of the American Medical Association* (August 5): 607.

Kravitz, L., and J. Mayo. 1997. Aquatic exercise: a review. *AKWA Letter* (October/November).

Lieber, D.C., R.L. Lieber, and W.C. Adams. 1989. Effects of run training and swim training at similar absolute intensities on treadmill VO$_2$max. *Medicine and Science in Sports and Exercise* 21(6): 655–661.

McArdle, W., R. Katch, and V. Katch. 1991. *Exercise physiology, energy, nutrition and human performance.* 3rd ed. Philadelphia: Lea & Febiger.

Nielson, M. 1996. *Strong women stay young.* New York: Bantam Books.

Nieman, D. 1995. *Fitness and sports medicine, a health related approach.* Los Altos: Bull Publishing.

Otis, C.L. 1990. When a cooldown is undesirable. *Women's Sports and Fitness* (March).

Ruoti, R.G., J.T. Troup, and R.A. Berger. 1994. The effects of nonswimming water exercises on older adults. *Journal of Orthopaedic and Sports Physical Therapy* 19(3): 140–145.

Sanders, M., and C. Maloney-Hills. 1998. Aquatic exercise for better living on land. *ACSM's Health Fitness Journal* 2(3): 16–23.

Sanders, M., and N. Rippee. 1994. *Speedo aquatic fitness system, instructor training manual.* London: Speedo International Ltd.

Strauss, S. 1985. Adjusting nature's thermostat. *Runner's World.* (January): 52.

Study, M., ed. 1991. *Personal trainer manual, the resource for fitness instructors.* San Diego, CA: American Council on Exercise.

Thornton, J. 1990. Hypothermia shouldn't freeze out cold-weather athletes. *Physician and Sportsmedicine* (January): 109.

Tsukahara, N., A. Toda, J. Goto, and I. Ezawa. 1994. Cross-sectional and longitudinal studies on the effects of water exercise in controlling bone loss in Japanese postmenopausal women. *Journal of Nutrition and Science Vitaminology* 40(1): 37–47.

YMCA. 1997. *Principles of YMCA aquatics.* Champaign, IL: Human Kinetics.

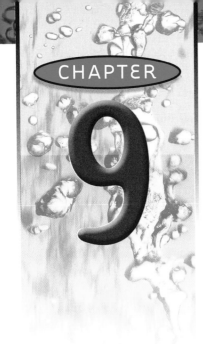

CHAPTER 9

Specificity of Training and Training Guidelines

MARY E. SANDERS

Objectives:

◎ To define "specificity of training" for purposeful exercises that effectively target cardiorespiratory endurance, muscular strength and endurance, flexibility, body composition, and functional activities of daily living (ADL) training.

◎ To examine training guidelines targeting specific training objectives: cardiorespiratory fitness and body composition; muscular strength and endurance and body composition; flexibility and active range of motion; weight management and healthy body composition; and functional ADL training.

◎ To examine the 1998 training guidelines from the American College of Sports Medicine (ACSM) for healthy adults and review recommendations for older adults and very old or frail adults.

◎ To apply the guidelines to water exercise progressions using the S.W.E.A.T. formula.

The specificity of training principle is that the body adapts specifically to whatever type of overload it is given during an activity. For example, a person who trains for high aerobic endurance by running may not exhibit the same amount of endurance when swimming. The movement patterns, muscle groups, and specific metabolic systems (chemical processes in the body) used for each activity are different. To become a better swimmer, athletes must train by swimming if they want to develop aerobic fitness for swimming. He or she must train the muscles for the cardiorespiratory fitness, muscular endurance, and flexibility needed to achieve the desired performance. "Specific exercise elicits specific adaptations creating specific training effects" (McArdle, Katch, and Katch, 1991, p. 425). Some areas of training can overlap; for example, cardiorespiratory endurance developed by running may make swimming easier for some individuals.

The specificity principle doesn't apply just to athletic training. Even functional activities of daily living can be improved with properly designed exercises that provide a progressive overload. Åstrand (1992) states that "if animals are built reasonably, they should build and maintain just enough, but no more, structure than they need to meet functional requirements" (p. 154).

People dream of the activities that will make their lives fulfilling and fun. By exercising purposefully, targeting their physical "dreams," people can succeed at physical activities that will enhance the quality of their lives for a lifetime.

In 1998, the ACSM released a position statement on the amount and quality of exercise recommended for developing and maintaining health in adults (see that statement in chapter 4). Specific types of training included were cardiorespiratory and muscular fitness, along with healthy body composition and flexibility training. The same types of exercise were recom-

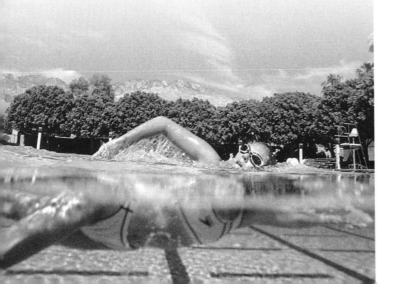

Parts of this chapter adapted with permission of IDEA, The Health and Fitness Source. (800) 999-IDEA or (619) 535-8979. See page x for complete source information.

mended for older adults, with the addition of specific exercises targeting postural stability.

In order to determine the proper amount and quality of exercise needed for improvement, we can apply the **F.I.T.T.** principle:

> **F. = Frequency** of exercise, which is how often a person exercises per day or week.
>
> **I. = Intensity,** which is how hard a person works. Intensity should be progressive in order to provide sufficient overload to create a training response that will produce healthy improvements. A few ways that intensity can be measured include a percentage of $\dot{V}O_2$ (oxygen uptake), percent of maximal heart rate (220 - age), rate of perceived exertion (RPE), and the talk test.

As mentioned earlier, heart rate responses to exercise in the water differ from those to exercise on land, especially when the chest is submerged. Due to a number of variables, including the effects of hydrostatic pressure, water depth, and water temperature (especially in cool water of 64 degrees to 77 degrees F.), heart rates may be 10 to 15 beats lower in the water when compared to a similar cardiorespiratory intensity on land (Craig and Dvorak, 1969; Svendenhag and Seger, 1992). Several researchers (Craig and Dvorak, 1969; Evans, Cureton, and Purvis, 1978) have concluded that water exercise conducted in shallow water, where the chest is not submerged (navel depth and below), and when the water temperature is approximately 86 degrees F or warmer, tends to elicit heart rates comparable to those on land. So, based on the wide variations in

heart rates and their unreliability, water exercise participants should be encouraged to use RPE to monitor intensity. A heart-rate monitor can be used periodically to help participants get in touch with how their bodies respond and to learn how to use RPE more effectively. Heart rates measured by a monitor should always be used as a training guide by those who require a precise measure because it is critical to their safety.

In this chapter, intensity is discussed in terms of maximal heart rate (MHR) and rate of perceived exertion. Table 9.1 shows how maximal heart rate and rate of perceived exertion relate to each other.

> **T. = Time** is the total continuous or accumulated time that a person spends performing some level of physical activity throughout the day or week.
>
> **T. = Type** of exercise describes the physical activity performed. Examples include the following:
>
> - *Rhythmic movement using primarily the large muscles of the lower body for cardiorespiratory and body composition training (running, bicycling, and jumping jacks on land or in the pool)*
>
> - *Resistance exercise that overloads muscle groups for muscular strength and endurance training and body composition improvements (free weights, resistance machines, moving through water and using water-specific equipment for overload)*
>
> - *Range-of-motion activities for flexibility, mobility, and ease of movement (Tai Chi, yoga, using the properties of water such as buoyancy to progressively stretch)*
>
> - *Postural exercises for better posture and stability through a variety of movements (balance boards on land and balancing against the currents of water in the pool)*
>
> - **Functional activities of daily living (ADL)** *exercises that combine many types of exercise into daily activity "drills" or "patterns" to improve ADL functioning (stair climbing on land or in the pool)*
>
> - *Sports-specific activities that combine a number of types of exercise into sports "drills" or "patterns" that train the body for competitive level performance (plyometric jumps on land or explosive jumping in shallow water)*

Table 9.1 **Intensity as Shown by MaxHR and RPE**

Intensity	MaxHR	RPE (Borg, 1982)
Very light	< 35%	< 10
Light	35—54%	10—11
Moderate	55—69%	12—13
Hard	60—89%	14—16
Very hard	≥ 90%	17—19
Maximal	100%	20

Adapted, by permission, from ACSM; Haskell and Pollock, 1998. "The recommended quantity and quality of exercise for developing and maintaining cardiorespiratory and muscular fitness, and flexibility in healthy adults." *Medicine & Science in Sports & Exercise* 30(6): 975—985.

According to ACSM (1998a), research suggests that exercising less than two days per week (frequency) at less than 55 to 65 percent of max HR (intensity) for less than 10 minutes (time) performing aerobic endurance training (type) is not sufficient to develop and maintain fitness in healthy adults. For people who are unfit or who are unable to exercise at a weak to moderate intensity, the research suggests that more frequent exercise that continues for a longer period of time at a lower intensity can still create improvements, especially when exercise intensity is increased progressively. One way to gradually increase an individual's frequency and duration of exercise, if single sessions of continuous exercise are not possible, is to accumulate 20 to 60 minutes of physical activity during the day in shorter bouts of 10-minute durations. This intermittent style of exercise could include a 10-minute walk to the pool, followed by a 30-minute water exercise class, along with a brisk 10-minute walk back to the office, and finally a 10-minute walk after dinner with the dogs.

The ACSM recommendations are designed to address individual goals, fitness levels, and health needs. For example, people whose primary objective is weight management need to adjust the time and intensity to achieve their own health gains in cardiorespiratory fitness, muscular strength and endurance, and flexibility while balancing kilocalories consumed with kilocalories expended. Athletes who want to improve their performance in competitive sports need to specifically address the performance objectives of their sport and the risk of injury with higher-intensity training. As part of a safe training program, current guidelines for training recommend appropriate warm-up and cool-down periods that include flexibility exercises.

As an instructor, you need to design effective programs that "provide the proper amount of physical activity to attain maximal benefit at the lowest risk" (ACSM, 1998a, p. 975). When participants understand the purpose of the exercises and why they are important for health, it's easier for them to make lifestyle changes that result in "a lifetime of physical activity" (ACSM, 1998a, p. 975). "As a result of specificity of training and the need for maintaining muscular strength and endurance, and flexibility of the major muscle groups, a well-rounded training program including aerobic and resistance training, and flexibility exercises is recommended" (ACSM, 1998a, p. 975).

Water exercise offers a low-risk environment where all the components of fitness can be targeted effectively through individual progressions. You must understand how to use the water effectively so participants can successfully meet the ACSM training guidelines. By combining exercise science with information on the properties of water and current knowledge from published research, we can effectively apply the guidelines for specific training. Research studies conducted in the water offer ideas on improving class format and exercise effectiveness to improve the components of fitness for better living on land.

In this chapter, we'll examine how to effectively target each of the components, keeping in mind that the most effective training occurs when the exercise is specific to the objective. For example, training guidelines for muscular improvements are different than those for cardiorespiratory or flexibility fitness. In order to provide an effective program that produces balanced results, both you and your participants must understand how to use water properly to target specific health objectives.

Let's now look at each of the sets of training guidelines targeting five specific training objectives:

1. Cardiorespiratory fitness and body composition
2. Muscular endurance and strength
3. Flexibility and active range of motion
4. Weight management and healthy body composition
5. Functional activities of daily living training

For all categories, except weight management, we will define some terms, describe ACSM guidelines, and give guidelines for designing water-specific exercises.

Cardiorespiratory Fitness and Body Composition

Before discussing the guidelines for cardiorespiratory fitness and body composition, we need to define some terms.

Fitness is defined as "the ability to perform moderate-to-vigorous levels of physical activity without undue fatigue and the capability of maintaining this capacity throughout life" (Wilmore, 1988).

Cardiorespiratory conditioning or *fitness* is the ability to perform large-muscle movements over a sustained period of time; the capacity of the heart-lung system to deliver oxygen for sustained energy production.

Cardiorespiratory endurance includes conditioning of the heart and lungs for an aerobic cardiorespiratory training effect. This type of exercise

ability of the body to meet the skeletal demands for oxygen. *Oxygen consumption*, or $\dot{V}O_2$max measures the ability of the body to maximize oxygen uptake and describes the arterial venous difference, which is an indicator of cardiorespiratory endurance capacity. **Arteriovenous difference** is the difference in oxygen content of arterial and mixed venous blood or the $(a-\bar{V})O_2$ difference (McArdle, Katch, and Katch, 1991). Potential health benefits of increased physical activity may include the following:

- Reduced risk of diabetes and coronary heart disease
- Management of hypertension and weight
- Management or prevention of osteoporosis
- Maintenance of functional activities of daily living and an active lifestyle

Body composition is the makeup of the body in terms of its relative percentages of lean body mass and body fat (Study, 1991). *Obesity* is defined as "positive energy balance" (Bouchard, 1997), due to a lack of exercise and activity in our lives. Studies suggest that the number of **kilocalories (kcal)** consumed per person per day has not increased over the last 50 years; however, the National Institutes of Health, using new guidelines, now classify 55 percent of the American population as overweight or obese. It is estimated by the National Institutes of Health that we are expending 200 to 800 kcals less per day than our ancestors. Based on trends from 1960 to 1991, 100 percent of U.S. adults will be overweight in two centuries. Children have demonstrated a threefold increase in obesity during the period 1960 to 1991, from 5 percent to 14 percent. According to Bouchard (1997), the current health care cost of obesity is $70 billion in the United States alone.

In 1998, the National Institutes of Health released clinical guidelines to define "overweight" and "obese." The old height/weight charts are being replaced with the Body Mass Index (BMI). For most people, BMI is related to fatness and its associated health risks, although very muscular people may have a high BMI without associated health risks. The new evidence suggests that, for the majority of the population, the risks for various cardiovascular and other diseases begin rising at a BMI of 25. Therefore, a BMI of 25 to less than 30 is now considered "overweight." Obesity is defined as a BMI of 30 or above.

Calculating BMI can help determine if you or your participants have a healthy body weight so you can use the information to design an effective lifestyle and weight management program if needed. Use the following formula to calculate BMI:

1. Multiply your weight in pounds by 700.
2. Divide the sum (weight × 700) by your height in inches.
3. Divide by your height in inches again.

For example, if you are 6 feet tall and weigh 220 pounds, the equation is computed like this:

$$220 \text{ lbs} \times 700 = 154,000 \text{ lbs}$$

$$\frac{154,000 \text{ lbs}}{72 \text{ in}} = 2,139$$

$$\frac{2,139}{72 \text{ in}} = 29.7 \text{ BMI (overweight)}$$

Refer to the BMI chart in appendix A for more information.

ACSM Guidelines for Cardiorespiratory Fitness

The 1998 ACSM guidelines for healthy adults (ACSM, 1998a) are as follows:

Frequency: Three to five days per week

Intensity: 55/65 percent to 90 percent of maximum heart rate or 40/50 percent to 85 percent of maximum oxygen uptake reserve or maximum heart rate reserve [The lower-intensity values, 55 to 64 percent of max HR or 40 to 49 percent of $\dot{V}O_2$ reserve, are most applicable to unfit people.]

Time/Duration: 20 to 60 continuous minutes or 10-minute bouts accumulated throughout the day to equal 20 to 60 minutes

Lower-intensity activity should be performed 30 minutes or more, while people doing higher-intensity training should train at least 20 minutes or longer.

"Total fitness" is achieved more effectively with exercise sessions of longer durations. Higher-intensity sessions may place participants at higher risk for injury and be perceived as being "too hard," resulting in poor attendance or high dropout rates. As a result, the ACSM recommends that adults who are not doing athletic training exercise at moderate intensity for a longer time period.

Mode: Any activity that uses large-muscle groups continuously and is rhythmical and aerobic in nature, such as walking, swimming, cross-country skiing, rowing, stair climbing, aerobic dance/group exercise, or endurance game activities.

ACSM (1998b) also recommends that aerobic exercise be integrated into older adults' lifestyles to maximize the quality and length of their lives. Such exercise helps reduce the rate of age-related decline in numerous physical functions. Although the Centers for Disease Control and the ACSM recommend that lifestyle physical activities be performed at a light to moderate intensity to optimize health, older adults may need to perform moderate-to-high intensity exercise in order to improve their cardiovascular systems and to reduce their risk of cardiovascular disease. We believe that water exercise programs provide a safe and effective environment in which older adults may be able to maximize their exercise intensity while minimizing the risk of injury.

The ACSM also has exercise recommendations for the very old and frail population (ACSM, 1998b). Aerobic training is the most difficult prescription for this age group due to the many physical challenges and difficulties in being able to move safely and effectively. Minimal muscle power must first be developed to perform tasks such as getting out of a chair and maintaining erect posture while moving through space. It is suggested that for these adults, in order to prepare their bodies for more aerobic activity, they first improve strength, joint stability, and balance. When moderate intensity aerobic training can begin, the guidelines are as follows:

Frequency: Three days per week

Intensity: 11 to 13 on the Borg scale *or* 40–60 percent of heart rate reserve

Duration: At least 20 minutes

Mode: Walking is preferred. Intensity can be increased by walking hills, inclines, or stairs. Additional overload can be achieved by performing arm or dance movements or pushing a weighted or occupied wheelchair. Alternatives may include arm or leg ergometry machines and seated stepping machines. Water exercise is also recommended.

Water-Specific Cardiorespiratory Fitness and Body Composition Exercise Design

Water exercise modes include movements in water similar to movements on land (such as cross-country skiing or walking) that are modified to produce training intensities similar to those generated when the movements are done on land. Land activities performed in the water without modification produce different training responses than they would on land (Brown et al, 1997; Byma, Craig, and Wilmore, 1996; Hered, Darby, and Yaekle, 1997; Napoletan and Hicks, 1995). Therefore, it cannot be assumed that walking on land and walking in the pool, at the same rate, using the same biomechanics, are equivalent training choices. (Refer to chapter 6 for what research reveals about land and water differences.) Effective water-specific modes are determined by designing water-specific exercises based on the guidelines and derived from land modes.

Begin with the basic moves for each depth—walking, scissors, jumping, jogging, bicycle, and kicking—and vary them using the **S.W.E.A.T.** formula as described in chapter 8. Focus on having participants use the large muscles of the legs to perform continuous, rhythmic movements. Hands or webbed gloves should be used primarily for balancing and assisting travel, with the legs performing most of the work. Upper-body work can contribute to the cardiorespiratory load, unless use of the arms slows the speed and decreases the intensity of the legs. Check that participants' bodies are balanced for effective lower-body work.

- **Use the "S" in the formula for speed and surface area variations.** Vary and surface areas and speed to adjust cardiorespiratory intensity (Brown et al., 1997; Byma, Craig, and Wilmore, 1996; Hered, Darby, and Yaekle, 1997; Napoletan and Hicks, 1995). Consider interval training, which has been shown to be effective in maintaining cardiorespiratory fitness for running on land (Bushman et al., 1997).

- **Use the "W" in the formula to change muscle groups and intensity.** Vary the basic moves through the working positions of rebound, neutral, and suspended to change muscle use, prevent local muscle fatigue, and decrease risk of injury. Rebounding adds body weight to lower extremities and increases the load. The neutral position reduces the body weight load but increases the ability to achieve a fuller range of motion (ROM) by allowing the arms and legs to work without weight. The suspended position involves the use of stabilizers and requires concentration to coordinate arms and legs through full ROM at a sufficient speed to maintain lift off the bottom!

- **Use the "E" in the formula to maximize muscle use.** Enlarge the size and surface area of the movement to increase intensity. Change the shape of the body as it moves through the water (such as dragging the arms during a jog) or simply exaggerate movements to increase the total surface area of the body as it works through the resistance and against buoyancy. Decrease intensity by making movements smaller in order to continue the work, increasing duration.

- **Use the "A" in the formula to keep "fresh" muscles engaged.** Due to water resistance, muscles will fatigue if they aren't changed frequently enough to prevent local fatigue (Hoeger et al., 1992).

- **Use the "T" in the formula to increase resistance and drag.** Research, common sense, and experience tell us that traveling through water creates the optimal cardiorespiratory response by fully engaging the properties of water.

Note that participants may have to develop muscular endurance first to be able to achieve optimal cardiorespiratory training. Include progressions that target muscular conditioning as a primary objective in your program so participants can develop their muscles in order to achieve training levels for cardiorespiratory fitness.

Use rate of perceived exertion and the talk test to monitor intensity. If you like, also use heart rate monitors for supplemental intensity feedback. Be sure to apply water-adjusted rates in water over xiphoid depth and in cool water.

Encourage participants to pace themselves, trying to work at an intensity of "somewhat hard" to "strong." When participants begin to fatigue, remind them to regulate their intensity using the 4 **S**'s so they can keep going for endurance:

To decrease intensity:

1. *Slow* down.
2. Make the move *Smaller*.
3. *Stabilize* with sculling.
4. *Substitute* a modified or different move.

To increase intensity:

1. *Stabilize* with sculling.
2. Enlarge the *Size* of the move.
3. Push with more force, increasing the *Speed*.
4. Continue to increase the intensity for participants by using the **S.W.E.A.T.** formula.

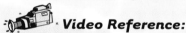 **Video Reference:**

Specificity of Training and Deep Water Program. Session 3.

Sample Cardiorespiratory Fitness and Healthy Body Composition Training Progressions

You can choose to use either continuous training or interval training for cardiorespiratory fitness. Here are some sample progressions, plus additional information on interval training.

Continuous Training (20–60 minutes)

One example of continuous training is shallow water walking. Shallow water walking can be defined as performing a traveling movement in a fairly consistent depth without changing working positions. One foot is always in contact with the pool bottom, with power and force initiated at the foot and directed through the water by the leg muscles. Arms work in conjunction with the lower body to assist movement.

To perform water walking cycles, place participants in mid-thigh to navel-high water. As they walk, have participants change directions. This creates water current patterns that can increase or decrease the effects of inertia currents and affect intensity. Travel should be continuous, but the movements can be varied using the tools from the **S.W.E.A.T.** formula, as in this example:

- Begin the pattern of movement desired.
- Walk faster (**S. T.**).
- Walk with "giant steps" (**E. T.**).
- Change the direction of travel (**T.**).
- Walk sideways and diagonally (**A. T.**).

You can then continue to use **S.E.A.T.** from the formula to create new moves (**W.** is working position, which should not change).

Interval Training

Interval training is used to vary workout intensity. The idea behind interval training is that an individual can produce a greater amount of work if rest periods are spaced between work bouts. For example, many people find the resistance of the water too difficult to continuously work through. We know that untrained water exercise participants (Frangolias & Rhodes, 1995), moving in the water, experience an initial increase in lactate that is higher than when the same movement is performed on land (lactate is thought to cause muscle soreness). If we use interval training for water exercise, we can help participants adapt to this change more easily and enjoy the activity more.

The following terms may help you understand interval training better (Kravitz, 1996):

Work interval: Time of the high-intensity work effort.

Recovery interval: Time between work intervals. The recovery interval may consist of light activity (sculling only) or moderate activity (easy jog).

Work/recovery ratio: Time ratio of the work and recovery intervals. A work/recovery ratio of one to three means the recovery interval is three times as long as the work interval. For example, jogging one minute and recovering three minutes represents a one-to-three work/recovery ratio.

Cycle/repetition: A work interval and a recovery interval represent one cycle. Since a recovery interval follows a work interval, some resources report the number of work intervals as repetitions.

Set: The specific number of cycles. A series of four work/recovery cycles represents one set of four cycles.

During a recovery interval you can introduce the next move and emphasize performing a full range of motion. Consider this to be the first set of the new movement and emphasize flexibility by having participants perform the movement through a full range of motion. Then go right into the work interval, as the neuromuscular pattern of movement has been set (Kennedy, 1998).

Benefits of Interval Training

Working and moving in intervals, or varying speed or effort over a period of time, have long been used for training by athletes. One of the benefits is that high-intensity bouts that push the body to the limit are followed by recovery periods, providing both mental and physical rest. Short bouts of high-intensity work also reduce the risk for injury by limiting the duration of potentially risky high-intensity work.

This type of training is not just for athletes; we live life in intervals, even in simple activities such as shopping. The sequence begins with a drive to the store, then a walk to the corner, followed by an increase in intensity as we run across the street. We then walk briskly to the store and begin browsing at a slower speed for our hot sale item! Finally, our rest/recovery phase comes as we stand in line for 15 minutes to purchase the item. Then we repeat the sequence to make it back to work on time! However, if we're using interval formats for training, we need to increase the intensity beyond "normal" activity to create physiological change, so the overload must be greater than a jog across the street!

Water is an excellent form of training for the athlete who wants to work hard and last longer in the anaerobic zone, which contributes to cardiorespiratory gains.

Interval training has been used for conditioning athletes in all sports from track and field to basketball and softball. Some athletes call them blocks, others train in descending or ascending sets, or pyramids, but all interval training sets come with well-deserved recovery time. The major advantage of this type of training in the pool is that water's viscosity provides accommodating resistance. Intensity levels can instantaneously be varied with small amounts of effort or power changes, allowing the athlete to individually rest or work on demand.

Research by Frangolias and Rhodes (1995) indicates that nonwater conditioned athletes who train anaerobically in the water will increase blood lactate level (a by-product of anaerobic metabolism) to higher levels than those achieved by comparable training on land. So water is an excellent form of training for the athlete who wants to work hard and last longer in the anaerobic zone, which contributes to cardiorespiratory gains.

At Indiana University–Bloomington, water training has been used as an effective tool for adding variety and fun to off-season training for varsity athletes in several sports. Athletes have the power to make the most out of the water if they are coached effectively. They enjoy working hard in this low-impact (or in deep water, nonimpact) medium that allows intense training without the jarring impact experienced on land. Additionally, since water is a giant resistance machine, athletes have the opportunity to overload muscles in almost every direction of movement, especially targeting the trunk stabilizers. When basketball players are given a few water polo balls in the deep water, they get into competitive battle zones and work hard. Indiana's wrestlers can power their bodies in a suspended mode longer than any other athletes, working in a fun way to improve cardiorespiratory endurance.

Interval Duration

While no absolute rules exist for interval duration, usually about 20–45 seconds' work and 30–75 seconds' rest seems adequate for water exercise. The resistance of water fatigues muscles more quickly than land work, so intervals may need to be shorter in the pool than they are on land in order to minimize muscular fatigue and maximize cardiorespiratory levels.

Interval lengths depend on these factors:

- Skills (how quickly the resistance of water can be effectively engaged against the body)
- Strength and endurance (muscular condition)
- In deep water, body composition (low body fat and high muscle mass increases the difficulty of suspended moves)
- Training objectives (endurance athletes may want to work longer and rest shorter, while sprinting athletes may want shorter bouts)

Use perceived exertion, heart rate monitors, and/or the talk test to check intensity. Remember, heart rates in water are variable and are only a part of the intensity story.

Add some interval sets to your training program:

Tug O'War

Pair up your participants and give each pair a five-foot resistance band. Have them get into the suspended position, one person facing the back of the other. The lead person runs forward while the partner tries to run backward. The direction they travel shows who is the strongest! Use intervals of 30 seconds of work and 15 seconds of rest. Have them perform about 10 sets, then switch positions.

 Video References:

The Golden Waves Program, Functional Water Fitness Training for Health, Golden Waves Video II, Advanced Progressions.

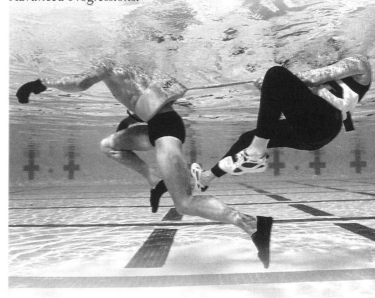

Scissors/Jax Combination

Use the scissors/jax moves to alternate muscle groups to maximize cardiorespiratory work. Begin with the scissors move in one of the working positions and gradually increase the intensity using the following progression:

- *Have participants practice the move (scissors or jax). Check their alignment and range of motion (lowest intensity).*
- *Work it! Add force. Begin the work phase.*
- *Increase speed.*
- *Change the working position.*
- *Have participants travel forward, sideways, and backward (highest intensity).*
- *Give participants an active rest/recovery period, such as an easy jog.*

Repeat the sequence using a jax.

Repeat, alternating the moves for about 45 seconds of work (includes the practice time for the move) and 30 seconds of active rest/recovery, and do 10 to 15 sets.

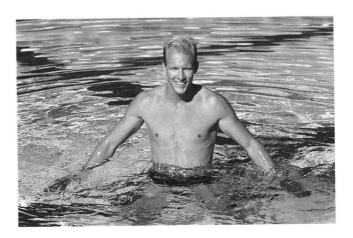

Jump Training

Give each participant a step and a pair of webbed gloves. Water depth should be up to the elbow when participants stand on their steps.

First have participants stabilize the upper body by working the hands on the surface, in front and to the sides. Occasionally cue participants to check step placement for safety. Then gradually increase the intensity of the move:

- *Have participants practice with only small jumps, then work it (lowest intensity)!*
- *Have them jump using both feet on the step for takeoff and landing.*
- *Have them work with one leg.*
- *Increase the height.*
- *Increase the speed.*
- *Work in shallower water if greater impact is required for training (highest intensity).*

Vary the work/rest ratios with fitness levels. Begin with 15 seconds of work and 30-second rest intervals for 8 to 10 sets on each leg.

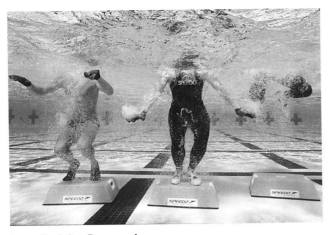
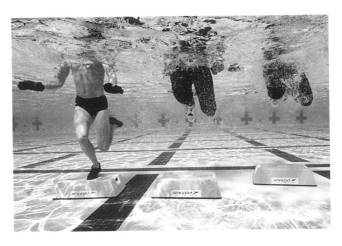

Jump Training Progression

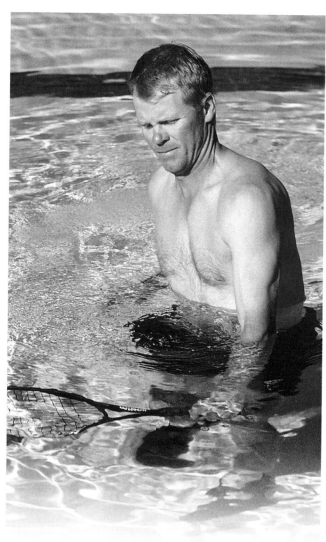

Deep Water Running

Hand out a flotation belt to each participant and have participants run in the suspended position. Choose the work/rest cycles you want to use and gradually increase the intensity using the following progression:

- *Have participants practice and develop a full range of motion. Check their posture, then work it (lowest intensity)!*
- *Add force and speed.*
- *Have them travel or pull against the tether.*
- *Tell them to hold their arms stationary, first one arm overhead, then two arms overhead (don't sink).*
- *Repeat without buoyancy gear (highest intensity).*

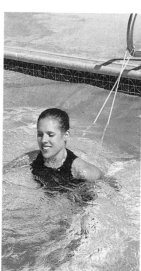

During the rest/ recovery interval, have participants do an easy jog or a quadriceps/ hamstrings stretch.

Liquid Tennis

Use work/rest sets to train participants to improve the power in their tennis games. This university tennis coach plays hard, then easy to create resistance drills in the water.

Participants should keep their wrists in neutral and use the slower speeds to check their biomechanics.

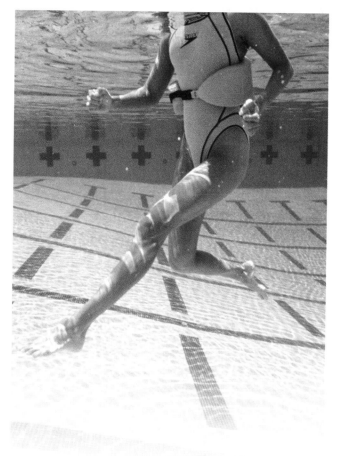

Muscular Strength and Endurance

Since 1990, the ACSM guidelines for training have included resistance training as an important part of an adult fitness program. Intensity should be high enough to improve muscular strength and endurance and to maintain fat-free mass. ACSM suggests that resistance be progressive, individualized, and provide work for all the major muscle groups.

Before we describe the guidelines for training for muscular strength and endurance, we need to define those two terms.

Muscular strength is the maximum force that a muscle can produce against resistance in a single, maximal effort (Study, 1991). Muscular strength is developed by using heavy weight (that requires maximum or nearly maximum tension development) with few repetitions.

Muscular endurance is the capacity of a muscle to exert force repeatedly against a resistance, or to hold a fixed or static contraction over time (Study, 1991). This type of training is best developed by using lighter weights with a greater number of repetitions.

ACSM Guidelines for Muscular Strength and Endurance

These are the 1998 ACSM guidelines for healthy adults (ACSM, 1998a):

Frequency: Two to three times per week

Intensity: *Repetition maximum* (RM) refers to the maximal number of times a load can be lifted before fatigue, using good form and technique. Perform the recommended repetitions at a repetition maximum load.

Modification: Low to moderate resistance repetition maximum using 10 to 15 repetitions for older, more frail participants

Type/Time: Major muscle groups resisted through full range of motion. Generally one set of 8 to 10 exercises for the major muscle groups or multiple sets if time allows.

More specifically: 8–12 reps < 50 years old and 10–15 reps > 50 years old

Major muscle groups: Arms, shoulders, chest, abdomen, back, hips, and legs

The ACSM (ACSM, 1998b) also recommends strength training for older adults to minimize muscle loss and weakness due to aging. Strength training can help increase levels of physical activity, increase energy metabolism, maintain bone density, improve insulin action, and improve functional status for a higher quality of life for older adults.

This is the ACSM recommendation for the frail and very old (ACSM, 1998b):

Strength training can help increase activity and reverse age-related muscle weakness, low muscle mass, low bone density, low cardiovascular conditioning, and poor balance and gait. It is therefore recommended that all exercise programs for this group include progressive resistance training, similar to the guidelines for younger adults:

Frequency: Two days, but preferably three days, per week

Intensity/Time: Higher-intensity training; two to three sets

Type: Standing postures with free weights and resistance sets targeting hip extensors, knee extensors, ankle plantar flexors and dorsiflexors, biceps, triceps, shoulders, back extensors, and abdominal muscles

Balance training should be included, either within strength training or as separate exercise. Balance exercises should progressively add more challenging postures, for example, a two-legged stand to a one-legged stand, and gradually add dynamic movements such as "walking on a line" and walking in a circle, or adding pivot turns to a walk sequence. Other important muscle groups can be challenged by performing heel stands (dorsiflexors) and by changing vision input (balance with eyes closed). In the water, balance training is safe and the water currents challenge the stabilizers constantly.

Training for Muscle Balance

To counteract muscle imbalances caused during daily living by poor posture habits or excessive time spent in front of computers, we need to focus on proper balance between strong and flexible muscles in our classes. We need to try to strengthen those muscles that are prone to weakness and stretch those muscles that are prone to tightness, as listed in table 9.2. (See figures 5.12 to 5.17 in chapter 5 for diagrams of the muscles.)

Water-Specific Training for Muscular Endurance and Strength

To target strength more specifically, the ACSM says that a "lower repetition range, with a heavier weight, e.g., six to eight repetitions, may better optimize strength and power" (ACSM, 1998a, p. 982). In order to have sufficient stimulus for training in water, most people need to

Table 9.2 *Location of Weak or Tight Muscles*

Muscles that need strengthening	Muscles that need stretching
Anterior tibialis	Gastrocnemius
Hamstrings	Quadriceps/Iliopsoas
Rhomboids	Upper trapezius
Trapezius	Pectorals
Triceps	Hamstrings
Latissimus dorsi	Sternocleidomastoid
Gluteals	Deltoids (anterior)
Deltoids (posterior)	Adductors
Erector spinae	Erector spinae
Abductors	Abductors
Abdominals	Obliques
Obliques	

use equipment with a large surface area at a sufficient speed to adequately overload the muscles. Handheld devices such as dumbbells or chutes progressively increase muscular load to a high-intensity level for most participants. However, remember that the risk of injury is higher with greater resistance, even in water. Check that participants use proper form and that the overload is appropriate for each individual's fitness level.

Muscular endurance and strength training in the water has two advantages over land work: Water provides variable resistance training and core stabilization.

Moving through the water is like lifting "liquid weight": The more force you use through the movement, the higher the resistance forces that act against you. Water's heaviness facilitates specific variable or accommodating work. This type of dynamic muscular endurance conditioning cannot be accomplished on variable resistance machines.

While variable resistance machines do help strengthen individual muscle groups, they also stabilize the trunk "corset" area, minimizing the work of the stabilizing muscles. In contrast, the water environment allows participants to strengthen muscles in a functional/upright position, especially within the trunk "corset" area. Performing basic locomotor patterns, such as walking and running, utilizing the water's resistance enhances function as the body stabilizes itself against resistance. The true power of water exercise lies in its ability to challenge the stabilizers and provide specific resistance in an upright, functional position.

Sports conditioning experts know that to improve performance, muscles must be trained with movements as close as possible to the desired movements or skills.

What are the actual skills needed for improved daily living? Those that enhance proper posture!

For example, does performing supine curl-ups on land prepare the abdominals to be strong in a functional, upright position? Not really. With curl-ups, the abdominals are strengthened in a forward flexed position. In the water, the abdominals are worked in an upright position by simply walking through the water. Using water's natural resistance can strengthen the abdominals specifically to improve daily functioning.

Let's look at training in water for muscular strength and endurance in more depth by considering some of the differences between training on land and in water and by discussing how to design a program.

Differences Between Strength Training on Land and in Water

Two major differences between strength training on land and in water are the effects of gravity versus buoyancy and the lessening of eccentric muscle contractions in water.

Gravity vs. Buoyancy

When you are standing on land in an upright position with your hands at your sides, certain muscle groups are assisted and resisted by gravity. (See table 9.3.) For example, when you perform a biceps curl, gravity resists the flexion, and when you extend your elbow, gravity assists the extension. Try this by doing a biceps curl and not resisting the extension action. Your arm naturally straightens due to the assistance of gravity. In water, triceps may have to work harder than biceps, creating an opportunity for muscular balance.

In water, buoyancy's upward force rather than gravity's downward force is the primary effect to be considered during muscular conditioning exercises. The arms and legs have a different degree of buoyancy depending on body composition and buoyancy resistance based on lever length.

Buoyancy assists upward movements and provides some resistance to downward movements (Fawcett, 1992). For example, during a biceps curl in chest-deep water, buoyancy assists the buoyant person. Test the effects of buoyancy by placing your hands at your sides in the water and watching how your arms float slowly to the surface. (Of course, the degree of assistance depends on individual body composition.) This floating action is due to the effects of buoyancy.

We've found that buoyancy in the water can affect muscle groups differently than gravity on land affects them. (See table 9.3.) The biceps are considered strong muscle groups on land. They can be assisted in water, while the weaker triceps can be resisted against buoyancy for natural overload. In summary, buoyancy can help create muscular balance, since water provides the opportunity for some weaker muscle groups to work more frequently during the workout.

Less Eccentric Muscle Contraction

Not only does water exercise automatically use some of the weaker muscle groups, but due to the loss of gravity it also decreases the effect of eccentric muscle contraction. **Eccentric muscle contraction** is a muscle contraction in which a muscle exerts force, lengthens (increases joint angle), and is overcome by resistance (Study, 1991). **Concentric muscle contraction** is a muscle contraction in which a muscle exerts force, shortens (decreases joint angle), and overcomes resistance (Study, 1991).

Table 9.3 **Assisted and Resisted Muscle Groups on Land and in Water in a Standing Position**

Land

Assisted	Resisted
Triceps	Biceps
Abdominals	Erector spinae
Adductors	Abductors
Lats	Deltoids

Water

Assisted	Resisted
Abductors	Adductors
Deltoids	Lats
Biceps	Triceps

Adapted from Kennedy, C., and M. Sanders. 1995. Strength training gets wet! *IDEA Today* (May): 24–30. Adapted with permission from IDEA, The Health & Fitness Source, (800) 999-IDEA, ext. 7.

For example, for a basic biceps curl in water, the flexion action is a concentric contraction of the biceps working with buoyancy, and the extension action is a concentric contraction of the triceps working against buoyancy. Because of the lack of gravity, there is little eccentric contraction in water unless equipment is used.

Table 9.4 summarizes the types of muscle contraction occurring during a basic biceps curl on land and in water. As you can see, concentric muscle contractions are the main action in water exercise. Unless a foam dumbbell is used, little to no eccentric muscle contraction occurs.

Nieman (1995) has suggested that eccentric muscle contraction is associated with muscle soreness.

Table 9.4 **Elbow Flexion/Extension Muscle Contraction on Land and in Water***

Environment	Equipment	Joint action	Biceps	Triceps
Land	None or dumbbell	Elbow flexion	Concentric	None
	None or dumbbell	Elbow extension	Eccentric	None
Water	None or webbed gloves	Elbow flexion	Concentric	None
	None or webbed gloves	Elbow extension**	None	Concentric
Water	Foam dumbbell	Elbow flexion**	None	Eccentric
	Foam dumbbell	Elbow extension	None	Concentric

*Perform this exercise standing upright with hands at sides and elbows at waist.
**Use slow speed to resist buoyancy.
Kennedy, C., and M. Sanders. 1995. Strength training gets wet! *IDEA Today* (May): 24–30.
Reprinted with permission from IDEA, The Health & Fitness Source, (800) 999-IDEA, ext. 7.

Couple this idea with the low-impact nature of water exercise and you have a very different environment than you have in land exercise. This helps explain why exercising in the water is so comfortable—aches and pains are rare the day after a water workout.

Designing Muscle Strength and Endurance Training Programs

When designing water exercise programs, you need to take into account the differences between muscular endurance training on land and muscular endurance training in the water. Land training involves the use of gravity as resistance and/or added external resistance, such as dumbbells or resistance bands. On land, we first use gravity and then move to adding resistance. In the water, we begin by using the effects of buoyancy and then add buoyancy-resistant devices (such as foam dumbbells), devices to increase surface area (such as webbed gloves), and speed of movement.

In water, speed can increase intensity, but range of motion really makes the most difference. Evans, Cureton, and Purvis (1978) have recommended that, in waist-deep water, the speed of a movement be decreased to one-half or one-third of what it would be on land for an equal energy expenditure. Slowing down movements actually enhances the muscular conditioning advantage of water exercise. Using force and the resulting speed to increase intensity is only one of several options, as can be seen in figure 9.1.

You can gradually take a move from low intensity to high intensity to accommodate different ability levels. The following example using cross-country ski moves is based on the model described in figure 9.1:

- Start with feet on the pool bottom (lowest intensity).
- Increase the speed.
- Increase the range of motion of all muscles by lengthening the moves.
- Increase the speed again using this wider range of motion.
- Travel forward.
- Travel forward faster.
- Suspend the move (lift feet entirely) so the abdominals and trunk stabilizers assist (highest intensity).

Figure 9.1 *Water Resistance Intensity Progression*

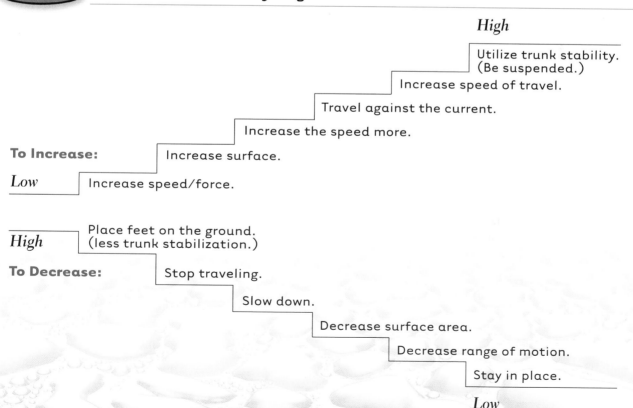

Kennedy, C., and M. Sanders. 1995. Strength training gets wet! *IDEA Today* (May): 24–30.
Reprinted with permission by IDEA, The Health & Fitness Source, (800)999-IDEA or (619) 535-8979.

You also can use the water resistance intensity progression model in figure 9.1 to individualize workouts for participants who are at different fitness levels. Using this model is the same as adjusting the setting on a variable resistance machine. Participants in a water exercise class should not all work with the same surface area or at the same speed, just as everyone should not use the same weight on a variable resistance machine. We must encourage individuals to move at their own pace.

To design an effective class, keep the progression model and the following tips in mind:

- So participants can keep their own pace, use background music rather than tempo (beat) music during the muscular strength and endurance training segment.

- Show different levels of range of motion and speed of movement from the deck.

- Have various pieces of buoyant and surface area equipment (see chapter 12) available to accommodate different fitness levels.

- Design the workout based on the daily activity needs of participants. Survey them before class to discover their needs.

- Switch upper- and lower-body work to use various joints.

Sometimes water fitness participants with excellent cardiorespiratory fitness on land find they are unable to get as hard a cardiorespiratory workout in the water as they do on land.

Participants might not possess the trunk muscular stability needed to get the same cardiorespiratory workout in the water as on land. Hoeger et al. (1993), comparing water aerobics to low-impact aerobic dance, found that muscular strength gains for the water aerobics group were greater than those for the low-impact group. Water is a resistant medium, so it takes some time and physiological adaptations for participants to develop the strength to perform the same cardiorespiratory task in water that they can perform on land, particularly with trunk stability exercises. Participants highly conditioned in cardiorespiratory fitness may need to develop greater muscular endurance to overload in water for additional aerobic conditioning or even to maintain the same level of cardiorespiratory conditioning. Therefore, we must consider water a resistance training medium as well as a place to gain cardiorespiratory fitness.

Water-Specific Muscular Endurance and Strength Exercise Design

To develop water-specific exercises, isolate the targeted muscles and practice the pattern of movement to target the muscle group(s). Examine the properties of water used to create work (which direction is buoyancy assisting?).

Stabilize the body using an active basic move such as jogging (see chapter 8) or a stationary stance such as a lunge. Try to submerge the joint being worked, and check alignment.

Determine the optimal overload: Work each muscle group through a progression so participants can find their own resistance level. Apply the **S.W.E.A.T.** formula to your moves.

- **Use the "S" in the formula to increase resistance.** Adjust surface area of the limbs or add surface area equipment for overload. Adjust the speed to increase or decrease resistance levels. Tell participants to find the speed, surface area, and resistance level where they feel the work is "hard" or "somewhat hard."

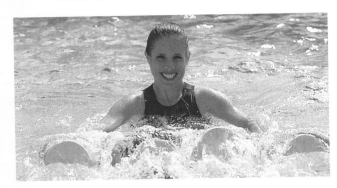

- **Use the "W" in the formula to gradually increase resistance.** Change working positions to target different lower-body muscle groups. In shallow water, use "squats" and fast "sit to stand ups" to overload upper-body groups such as the latissimus dorsi (squats) and deltoids (sit to stand up). In deep water, use "Power Pops" to overload the latissimus dorsi during upper-body work and the gluteus maximus during a "Power Pop" scissors.

- **Use the "E" in the formula for functional strength.** Enlarge the joint range of motion, contracting the muscles through a full range of motion. For maximum benefit and strength, muscles should be trained through the entire range (Graves et al., 1989).

• **Use the "A" in the formula to work around the joint, moving the lever in different planes.** Isolate the muscles targeted for work. Changing planes only slightly may still target the same muscle groups, but in a slightly different way, using slightly different fibers. Remember specificity of training. The muscles get stronger in the plane and range of motion in which they have been trained, so be sure to use ranges and planes that improve functioning on land.

For example, on an exercise machine, the rhomboids are targeted in a single plane. To train all the functional fibers in different planes of motion for the rhomboids, the movement should include downward action, using long levers. In the water, many planes can be targeted so all the functional fibers are worked. (See the sample exercise progressions for rhomboids later in this section.)

In cardiorespiratory training, the "A" is applied to exercise design to prevent local muscle fatigue, which would not be consistent with the training guidelines for muscular endurance/strength training.

• **Use the "T" in the formula to gradually increase resistance.** To overload farther after speed and surface area have been maximized or to overload stabilizing groups such as the abdominals, travel in the same direction as the power phase, or use the power phase effort to push or pull the body through the water, dragging the entire body for overload. For example, to increase the overload for the pectorals, walk forward during a pectoral press (arms power in across the chest).

 Video References:

Specificity of Training and Deep Water Program, Session 3.
The Golden Waves Video II, Sections 7 and 8.

For average adults who are beginning a strength training program, research indicates that one set of 8 to 10 exercises performed a minimum of twice a week is recommended because it is less time consuming and produces most of the health and fitness benefits of multiple-set programs (Feigenbaum & Pollock, 1997).

Give the following performance tips to your participants:

• Find your level and perform repetitions until muscles begin to fatigue.
• Exhale on exertion, inhale on recovery.
• If you perform both push and pull phases with effort, allow time between phases for inhalation before beginning the next work phase, or breathe rhythmically during the repetitions.
• Keep warm by working your legs (jogging, bicycling) during armwork.

You also can help participants keep warm by inserting thermal relaxation sets or a cardiorespiratory sequence between muscle conditioning sets.

Monitor exercise intensity and check participants' body form. Encourage participants to adjust exercise intensity by using the 4 **S**'s for muscular strength and endurance training:

To decrease intensity:

1. *Slow* down.
2. Make the move *Smaller.*
3. *Stabilize* the body and working joints, and let go of the equipment.
4. *Substitute* lower-resistance equipment.

To increase intensity:

1. *Stabilize* the body position and working joints (submerge the joints).
2. Practice and use the functional range or appropriate *Size* of the pattern for the muscle groups being targeted.
3. Adjust resistance by choosing the proper *Surface* area overload.
4. Add force and increase *Speed* for higher resistance.

When you add equipment, be sure to teach participants the purpose of the equipment and its proper use and safety.

Sample Muscular Endurance and Strength Training Progression

This section describes a sample muscular strength and endurance training workout. It specifies the muscles being worked, the joint that is loaded, and equipment that can be used to overload the muscles. It includes tips for using the movements in shallow, transitional, and deep water and has cues for the movements. Water depths are defined as follows:

Shallow: Navel to nipple

Transitional: Nipple to neck (lungs fully submerged)

Deep: Neck depth and deeper (use buoyancy gear)

Choose the proper working depth based on the percentage of weight bearing desired for training, the equipment used, and the skill of the participants.

Thermal relaxation and a brief cardiorespiratory sequence follow each muscle conditioning set.

Thermal Warm-Up (3–5 minutes)

Have participants perform light, easy moves, beginning with short levers and slowly extending to longer arms and legs. Cue participants to press their heels to the bottom and scull for balance. Pace your warm-up according to the water temperature. Allow participants to accommodate to buoyancy, adjusting to the resistance by slowly enlarging movements, then gradually increasing speed. Use travel moves for additional cardiorespiratory and stabilization work and to increase body warmth.

Rhomboids and Trapezius

The joint loaded is the shoulders. Use equipment that increases surface area.

Cue: Make "back cleavage" by squeezing the shoulder blades together, then relax forward.

For shallow: Jog backward and press back to maximize the load.

For transitional: Use the press to push the body forward. Check that the body has traveled.

For deep: Use flutter kicks to propel the body backward while using the press to counteract this action. The body should remain stationary.

Thermal relaxation (30–60 seconds): Jog easily, reaching forward to relax the back.

Cardio sequence (3 minutes): Jog and travel in different working positions using the **S.W.E.A.T.** formula.

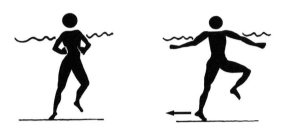

Shallow and transitional depths

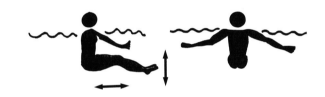

Deep water

Gluteals

The joint loaded is the hips. Use equipment that increases surface area and/or buoyancy.

Cue: Add power on hip extension, relax on hip flexion.

For shallow: Travel backward and power down.

For transitional: Lift the body upward (don't jump).

For deep: Maintain the neutral position. Look at the bottom, flex the toes, and bring the knee to the chest on recovery. Use the hands to scull, pushing and pulling underwater in opposition to the legs for balance.

Thermal relaxation (30–60 seconds): Perform easy jumping jax in a flexuous mode.

Cardio sequence (3 minutes): Perform scissors/jax through the **S.W.E.A.T.** formula and working positions.

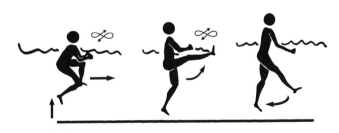

Shallow and transitional depths

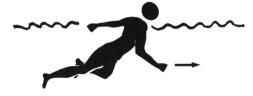

Deep water

Triceps

The joint loaded is the elbows. Use equipment that increases surface area and/or buoyancy.

Cue: Begin the curl, palm up or down, near the surface. Slice on recovery.

For shallow: Travel backward during elbow extension for overload.

For transitional and deep: Lift the body upward during the pressdown.

Thermal relaxation (30–60 seconds): Rock sideways, lifting the elbows high and reaching.

Cardio sequence (3 minutes): Rock and jump, using the progression and working positions.

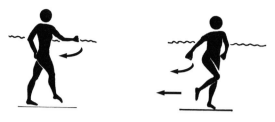

Shallow and transitional depths

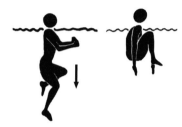

Deep water

Hamstrings

The joint loaded is the knees. Use equipment such as a step or fins in deep water.

Cues: Check your range of motion. Develop speed to minimize buoyancy during the curl.

For shallow: Flex fully to maximize speed during the curl. Scull for balance.

For transitional: To prevent submersion, land tall, then slowly get into position to curl under. Powerful curls will pull you downward; scull for lift.

For deep: Lean slightly forward and keep the knees "quiet." Check to see that you travel forward as a result of the curl. Put your hands on the hamstring and feel it.

Thermal relaxation (30–60 seconds): Perform easy kicks to the front, side, and back.

Cardio sequence (3 minutes): Kick and change planes, using the progression and working positions.

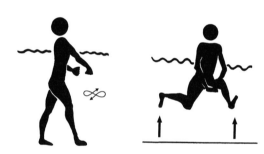

Shallow and transitional depths

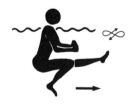

Deep water

Latissimus Dorsi

The joint loaded is the shoulders. Use equipment that increases surface area and/or buoyancy.

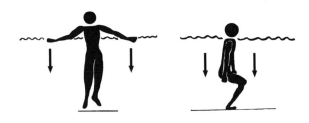

Cue: Allow buoyancy to assist rest during recovery.

For shallow: Squat down during the pull down to overload (use action/reaction).

For transitional and deep: Lift the body upward during the press and scull to "catch" your descent. A straddle leg position helps keep the hips in alignment.

Thermal relaxation (30–60 seconds): Softly rock forward and back, reaching with the arms.

Cardio sequence (3 minutes): Go from walking to leaping. Change planes and use progression.

Shallow water

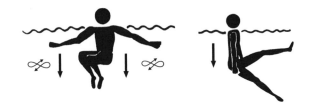

Transitional and deep water

Abductors or Adductors

The joint loaded is the hips. Use equipment that increases buoyancy to work the adductors.

Abductors

Cue: Power "in" to target adductors, power "out" to target abductors, toes forward.

For shallow: Use buoyancy to increase range of motion.

For transitional: Land tall between the power phases. Adduction may lift the body upward, and abduction may pull you down. Use hands in opposition to the legs to prevent bobbing (not shown).

For deep: Change body positions from vertical to horizontal for fun. On your back, you'll move head first during adduction and feet first during abduction!

Thermal relaxation (30–60 seconds): Perform easy scissors (cross-country ski) with hands slicing.

Cardio sequence (3 minutes): Perform intervals of scissors and jax, going through the working positions.

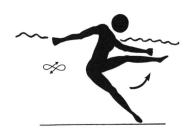

Shallow water

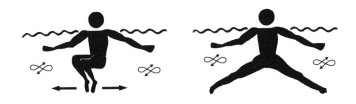

Transitional and deep water

Trunk Corset (*Latissimus Dorsi, Erector Spinae, Abdominals*)

The joints loaded are the knees, shoulders, and hips. Use equipment such as a kickboard, fins (optional), or flotation belt (optional).

Cues:

- Flutter kick to move backward. Using fins increases speed and resistance against the entire body, making the exercise more effective.
- Relax the neck and pull your navel to the spine as you reverse curl slowly.
- In vertical, push the spine into neutral stance, contract the lats to hold the board submerged (don't shrug your shoulders), and travel backward. Stand tall!
- Resist buoyancy by moving from vertical slowly back to horizontal.

Warm-Down

Before exiting the pool, have participants perform active range-of-motion exercises to relax the muscles worked and keep them warm. If the workout was in deep water, move into the shallow end to slowly add gravity to the movements.

 Video Reference:

The Aquatic Step Program. (Exercises are shown using the step but can be performed without it.)

Sample Combination Training Progression (Muscular Endurance/Strength, Cardiorespiratory fitness, and Body Composition)

Figure 9.2 shows two sample combination workouts that use circuit training.

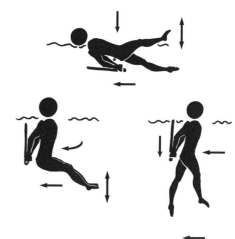

Shallow to deep or deep water only

In circuit training, exercises are sequenced to alternately challenge different muscle groups. Sets can be designed with or without equipment.

 Video Reference:

Tidal Waves

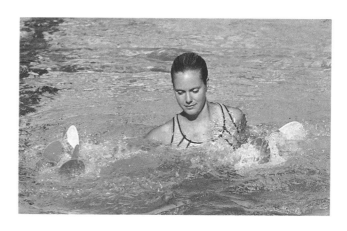

Figure 9.2 *Sample combination training progressions*

Circuit Cycle, No Equipment

Stationary muscular conditioning	3—4 min
Basic moves (**S.W.E.A.**)	3—4 min
Cardio travel: Basic moves (**S.W.E.A.T.**)	3—4 min

One cycle lasts 6 to 8 minutes. Perform four to five cycles totaling 24—40 minutes.

Circuit Cycle, With Equipment

Cardio travel: Basic moves (**S.W.E.A.T.**)	3—4 min
Transition to the equipment sites	30 sec
Muscular conditioning station work using equipment	3—4 min
Transition to the center of the pool for cardio traveling	30 sec

One cycle lasts 7 to 9 minutes. Perform four cycles totaling 28—36 minutes.

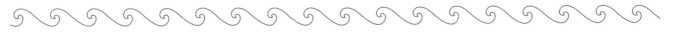

Flexibility and Active Range of Motion

Another aspect of fitness that water exercise can address is flexibility. Let's define some terms related to flexibility before we look at the ACSM guidelines for flexibility training.

Flexibility is the range of motion possible about a joint (Study, 1991).

Range of motion is the number of degrees that a joint allows one of its segments to move (Study, 1991).

Dynamic stretching (also referred to as *active stretching*) requires muscle contraction through a range of motion, where it has a tendency to load, strengthen, and prepare muscles and connective tissues for functional activities (Study, 1991).

Static stretching is also referred to as *passive stretching*, which is a low-force, long-duration stretch that holds the desired muscles at their greatest possible length for 15 to 30 seconds (Study, 1991).

During an active or a passive stretch, the elastic components of the muscle are usually relaxed, and the portion of the muscle most likely to be loaded is the connective tissue structures (Study, 1991).

ACSM Guidelines for Flexibility

According to the ACSM, flexibility exercises should be incorporated into a general fitness program. The exercises should provide enough stimulus to develop and maintain range of motion (ROM).

The 1998 ACSM guidelines for flexibility training for healthy adults (ACSM, 1998a) are as follows:

Frequency: two to three times per week

Intensity: Sufficient to develop and maintain ROM

Type: Static and/or dynamic stretching techniques

The ACSM (1998b) finds that currently there is very little research to indicate the best exercises to improve flexibility in the older adult, despite apparent age-related decline in joint range of motion. Their recommendations include exercises such as walking, aerobic dance, and stretching as part of a general exercise program for older adults. The exact amount or intensity has not yet been determined; however, it appears that a variety of movements, even performed for only a short duration, may have a positive effect on flexibility.

Water-Specific Flexibility Exercise Design

You can use static stretches in warm water. In cooler water, either alternate static stretching with moderate aerobic movements to keep participants warm, or use dynamic stretches instead. Dynamic stretches are appropriate for most community and YMCA pool temperatures. Encourage participants to keep their legs moving (jogging) during upper-body stretches.

Try to obtain a functional range of motion for each joint through exercises. Check participants' balance, alignment, and comfort as they exercise.

Encourage older adults to perform movements that are related to activities of daily living (such as walking, dancing, or reaching) while using the support of buoyancy to allow them to exaggerate the movements' size. This allows them to train for both range-of-motion and balance/recovery skills.

- **Use the "S" in the formula for buoyancy assistance.** Slow down the basic movements. Use surface area variations to act as "table top" support. Participants can lean on this to sustain correct joint positions and to support the body through large ranges of motion. For example, participants can hold kickboards at the surface for support as they lean or fall forward into a calf stretch, then recover to a stand. They can repeat leaning, stretching, and recovering as they travel across the pool.

- **Use the "W" to vary impact and range of motion.** Use moves such as scissors and jax in neutral or suspended positions (participants can wear flotation belts) to focus on range of motion and minimize impact.

- **Use the "E" to maximize range of motion.** Vary the size of moves, focusing on lengthening to full range. Use buoyancy to assist with lower-body ranges of motion while using moves such as "leaping" across the pool. Also, add buoyancy equipment to the limbs for enhancement. For example, use a buoyant dumbbell under the leg to assist with a hamstring stretch.

- **Use the "A" to ensure flexibility balance.** Refer back to table 9.2 for muscles that need strengthening or stretching. Work around the body and the joints to maintain functional ranges for a wide variety of activities. Target muscles that need to be stretched during exercise class.

- **Use the "T" to assist with dynamic stretches and to keep the body warm.** Participants can perform dynamic stretches while moving for warmth. Walking through the water while dragging the arms, for example, can stretch the muscles of the chest. Use the water currents created by travel and movement through the water to "push" or assist limbs into fuller stretches.

 Video References:

Introduction to the Waterfit Aquatic Fitness System, Shallow Water
Specificity of Training and Deep Water Program
The Aquatic Step Program
The Golden Waves Program, Functional Water Training for Health
The Golden Waves Program, Video II
Tidal Waves

Sample Progression for Flexibility

Figure 5.18 in chapter 5 illustrates normal, functional ranges of motion for healthy adults. While individuals may need to modify their ranges of motion according to their own body types, use these figures as a guideline. Many times buoyancy pushes a limb beyond a safe, normal range by assisting too much! Also, you need to know the appropriate joint range of motion to effectively train weaker muscle groups. For example, if a person stands in the water and abducts a leg past a 45-degree angle, the hip flexors take over and perform the movement, instead of the targeted abductors! Check to see that participants are working appropriately so they develop flexibility that keeps them moving in all the directions they'll need for an active life.

Here are two sample stretch progressions for use in shallow water:

HAMSTRINGS STRETCH PROGRESSION

- In shallow water, extend the leg forward, heel on the floor, hips back (lowest intensity).
- Hop on one leg in the neutral position, moving backward (**T.**).
- Extend a leg forward, push the hips back, and "crawl hips up the wall" (**E. T.**).
- Stop traveling and assist the stretch with a step, push down, and release.
- Assist the stretch with stable buoyancy equipment placed under the thigh (**S.**).
- Assist the stretch with stable buoyancy equipment placed near the ankle (**S. E.**).
- Leap sideways in the neutral position, traveling across the pool, enlarging the leap each time.
- Leap diagonally and repeat (**S.W.E.A.T.**) (highest intensity).

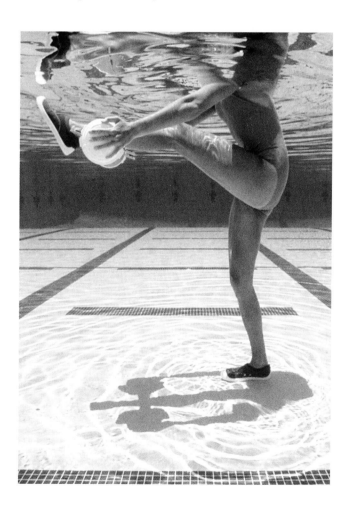

OBLIQUE STRETCH PROGRESSION

- Lean on a kickboard extended to the side (**S.**)(lowest intensity).
- "Fall" sideways, reaching as far as possible with the board. Recover to a stand (**S.E.T.**).
- Reach farther, lifting the feet off the bottom to become suspended, then recover to a stand.
- Increase the speed and number of repetitions.
- Reach out slightly on a diagonal and repeat the sequence (**S.W.E.A.T.**) (highest intensity).

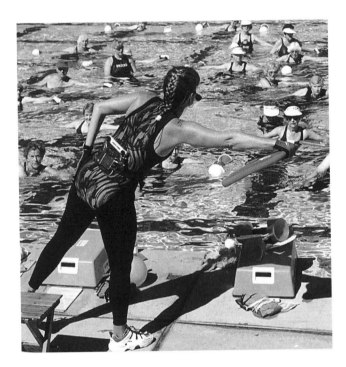

Weight Management and Healthy Body Composition

Many of our participants come to class only to lose weight. Their two objectives are to see results and to do it as soon as possible! In this section, we'll examine how to target weight loss as a training objective, one that has to become a lifestyle change, and examine how to maximize results.

According to the ACSM (1998a), people who engage in physical activity alone without dieting (limiting the number of kilocalories consumed) have only modest changes in total body mass and body fat loss. Combining diet and exercise is most effective in bringing about lasting body composition changes. Cardiorespiratory fitness programs appear to promote body fat loss while maintaining or even increasing fat-free mass (primarily muscle). Weight-loss programs using "diet only" result in loss of both fat and lean mass.

Refer to the BMI formula discussed in the cardiorespiratory and body composition section of this chapter and to the BMI chart in appendix A to determine if you or your participants have healthy weights.

One of the greatest benefits of water is that its natural resistance can stimulate both cardiorespiratory and muscular endurance conditioning. As discussed in chapter 6, a number of training studies conducted in the water indicated significant body fat loss along with significant muscular strength/endurance gains (Barretta, 1993; Hoeger et al., 1993; Sanders, 1993). Other benefits of water exercise include the ability for you to regulate impact by changing depths and for participants to instantly regulate their intensity for their own comfort. Because slowing down or stopping movement safely reduces or removes overload, participants are in control of their workout.

Research by Grediagin et al. (1995) suggests that if fat loss is the goal of a program and time is limited, people should be encouraged to exercise safely at as high an intensity as tolerable to expend as much energy (kcal) as possible during their allotted time. Water provides a safe and effective environment to work at high intensity without some of the risks associated with exercising on land. Workouts in the pool can be designed to be fun, using play to deliver serious results and encourage an active lifestyle.

Cardiorespiratory training promotes fat loss by using the stored energy of body fat for fuel. A lot of debate has gone on regarding what the ideal exercise intensity is to accelerate the use of fat. Many people believe that working out at low intensities is the best way to utilize fat. However, William Haskell (1999) has stated that, while lower intensity work does draw on fat for energy, unlike higher intensity work that draws more on sugars for energy, this difference occurs only *during* exercise. In the 24-hour period following exercise, the body replenishes its stored muscle glycogen and, if the energy expenditure during exercise was greater than energy consumption, fat will be used to do this. Higher intensity work ultimately burns more fat off the body because it burns more calories.

ACSM Guidelines for Weight Management and Body Composition

The following are the ACSM guidelines for weight management and body composition (ACSM, 1998a):

Frequency: Three days per week

Intensity: High enough to expend 250–300 kcal per session

Type/Mode: Cardiorespiratory fitness

Time: Approximately 30–45 minutes for a person of average fitness

For people who want to target weight loss as their primary training objective, the ACSM recommends programs that are conducted more frequently for a longer duration and performed at a moderate intensity (ACSM, 1998a). Sample training guidelines for such a program could be:

Frequency: Four days per week

Intensity: High enough to expend 200 kcal per session

Type/Mode: Cardiorespiratory fitness

Time: 30–45 minutes

Now that you know the guidelines, let's discuss how to plan exercise sessions to expend sufficient energy for weight loss and what to recommend about good nutrition.

Exercise Intensity and Estimated Energy Expenditure

Table 9.5, adapted from Kravitz and Mayo (1997) with additions from McArdle, Katch, and Katch (1991), shows predicted kilocalorie expenditures for a variety of activities. Some of the kilocalories have been estimated from research studies that measured MET equivalents.

A number of water-based studies can be used to predict kilocalorie expenditures based on documented MET measures (1 MET equals 3.5 ml·kg^{-1}·min^{-1}). Table 9.6, adapted from ACSM, shows MET levels to determine intensity and estimates the number of kcal per minute that could be expended during the activity. Compare the MET levels in this table with those in the previous table to relate how hard participants must work in order to expend the predicted kcals in the range. During class, use the intensity levels to help your participants apply RPE effectively to target their individual training objectives.

METs, or the metabolic energy cost of activities, is a means of measuring physical energy expenditure. A MET is a unit of oxygen expended, with one MET being the energy (measured as kilocalories) needed while the body is in a resting state (Study, 1991). A kilocalorie (kcal) is a measure of heat used to express the energy value of food (McArdle, Katch, and Katch, 1991). For example, an activity that uses seven METs

Table 9.5 *Predicted Kilocalorie Expenditures for Various Activities*

Activity	kcal/min
Aquatic exercise	5.7–6.5
Aerobic dance on land, moderate intensity (130–143 lb person)	6.2–6.6
Walking on land, normal pace on asphalt (123–150 lb person)	4.5–5.4
Deep water walking	8.8
Running 11 min/mile on land (130 lb person)	8.0
Deep water running	11.5
Golf (130–150 lb person)	5.0–5.8
Circuit training, free weights (150 lb person)	5.8
Skiing on soft snow, leisurely pace (143 lb woman)	6.4
Sitting quietly (123–150 lb person)	1.2–1.4

Adapted from tables in Kravitz, L., and J. Mayo. 1997. Aquatic exercise: A review. *AKWA Letter*, (October/November): 7,12,31.and McArdle, W., R. Katch, and V. Katch. 1991. *Exercise physiology, energy, nutrition and human performance* (3rd ed.). Philadelphia: Lea & Febiger.

Table 9.6 *Exercise Intensity and Estimated METs for Healthy Adult Men and Women of Varying Ages*

Men

Intensity	20–39 yrs	40–64 yrs	65–79 yrs	80+ yrs
Very light	< 2.4	< 2.0	< 1.6	≤ 1.0
Light	2.4–4.7	2.0–3.9	1.6–3.1	1.1–1.9
Moderate	4.8–7.1	4.0–5.9	3.2–4.7	2.0–2.9
Hard	7.2–10.1	6.0–8.4	4.8–6.7	3.0–4.25
Very hard	≥ 10.2	≥ 8.5	≥ 6.8	≥ 4.25
Maximal	12.0	10.0	8.0	5.0

Women*

Intensity	20–39 yrs	40–64 yrs	65–79 yrs	80+ yrs
Very light	< 1.4	< 1.0	< .6	≤ .5
Light	1.4–3.7	1.0–2.9	.6–2.1	.1–.9
Moderate	3.8–6.1	3.0–4.9	2.2–3.7	1.0–1.9
Hard	6.2–9.1	5.0–7.4	3.8–5.7	2.0–3.25
Very hard	≥ 9.2	≥ 7.5	≥ 5.8	≥ 3.25
Maximal	11.0	9.0	7.0	4.0

* Mean MET values for women are approximately one to two METs lower than those for men. To estimate values for this chart, the women's range was calculated by subtracting 1.0 from the men's METs estimate.

Adapted, by permission, from ACSM, 1998a. "The recommended quantity and quality of exercise for developing and maintaining cardiorespiratory and muscular fitness in healthy adults." *Medicine & Science in Sports & Exercise* 30(6): 975–985.

requires seven times more energy (and kcals) than does a state of rest.

A heavier person requires more energy both at rest and during exercise. Additionally, the energy required to perform an activity changes with age. Table 9.7 illustrates intensity levels and estimated METs based on gender and age.

As you can see, the predicted kcal expenditure varies with the type of aquatic exercise, gender, and age, and the estimated kcal for water exercise is comparable to estimates for land-based activities.

Let's estimate kcal expenditure during some sample workouts, comparing water exercise with land-based exercise. Three comparisons are provided in figure 9.3. Each class begins with a warm-up (5–10 minutes) and ends with a warm-down (5–10 minutes). To make the workout time and kcal calculations simpler, these sets are combined at the beginning of each workout.

By looking at these sample training progressions, you can see that water exercise classes can meet the minimal weight loss threshold criteria of approximately 250–300 kcal per exercise session (30–45 minutes) for three days per week or 200 kcal per session (30–45 minutes) for four days per week (ACSM, 1998a). Water exercise compares favorably to land exercise and should be promoted to participants as a viable choice for healthy weight loss and management.

As the number of studies increases, we'll be able to predict kcal expenditures for a greater variety of exercises. For example, the effect of wearing webbed gloves on intensity levels is of interest. The gloves help stabilize the body so the legs can work at maximal range of motion, but data to support their use in cardiorespiratory training are not yet available. This information is important to help quantify exercise intensity in order to give specific feedback to medical providers and advise participants on appropriate exercise for a healthy weight. (Mainstreaming with health care providers is a trend in the fitness and health care industry. See chapter 12 for more information on how to work with the medical community.)

Remember that the number of kilocalories used during activity is only an estimate. Wide variations may occur among individuals based on their body composition and body surface area. For example, a person with a high fat mass may find water running

Table 9.7 *Aquatic Exercise Estimated METs and kcals for Men and Women*

Type of aquatic exercise	MET Levels		Estimated kcal/min based on MET equivalents	
	Women	*Men*	*Women*	*Men*
Upper extremity only	2.9–4.1	3.3–5.7	3–5	5–7
Lower extremity only (Cassady and Nielsen, 1992)	4.0–7.0	4.6–9.2	5–9	4–7
Water exercise in 1 m (3.25 ft) water (Eckerson and Anderson, 1992)	5.25	No data	6	No data
Waist-to-chest deep water, calisthenics (Vickery, Cureton, and Langstaff, 1983)	6.7–8.3	No data	8>9.5	No data
Chest-deep exercise using arms and legs (Hered, Darby, and Yaekle, 1997)	4.8–6.8	No data	6–8	No data
Bench exercise, 7 in. step: Speedo System (Evans and Cureton, 1998)	4.2–7.4	No data	5–9	No data
Bench exercise, 12 in. step: Speedo System (Evans and Cureton, 1998)	6.5–9.9	No data	8–13	No data
Running in chest-deep water (Kirby, Balch, and Kriellaars, 1984)	7.1	7.1	9	8
Aqua exercise in chest-deep water (Heberlein et al., 1987)	5.4	No data	7	No data
Deep water running at 76% HRmax (Michaud et al., 1995)	No data	11	No data	13 (or higher)
Deep water running at 83% HRmax (Richie and Hopkins, 1991)	No data	13.1	No data	15 (approx.)

Adapted with permission from the Aquatic Exercise Association (1-941-486-8600).

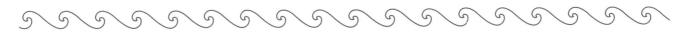

Figure 9.3 *Three comparisons of water and land exercise kcal estimates*

Comparison 1

Deep Water Interval Training for Women

Warm-up and warm-down
(6 kcal/min)   15 min

Training phase (30 min)
Walking (8.8 kcal/min)   10 min
Recovery (4 kcal/min)   1 min
Running (11.5 kcal/min)   3 min
Recovery (4 kcal/min)   1 min

Repeat the training phase twice
for a total workout time of 45 min.

Estimated kcals for training phase   261

Estimated kcals for total workout   351

Interval Training on Land (130-lb person)
Walking warm-up and cool-down
(5 kcal/min)   15 min

Training phase (30 min)
Running at 11 min-mile pace
(8 kcal/min)   10 min
Walking recovery (5 kcal/min)   1 min
Running at 9 min-mile pace
(11.4 kcal/min)   3 min
Walking recovery (5 kcal/min)   1 min

Repeat the training phase twice for
a total workout time of 45 min.

Estimated kcals for total workout   324

Comparison 2

Shallow Water Interval Training for Women

Warm-up and warm-down
(6 kcal/min)   15 min

Training phase (30 min)
Running in chest-deep water
(9 kcal/min)   2 min
Recovery (4 kcal/min)   1 min
Rebound jax on step (9 kcal/min)   1 min
Active recovery (4 kcal/min.)   1 min
Chest-deep exercise with arms
and legs (stationary work)
(7 kcal/min)   10 min

Repeat the run/recovery, step/recovery
cycle four times for a total workout
time of 45 min.

Estimated kcals for training phase   210

Estimated kcals for total workout   300

Interval Training on Land (123-lb person)
Walking warm-up and cool-down
(4.5 kcal/min)   15 min

Training phase (20 min)
Running at 11 min-mile pace
(8 kcal/min)   2 min
Active recovery
(walking, 4.5 kcal/min)   1 min
Jumping jax using a bench
or step (9.5 kcal/min)
(Evans and Cureton, 1998)   1 min
Active recovery
(walking, 4.5 kcal/min)   1 min
Aerobic dance on land at
moderate intensity (5.8 kcal/min) 10 min

Repeat the training phase without
aerobic dance four times for a total
workout time of 45 min.

Estimated kcals for total workout   264

Comparison 3

Combination Shallow and Deep Water Interval Training for Women

Participants wear a flotation belt so they can move between depths without interruption.

Warm-up and warm-down
(6 kcal/min)   10 min

Training phase (20 min)

Run shallow to deep for transition
(9 kcal/min)   1 min

Deep water (suspended) running with an interval cycle of 1 min work/30 sec active rest (11.5 kcal/4 kcal or 15.5 kcal each cycle), repeat for 6 cycles   9 min

Run deep to shallow to transition (9 kcal/min)   1 min

Shallow water (chest-deep) running with an interval cycle of 1 min work/30 sec active rest (9 kcal/4 kcal or 13 kcal each cycle), repeat for 6 cycles   9 min

The total training time is 30 min.

Estimated kcals for training phase   189

Estimated kcals for total workout   249

Interval Training on Land (130-lb person)
Warm-up and cool-down

Walking (5 kcal/min)   2 min

Running at 11 min-mile pace
(8 kcal/min)   10 min

Training phase (18 min)

Running at 8 min-mile pace
(12.5 kcal/min)   1 min

Walk recovery (5 kcal/min)   1 min

Repeat the training phase nine times
(17.5 kcal/cycle).

Total workout time is 30 min.

Estimated kcals for total workout   248

in shallow water easier than a lean individual. Body fat is buoyant, adding extra time for the body to float between foot strikes, slowing cadence and perhaps intensity. However, larger people may be working harder than smaller people when running at a matched pace. Additionally, Frangolias and Rhodes (1995) suggested that "water skills" are important to maximizing results. The subjects in their study who were "water trained" achieved higher intensities than those who apparently did not know how to use the water effectively.

Good Nutrition

According to Kosich (1995), losing weight is not just about food, but rather about the balance among exercise, sensible eating, and self-empowerment. His book *Get Real: A Personal Guide to Real-Life Management* can provide you and your participants with simple steps to achieve a healthy balance for weight management. This book is the participants' text for the YMCA's weight management program, and you may want to encourage those water exercise participants who want to manage their weight to take part in this program.

The U.S. Department of Agriculture recently released a simple chart to help guide people to make healthy dietary choices without having to calculate percentages of carbohydrates, fats, and proteins (figure 9.4). Eating within the pyramid guidelines should provide a healthy diet throughout a lifetime.

Figure 9.4   *The Food Guide Pyramid*

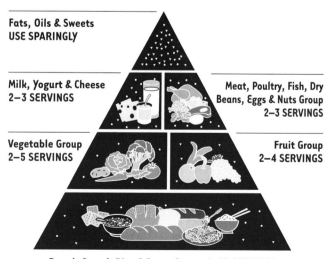

Source: U.S. Department of Agriculture/U.S. Department of Health and Human Services.

Functional Activities of Daily Living Training

Functional activities of daily living (ADL) water fitness training consists of exercises performed in the pool that target improvement of activities of daily living on the land, such as walking, getting up and down from a chair, climbing stairs, and lifting items. These exercises should be designed to most closely simulate each individual's identified functional activities. Each exercise must be specific to the targeted task and must gradually increase in intensity for training overload.

Most people who need ADL training are older adults or those who have been injured and have lost the ability to perform daily tasks. Ellen Gold and her colleagues at the University of California Medical School at Davis are studying the "functional fitness" of 10,000 women as part of the Study of Women Across the Nation (SWAN) project. Preliminary findings indicate that 20 percent of the women in this group, 40 to 55 years old, have trouble with simple physical tasks such as walking one block, climbing a flight of stairs, bathing, or dressing (Gold, in press). Fifty-five percent say they've felt stiffness or soreness in their joints, necks, or shoulders in the last two weeks. Impairment rates are highest for women who are overweight, sedentary, or poor. Baby boomers will expand this age group, and such a high prevalence of physical limits could predict greater disability-related costs. Exercise professionals can help ease the burden to the health care system and keep people independent by teaching them how to manage their weight and include activity and exercise as part of a healthy lifestyle. Functionally targeted exercises that are specific to tasks such as climbing stairs can help people minimize disability and improve their quality of life by encouraging activity and independence.

Loss of function can occur at any age from to the effects of injury and disease. Functional rehabilitation is managed by health care providers; however, as the healing progresses, professional exercise instructors can guide people through post-rehabilitation programs.

ACSM Guidelines on ADL Training

In 1998, the ACSM published a Position Stand on "Exercise and Physical Activity for Older Adults" (ACSM, 1998b). Some training recommendations for older adults already have been included in this chapter that cover cardiorespiratory endurance, muscular strength and endurance, and flexibility. In addition to these, ACSM recommends exercises that improve postural stability in order to reduce the incidence of falls. Exercise programs that can provide a wide variety of exercises should include balance training, resistive exercises, walking, and weight transfer, all suggested ways to improve postural stability in older adults.

Older adults frequently report depression. It can be a result of some of the aging processes. With aging, comes a loss of function (Haskell and Philips, 1995; Spirduso, 1995), and with this loss comes a reduction in activities of daily living and independence, resulting in a perceived loss of control. Perceptions of personal control and self-efficacy can influence how people feel about themselves and how well they can function. According to the ACSM (1998b), "it is well established that physical activity and psychological function are related" (p. 1000), therefore regular activity is recommended for this age group to "greatly improve the functional capacity of older men and women, thereby improving the quality of life in this population" (p. 1002).

For the very old and frail, the ACSM (1998b) recommends exercises that focus on scientifically proven strategies for reversing strength deficits instead of non-specific "movement" programs. Strength training has been shown to improve gait, velocity, balance, ability to rise from a chair, stair climbing power, aerobic capacity, and performance-based tests of functional independence. These gains were also suggested in the Golden Waves, a water-based study conducted by Sanders, Constantino, and Rippee (1997).

Strength training also contributed to improvements in morale, reduced depression, and better nutrition. Healthier elderly people found that strength training maintained or increased bone density, resting metabolic rate, and insulin sensitivity, improved digestion, decreased pain from arthritis, reduced body fat, and improved sleep quality.

Walking can improve both functional capacity to walk and contribute to cardiorespiratory endurance.

Water-Specific Functional ADL Exercise Design

In addition to following the recommendations by the ACSM for cardiorespiratory and muscular conditioning plus postural and flexibility training, we can design specific pool exercises to improve daily living skills on land. The following training recommendations are based on a study by Sanders et al. (1997), which used aquatic exercise exclusively for ADL training (Maloney-Hills, Sanders, 1998).

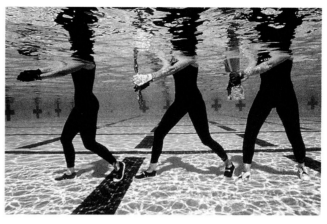

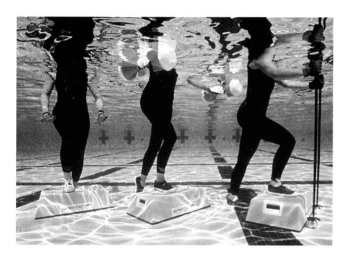

(glenohumeral and scapular muscles pectoralis, rotators of shoulder).

- **Include stabilization and dynamic trunk work:** trunk extension, flexion, lateral flexion.

- Train the neurological system how to "fire" and the muscles how to contract by training through real patterns of movement for ADL.

- Target neurological reflex patterns by practicing to improve proprioception for activity, balance, and recovery:

- **Use both gravity and the properties of water for overload.** For activities on land, the hips should be the center of balance for most of the work. Think about the specific application of the water progressions to the land task. Equipment such as the aquatic step for stair climbing and balance skills is important for gradually increasing exercise intensity and for making water exercise training more applicable to specific land skills.

- **Teach proper body alignment and emphasize it frequently.**

- **Adjust weight bearing by regulating water depth.** Progressively add weight (mimicking land impact) and reduce buoyancy's support of the body by working in shallower water.

- **Regulate intensity by allowing individuals to use an intensity progression.** For sufficient overload, encourage participants to work at moderate to high intensity without pain.

- **Include daily patterns of movement through various ranges of motion,** especially lower-body work targeting "power" training for walking and upper-body work targeting reaching and balance

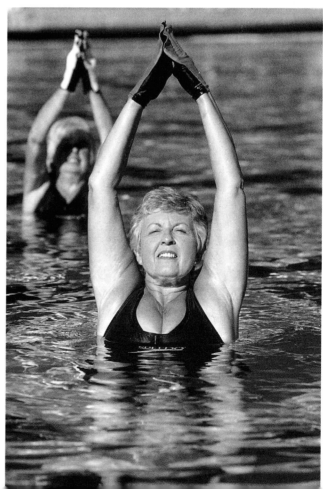

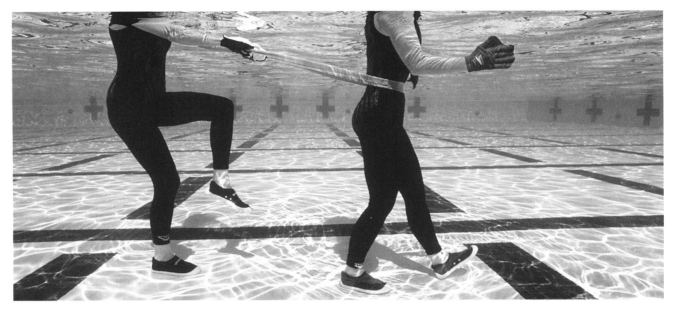

➤ Train for fast-twitch muscle improvement.

➤ Practice functional rotation movements.

➤ Use water's resistance for gait and stride training for improved walking, and use water's buoyancy for support and safety.

• **Include muscular endurance, strength, and "power" exercises,** using progressive resistance and speeds that mimic ADL.

• **Combine both isometric and eccentric work for land activity improvement.**

• **Emphasize exercises targeting strength, agility, and balance for stabilization to prevent falling and to manage a fall with safe recovery if one occurs:**

➤ Include exercises that mimic falling with the important training for recovery.

➤ Incorporate balance exercises using progressions to challenge individually.

➤ Practice responses and recovery to "surprises" to prevent falls, improve balance, and enhance recovery skills. For example, give participants cues to move in unanticipated directions.

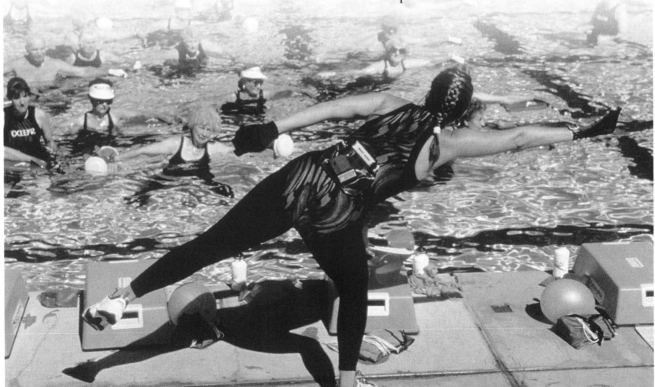

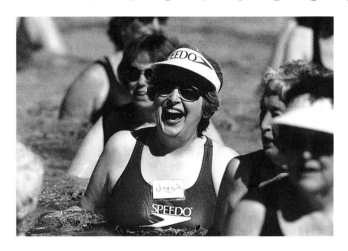

- **Include flexibility and active range-of-motion training that will improve overall mobility,** especially for the hip and knee (ACSM, 1998b).
- **Make it FUN!** Encourage playful sports and dance movements with "free time" to socialize, interact, and build relationships.
- **Make it purposeful!** Periodically provide participants with assessments of function to help them track progress and make them aware of the positive results of their lifestyle exercise commitment.

Refer to part IV for an in-depth examination of functional ADL training and sample progressions.

 Video References:

The Golden Waves Functional Water Fitness Program Golden Waves Leadership Program.

Bibliography

American Academy of Orthopaedic Surgeons. 1991. *Athletic Training and Sports Medicine.* Rosemont, IL: American Academy of Orthopaedic Surgeons.

American College of Sports Medicine. 1998a. The recommended quantity and quality of exercise for developing and maintaining cardiorespiratory and muscular fitness, and flexibility in healthy adults. *Medicine and Science in Sports and Exercise* 30(6): 975–991.

American College of Sports Medicine. 1998b. Exercise and physical activity for older adults. *Medicine and Science in Sports and Exercise* 30(6): 992–1008.

American College of Sports Medicine. 1992. *ACSM Fitness Book.* 2nd ed. Champaign, IL: Human Kinetics.

American College of Sports Medicine. 1990. The recommended quantity and quality of exercise for developing and maintaining cardiorespiratory and muscular fitness in healthy adults. *Medicine and Science in Sports and Exercise* 22: 265–274.

American College of Sports Medicine. 1986. *Resource manual for guidelines for exercise testing and prescription.* 3rd ed. Philadelphia: Lea & Febiger.

Astrand, P. 1992. Why exercise? *Medicine and Science in Sports and Exercise* 4(2): 153–162.

Baretta, R. 1993. Physiological training adaptations to a 14 week deep water exercise program. Unpublished dissertation, University of New Mexico, Albuquerque.

Barretta, R., and R. Robergs. 1995. Physiological training adaptations to a 14 week, deep water exercise program. *APTR* 3(3).

Borg, G.A. 1982. Psychophysical bases of perceived exertion. *Medicine and Science in Sports and Exercise* 14: 377.

Bouchard, C. 1997. The current obesity epidemic: Chaos, gluttony, sloth or nature? Joseph Wolffe Lecture, ACSM Annual Meeting. Denver, CO.

Brown, S., L. Chitwood, K. Beason, and D. McLemore. 1997. Deep water running physiologic responses: Gender differences at treadmill-matched walking/running cadences. *Journal of Strength and Conditioning Research* 11(2): 107–114.

Burns, N., ed. 1990. Unusual environments and human behavior. *Physiological and Psychological Problems of Man in Space* 13: 321–334.

Bushman, B., M. Flynn, F. Andres, C. Lambert, M. Taylor, and W. Braun. 1997. Effect of 4 weeks of deep water run training on running performance. *Medicine and Science in Sports and Exercise* 29(5): 694–699.

Byma, H.K., J.N. Craig, and J.H. Wilmore. 1996. A comparison of the effects of underwater treadmill walking on oxygen consumption, heart rate and cardiac output. *Journal of Aquatic Physical Therapy* (November): 4–11.

Cassady, S.L., and D.H. Nielsen. 1992. Cardiorespiratory responses of healthy subjects to calisthenics performed on land versus in water. *Physical Therapy* 72(7): 62/532–68/538.

Cole, A., M. Moschetti, and R.E. Eagleston (in press). Lumbar spine aquatic rehabilitation. In *A Sports Medicine Approach, Handbook of Pain Management,* ed. A. Cole, 2nd. ed. Baltimore: Williams & Wilkins.

Collins, R.L., ed. 1989. *AOPA's Handbook For Pilots.* Frederick, MD: AOPA.

Craig, A., and M. Dvorak. 1969. Comparison of exercise in air and in water of different temperatures. *Medicine and Science in Sports and Exercise* 1(3): 124–130.

Craig, A.B. Jr., and M. Dvorak. 1968. Thermal regulation of man during water immersion. *Journal of Applied Physiology* 25: 23–35.

Delhagen, K. 1987. Cold water survival. *Runner's World* (May).

Eckerson, J., and T. Anderson. 1992. Physiological response to water aerobics. *Journal of Sports Medicine and Physical Fitness* 32(3): 255–261.

Evans, E. 1996. Can water exercise tip the scale? *IDEA Today* (May): 27–31.

Evans, E., and K. Cureton. 1998. Metabolic, circulatory and perceptual responses to bench stepping in water. *Journal of Strength and Conditioning Research* (Summer).

Evans, F., K. Cureton, and J. Purvis. 1978. Metabolic and circulatory responses to walking and jogging in water. *Research Quarterly* 49: 442–449.

Fawcett, C. 1992. Principles of aquatic rehab: A new look at hydrotherapy. *Sports Medicine* 7(2): 6–9.

Feigenbaum, M., and M. Pollock. 1997. Strength training: Rationale for current guidelines for adult fitness programs. *Physician and Sports Medicine* 25(2): 44–64.

Frangolias, D., and E. Rhodes. 1995. Maximal and ventilatory threshold responses to treadmill and water immersion running. *Medicine and Science in Sports and Exercise* 27(7): 1007–1013.

Fox, M. 1998. The Hunger. *Fitness Swimmer Magazine* (April/May): 18.

Gold, E. 1998. Interview by author. University of California, Medical School, Davis, The study of women across the nation (SWAN)

Graves, J.E., M.L. Pollock, A.E. Jones, A.B. Colvin, and S.H. Leggett. 1989. Specificity of limited range of motion variable resistance training. *Medicine and Science in Sports and Exercise* 21: 84–89.

Grediagin, M., M. Cody, J. Rupp, D. Benardot, and R. Shern. 1995. Exercise intensity does not effect body composition change in untrained, moderately overfat women. *Journal of the American Dietetic Association* 95: 661–665.

Haskell, W.L., and W.T. Phillips. 1995. Exercise training, fitness, health, and longevity. Chap. 2 in *Perspectives in exercise science and sports medicine.* Vol. 8 of *Exercise in older adults,* edited by C.V. Gisolfi, D.R. Lamb, and E. Nadel. Carmel, IN: Cooper Publishing.

Hayward, J.S. 1990. Hypothermia, frostbite and other cold injuries, immersion hypothermia. *Physician and Sportsmedicine* (January): 66–73.

Heberlein, T., H. Perez, J. Wygand, and K. Connor. 1987. The metabolic cost of high impact aerobics and hydroaerobic exercise in middle-aged females. *Medicine and Science in Sports and Exercise* 19(2): Supplement, S89, 531.

Hered, S.L., L.A. Darby, and B.C. Yaekle. 1997. Comparison of physiological responses to comparable land and water exercises. *Medicine and Science in Sports and Exercise.* Abstract: 24(5) 523.

Hoeger, W.K., D.R. Hopkins, D.J. Barber, and T. Gibson. 1992. Comparison of maximal VO_2, HR and RPE between treadmill running and water aerobics. *Medicine and Science in Sports and Exercise* 24(5): S96.

Hoeger, W., T. Gibson, J. Moore, and D. Hopkins. 1993. A comparison of selected training responses to water aerobics and low-impact aerobic dance. *National Aquatics Journal* (Winter): 13–16.

JAMA, Journal of the American Medical Association. 1989. Hypothermia Prevention (Morbidity & Mortality Report) (January 27): 513.

Jull G., and V. Janda. 1987. Muscles and motor control in low back pain. In *Physical Therapy of the Low Back,* eds. L. Twomey and J. Taylor. New York: Churchill Livingstone.

Kennedy, C. 1998. Physiology of interval training. IDEA, The Health & Fitness Source, Water Fitness Specialty Conference Presentation, July 21–22, Orlando, FL.

Kennedy, C., and D. Legel. 1992. Anatomy of an exercise class: An exercise educator's handbook. Champaign, IL: Sagamore.

Kennedy, C., and Sanders, M. (1995). Strength training gets wet. *IDEA Today* (May).

Kirby, R.L., D.E. Balch, and D.J. Kriellaars. 1984. Oxygen consumption during exercise in a heated pool. *Archives of Physical Medicine and Rehabilitation* 65: 21–23.

Kirn, T. 1988. Do low levels of iron affect body's ability to regulate temperature, experience cold? *Journal of the American Medical Association* (August 5).

Kosich, D. 1995. *Get real, a personal guide to real-life weight management.* IDEA, The Health & Fitness Source. San Diego, CA.

Kravitz, L. 1996. The fitness professional's complete guide to circuits and intervals. *IDEA Today* 14(1): 32–43.

Kravitz, L., and J. Mayo 1997. Aquatic exercise: A review. *AKWA Letter* (October/November).

McArdle, W., R. Katch, and V. Katch. 1991. *Exercise physiology, energy, nutrition and human performance.* 3rd ed. Philadelphia: Lea & Febiger.

Michaud, T., J. Rodriguez-Zayas, F. Andres, M. Flynn, and C. Lambert. 1995. Comparative exercise responses of deep water and treadmill running. *Journal of Strength and Conditioning* 9(2): 104–109.

Morlock, J.F., and R.H. Dressendorfer. 1974. Modification of a standard bicycle ergometer for underwater use. *Undersea Biomedical Research* 1: 335.

Moody, D., J. Kollias, and E.R. Buskirk. 1969. The effect of moderate exercise program on body weight and skinfold thickness in overweight college women. *Medicine and Science in Sports and Exercise* 1: 75.

Napoletan, J.C., and R.W. Hicks. 1995. The metabolic effects of underwater treadmill exercise at two departments. *APTR* 3(2): 9–14.

Nielson, M. 1996. *Strong women stay young.* New York: Bantam Books.

Nieman, D. 1995. *Fitness and sports medicine, a health related approach*: Palo Alto, CA: Bull Publishing.

Otis, C.L. 1990. When a cooldown is undesirable. *Women's Sports and Fitness* (March).

Ritchie, S., and W. Hopkins. 1991. The intensity of deep water running. *International Journal of Sports Medicine* 12: 27–29.

Sanders, M.E. 1993. Selected physiological training adaptations during a water fitness program called Wave Aerobics. Thesis, University of Nevada, Reno, Microform Publications, University of Oregon, Eugene.

Sanders, M. 1999. *WaterFit instructor training and Speedo's aquatic fitness system* (2nd ed.). Reno, NV: WaterFit International/Wave Aerobics®.

Sanders, M., and C. Maloney-Hills. 1998. Aquatic exercise for better living on land. *ACSM's Health Fitness Journal* 2(3): 16–23.

Sanders, M.E., and C. Maloney-Hills. 1999. *The Golden Waves Program, Functional Water Training For Health: Aging Adults Leadership Course Manual.* Reno, NV: WaterFit/Wave Aerobics.

Sanders, M., N. Constantino, and N. Rippee. 1997. A comparison of results of functional water training on field and laboratory measures in older women. *Medicine and Science in Sports and Exercise* 29(5): Supplement to MSSE, p. S110, Abstract, 630.

Sanders, M., and N. Rippee. 1994. Speedo aquatic fitness system, instructor training manual, London: Speedo International Ltd.

Sanders, M., and N. Rippee. 1994. Speedo's Aquatic Fitness Instructor Course, 3 videos and manual.

Sanders, M., and N. Rippee. 1993. Selected physiological training adaptations during a water fitness program called wave aerobics. Thesis, University of Nevada, Reno.

Schoedinger, P. 1992. Aquatic Therapy Seminar, presented in Reno, Nevada, 1996.

Skinner, J.S. 1993. Exercise Testing and Exercise Prescription for Special Cases. 2nd ed. Philadelphia/London: Lea & Febiger.

Spirduso, W. 1995. Physical dimensions of aging. Champaign, IL: Human Kinetics.

Study, M., ed. 1991. *Personal trainer manual, the resource for fitness instructors.* San Diego, CA: American Council on Exercise.

Svendenhag, J., and J. Seger. 1992. Running on land and in water: Comparative exercise physiology. *Medicine and Science in Sports and Exercise* 24: 1155–1160.

Vickery, S.R., K.J. Cureton, and J.L. Langstaff. 1983. Heart rate and energy expenditure during aqua dynamics. *Physician and Sports Medicine* 11: 67–72.

Wilmore, J.H. 1988. Design issues and alternatives in assessing physical fitness among apparently healthy adults in a health examination survey of the general population. In *Assessing Physical Fitness and Activity in General Populations Studies,* ed. T.F. Drury. Washington, DC: U.S. Public Health Service, National Center for Health Statistics, pp. 107–140.

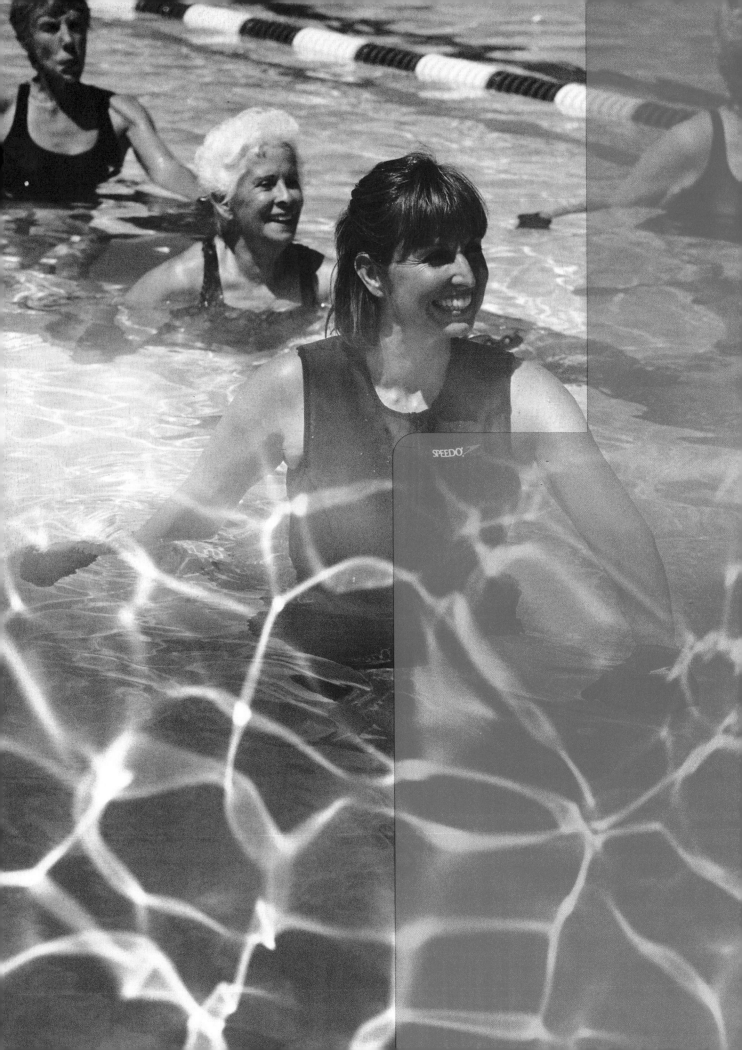

Part IV

Water Fitness Class Design

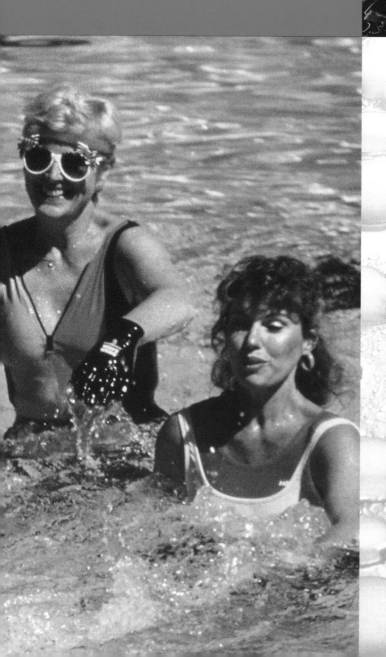

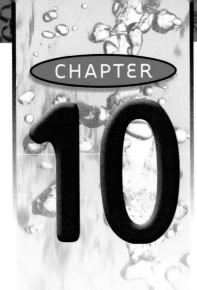

Designing a Workout:
A "Blueprint" for Success!

MARY CURRY

Objectives:

- To discuss four important components in water fitness programs

- To examine workout essentials and training options using a "blueprint" to design effective classes in shallow, transitional, and deep water

- To explore how to use music effectively during class

very day in life is different! Every water fitness class is guaranteed to be different, challenging, and as much fun as life, if we know what to do! Developing a successful class or workout is not done once and then considered complete. We have to respond to participants' needs by stepping back and evaluating the situation, then adjusting as necessary.

In this chapter, we will examine the workout components and training options and learn how to blend them together for a customized workout in one of three water depths. We also will discuss how best to use music to make water fitness more effective and fun.

Components of a Program

Let's begin by examining two components of any water fitness program: the environment and the equipment.

The Environment

Everyone's water environment is different. The pool's size and working space, water depth, deck floor, water and air temperature, deck space, entries and exits, as well as the availability and use of support facilities, are some of the many variables. Each one of these variables can make a difference when designing your class. We need to know how to work safely and effectively within whatever situation you have at your facility. Let's examine some of these variables and see what they mean to you and your water fitness program.

The Pool Tank

Pool area is the product of the length times the width of the tank. Pool space is the area around the participant in the appropriate working depth. We suggest you have a minimum of six to eight feet of pool space per person in all pool depths. This allows for traveling moves, which need space for the water to act against the body, thus increasing work intensity.

Working space is the total amount of pool space in any one depth. Calculate your class capacity based on providing at least the minimum pool space for each participant, given the surface area of one pool depth

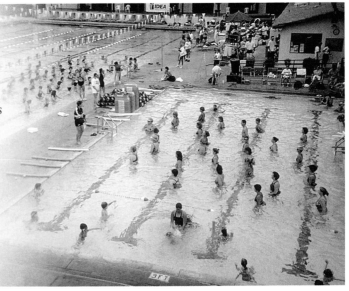

(for example, length × width in shallow water space). Find out if you will be sharing the pool with other programs that might limit your working space, and look for obstacles or depth changes that reduce traveling space.

Depths

In water fitness, water depths are defined as follows:

- **Shallow** is where the water level is between the navel and nipple.
- **Transitional** is where the water level is between the nipple and the shoulder depth. Participants can still touch the pool bottom.
- **Deep** is where the water level is above the nipple. Participants cannot touch the pool bottom.

You need to understand the different effects each depth has on the body so you can modify exercises or movements accordingly. Make sure that your exercise design is depth specific.

Deck and Pool Floor

You should recommend that participants wear water shoes to and from the locker room and in the pool to prevent slipping. Be sure to check for obstacles that might keep participants from seeing you clearly, such as diving boards, slides, or a lift for people with disabilities.

The Water

If the pool water feels cool, have participants jog or move continuously after entering the pool to maintain thermoregulation. Encourage participants to stay warm by layering extra clothing and increase their work intensity.

Make sure that your pool water is kept clear. You can't mirror your participants and you can't give them feedback if you can't see their movements underwater. You also can't see if someone is in trouble underwater.

Surrounding Area

Two characteristics of the pool area that may affect your water fitness classes are available deck space and placement and type of pool entries and exits.

Deck Space

Deck space is the total square feet of clear, unobstructed deck available for participants to enter and exit the pool and locker rooms and for you to demonstrate exercises. To make that space most usable, think about traffic flow and how it is affected by obstacles

such as the locker room door or equipment storage. Clear the space of lane lines, water bottles, equipment, and towels. Make sure you have enough space to teach safely on the deck and are far enough away from the water that the floor is not slippery.

Entries and Exits

The entries and exits define the areas where participants get into and out of the pool. Graded stairs into the pool with handrails are the most convenient and safe. However, many pools have vertical pool ladders, which may be difficult for participants with physical limitations to use. If your pool has vertical ladders, you may want to include the skill of using a vertical ladder unassisted as a prerequisite for participation. A better solution is to outfit your pool with a portable

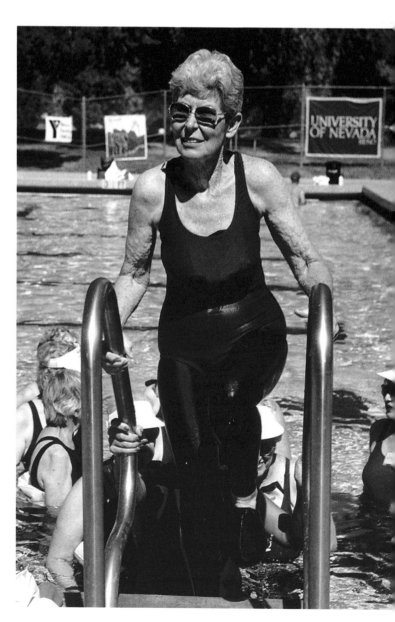

staircase. Lifts are effective if only a small number of participants require this type of assistance, but can be difficult for use with large groups and takes time.

When using vertical ladders, place spotters in the pool and on the deck to assist participants with entries and exits. If participants wear webbed gloves during class, have them put the gloves on *after* they enter the pool to ensure they have a safe grip on the ladder during entry.

The Equipment

Water fitness equipment has taken a giant leap forward. We have endurance fabric for our swimming suits and thermal vests and shoes specifically designed for our sport. Innovative and technical equipment has been developed to enhance and improve our water fitness programs. Let's evaluate equipment use by asking What, Why, When, and How.

What Are the Types of Equipment?

Equipment can be divided into four categories:

1. Buoyancy, such as buoyancy belts, buoyancy ankle cuffs, kickboards, and handheld buoyancy devices

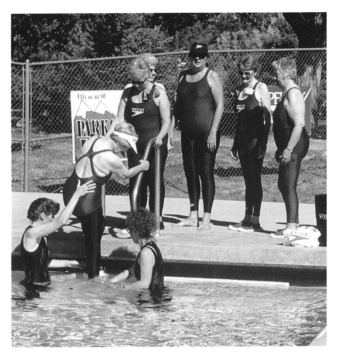

3. Integrated land/water, such as resistance bands or steps

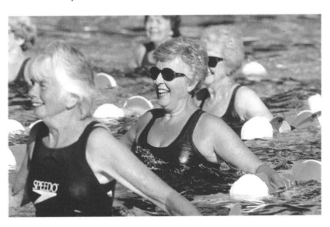

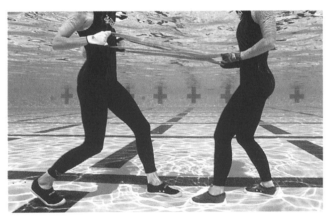

2. Surface area, such as webbed gloves, power buoys, kickboards, paddles, and leg fins

4. Gravity, such as a step

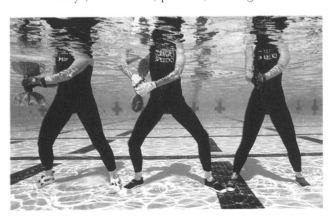

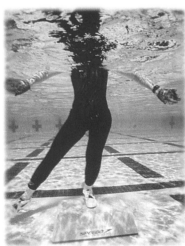

Why Use Equipment?

Adding equipment allows you to help your participants and your program advance.

- It can help optimize the water's resistance and buoyancy.
- It provides a broader range of intensity levels to participants.
- It can help older adults train functionally in the water to improve or maintain activities of daily living (ADL) on the land.
- It adds variety.

When Should Equipment Be Used?

Equipment gives us flexibility to respond to the characteristics of our water environment and the needs of our participants. For example, if a pool with deep water had no buoyancy equipment, you would not be able to utilize the full potential of the facility. Also, with the help of added equipment, a class of participants with mixed skill and fitness levels may all work on the same training objective at the same time.

How Should Equipment Be Used?

You will need education on equipment use to properly integrate it into your program. Manufacturers offer instructional videos and literature. Also seek out information on equipment use from the professionals at workshops and trainings.

Water exercise equipment may be more expensive than "pool toys" that are fun for children, but it should be evaluated differently. Such equipment can provide safety, variety, and increased challenges for our diverse population. Evaluate equipment for how it meets your needs and how it can improve your program.

For more on equipment, see chapter 12.

The Class Blueprint

A class blueprint should include these workout essentials: pre-class instruction (the teaching skills and safety), a warm-up, a workout, and a warm-down. The workout should offer a variety of training options, from targeting cardiorespiratory or muscular conditioning objectives to trying to improve ADL so people can function better in daily life. Creating a class means designing effective exercises that help participants meet specific objectives and individualizing training to make the sessions more effective. The goal is to deliver a class that reflects the needs of the participants and optimally uses the pool, blending all the components into the best experience for participants. Figure 10.1 provides some evaluation criteria questions you can use to develop safe and effective classes. Now let's examine each of the components of the blueprint.

Pre-Class Instruction (All Depths)

The first few minutes with your participants can be the best opportunity to have them "hear" what you have to say. Keep the music off and make your announcements clear and concise. Observe your class and use what you learn to teach responsively. Remember to tell them how to stay warm until the warm-up begins!

Always start off the class by saying your name. If you have any new participants, be sure to ask them quickly if they have any health issues you need to know about, such as pregnancy, or orthopedic concerns. State the type of class it is, such as "shallow and deep water class" or "interval training." Review the types of equipment used, including gloves or shoes, and remind the class of the proper depth for participation and any modifications that might be necessary because of special considerations.

For deep water classes, be sure to check that participants are comfortable in deep water. Make sure they can perform basic, personal safety skills such as treading water without a buoyancy device and changing body position from horizontal to vertical. (Refer to the video *Specificity of Training and Deep Water Program*.)

In transitional depth, check that participants are comfortable with the water depth and that they know how to stabilize using a **sculling** and scooping action with their hands to help maintain good posture. Show them how to scull, using a visual example such as "smoothing sand on a beach."

At all depths, help participants adjust to buoyancy and find proper body alignment. At shallow and **transitional depths**, review, demonstrate, and have them practice recovery to a stand. In deep and transitional depths, if participants are wearing buoyancy belts, practice and check the skills in the **A.B.y.S.S.S.** formula (see chapter 8 for the **A.B.y.S.S.S.** formula).

Before you begin, review and demonstrate basic moves, working positions, and visual cues used often in class. Have a "Water Fitness Basics" handout ready to distribute at the end of class for review and reinforcement in case participants missed something.

Warm-Up (All Depths)

In this section, we describe two warm-ups that can be used at any depth, one stationary and one traveling. Ideas for accompanying music appear at the end.

Stationary Buoyancy Warm-Up (3–5 Minutes)

The purpose of the warm-up is to elevate the heart rate slightly, warm up the muscles and joints, and help participants get comfortable in the water.

Objective Checklist

- Find the proper water depth. Direct your participants to a good working depth for the workout. Shallow water depth is between the navel and nipple; transitional depth is between the nipple and shoulder. You also can direct participants to move gradually to the deep water.

- Start warm and stay warm. Teach participants to move to stay warm, especially their legs.

- Help participants adjust their balance and practice good alignment. Cue them and remind them!

- Teach participants sculling. This helps them with balance and stabilization and also assists them when moving.

- Have participants rehearse. This is an opportunity to practice, at low intensity, the movements being used in the workout. Review the basic moves and any new skills. Make every moment a teaching moment!

- Keep the warm-up active. Warm up the major muscle groups.

- Slowly increase the range of motion and adjust to the water temperature. Participants should be getting warm.

- Remind participants to breathe normally. Cue them to breathe and not hold their breath.

- Check participants' comfort level and the music volume level.

Suggested Movements

Try the following stationary moves, starting at a lower intensity and gradually increasing it by enlarging the area covered and the force used:

- Scull and jog around the body. Slowly enlarge the area covered.

- Jog with breaststroke arms slicing through the water while wearing gloves (stretches the pectorals).

- Push and pull with a kick around the body. Slowly enlarge the area covered.

- Wearing gloves, push down, first slicing through the water, then with hands flat, and rock (for shallow water).

- Use "stir it up" arms (move arms as if stirring a pot of soup) and jog.

- Do easy scissors and jax.

Figure 10.1 Evaluation Criteria Questions

Using evaluation criteria questions can help you build the foundation for safe and effective class or exercise design. As an instructor, you should constantly evaluate exercises and programs to check that your objectives are being met effectively and that the exercises serve their chosen purposes. Here are some questions you can use to systematically evaluate a program or an exercise:

- What are the objectives for this class, exercise, or participant? Can I clearly identify the purpose of the exercises? For example, if an instructor says the objective of an exercise is cardiorespiratory training but the exercise has participants standing and pumping their arms overhead, out of the water, is the objective being met?

- What property of water creates the work? Examine the environment. Do the exercises fully engage resistance by using inertia currents and the water's buoyancy? How?

- Is the exercise or program safe and effective? While people often assume that injuries can't occur in the water, swimmers have the highest incidence of shoulder injury among competitive athletes. The buoyant water environment can help reduce the potential for joint and muscle injury, but using proper body mechanics during exercise is critical to injury prevention. Check each exercise for proper body alignment and body mechanics to ensure that the resistance of water is used to develop healthy gains, not reduce function.

- Assess the effectiveness of an exercise by asking participants "Where do you feel it?" as they perform an exercise. If the objective of an exercise is to develop the muscular endurance of the triceps and participants say they feel the workout in their chests when they perform the exercise, then the exercise is not reaching the objective effectively. Also, be sure you teach participants progressions for exercise intensity, so each participant can achieve a sufficient overload to gain a training effect.

- Are participants staying warm during class? This question relates to both safety and program adherence. If the body is cold, the muscles don't contract efficiently and the body doesn't perform optimally. Also, if your participants are doing "shiver aerobics," will they want to come back? Since you can't always turn up the heat in the pool, show participants how to control their own comfort by teaching them fundamental skills for maintaining their own thermoregulation.

- Can this be done better or differently? Asking this question makes you a more responsive exercise designer. By thinking beyond what you already thought was a good idea, you can design even better new exercises. Also, reconsidering exercises will help you identify poorly designed or less-effective exercises and replace them with better choices based on the most recent research-based information.

To actively warm up the major muscles, try these movements:

- For the quadriceps, jog with the heels coming up behind (knee flexion).
- For the hamstrings, first kick in front, then move to a comfortable working position while pressing the arms back.
- For the abductors and adductors, do a wide jog and easy jumping jacks.
- For the pectorals, move the arms in a breast-stroke motion, thumbs up.
- For the upper back, move the arms in a reverse breaststroke motion.
- For the ankles and shins, do ankle pops (small jumps in neutral) or rotate the ankles around in circles.

Water Temperature Alert!

Here are some suggestions for modifying the movement design for various water temperatures:

- In warm water (85 degrees F and up), use stationary range-of-motion movements, including self-massage exercises.
- In medium water (83–84 degrees F), use a stationary buoyancy warm-up, jogging, kicking, rocking, and sculling.
- In cool water (82 degrees F and below), use light and easy traveling, jogging, and active stretching . . . get them moving!

Cardiorespiratory and Traveling Warm-Up (2–3 Minutes)

The cardiorespiratory warm-up specifically addresses the changes and safety concerns occurring with traveling moves. Buoyancy, balance, and stabilization of postural alignment are affected to a greater degree by the increased resistance of travel, so participants need to practice traveling at a lower intensity before they begin the workout phase. The objective is to increase intensity progressively to increase deep muscle temperature and elevate heart rate into the lower end of the training zone.

Objective Checklist

- Teach participants assisting and resisting sculling for traveling moves so they feel the water.
- Observe how your participants move through the water and respond by adjusting water depth or participants' positions in class.

- Focus on leg moves and on increasing speed to raise the heart rate and core temperature gradually.
- Help participants adjust to buoyancy during travel, and regulate water depth as necessary.
- Check that participants can balance and use proper movement coordination.

Suggested Movements

Try the following stationary moves, starting with low-intensity movements, then moving to more intense ones.

Low Intensity

SHALLOW WATER

- Jog with assisting arm movement (sculling, breaststroke, scooping), traveling forward, backward, and sideways.
- Side step or do an easy grapevine with assisting arm movements.

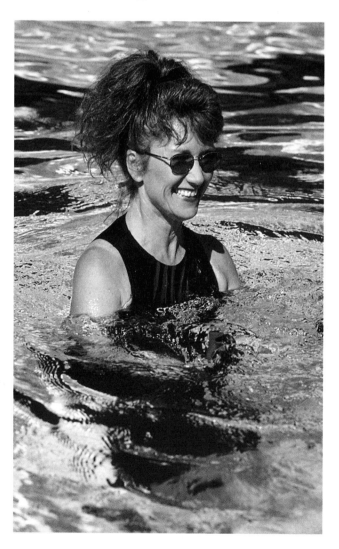

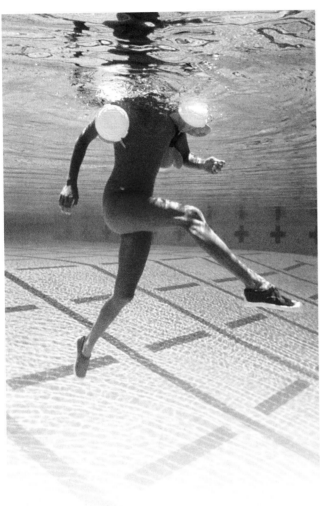

Transitional Water

- Jog easily, adding vertical propulsion by pushing off the bottom or rebounding.

Deep Water

- Bicycle (move legs in an "around and down" pattern) with assisting arm movements, traveling forward, backward, and sideways.

Higher Intensity

Shallow Water

- Jog with arm movement that assists traveling, then resists traveling. Work around the body.
- Do an easy kick, traveling backward, forward, and sideways.
- Rock, traveling forward, backward, and side to side.

Transitional Water

- Do a tuck jump.

Deep water

- Bicycle with arms behind the back (no assistance).
- Kick easily, traveling backward and sideways.

Turbulence Alert!

When participants travel through the water, the inertia their currents create can literally knock them off their feet! The traveling in this set is done at a slower pace. Allow enough time for directional change so participants feel in control of their movements. Cue and coach your participants to adjust their water depth and to stabilize their body alignment.

A Music Note

The warm-up music should be something that makes you want to move and be uplifting and stimulating. Instrumentals may be a good choice so you can be heard when teaching some of the basic skills. If the water is warm, slower tempo music (perhaps classical) is appropriate for a nice beginning. Using a song for each set objective, such as for the buoyancy warm-up, can help you piece together your workout.

Workout (20–40 Minutes)

This section describes a complete workout usable at all depths. A wide range of training objectives can be targeted in any workout. The specific ones addressed here include cardiorespiratory training, muscular endurance and strength training, flexibility training, functional conditioning, and general activity and fun.

Cardiorespiratory Training

Here are sample objectives, suggested movements, and music recommendations for cardiorespiratory training.

Objective Checklist

- Focus on using the large muscles of the legs, performing continuous, rhythmic movements.
- Change movements frequently. Due to the increased resistance caused by working in water rather than air, muscles will fatigue if movements aren't changed frequently enough to prevent local fatigue.
- Remember that participants may have to develop muscular endurance first to be able to achieve optimal cardiorespiratory training.
- Hands (perhaps with gloves) must be used to balance and to assist travel.

- Use the talk test and perceived exertion tests to monitor intensity during exercise in depths above the xiphoid process. A heart rate check may be used when the water is below this depth (where lungs are not submerged).
- Use basic moves appropriate to the working water depth, and increase intensity gradually by enlarging the range of motion and manipulating speed, surface area, working positions, and travel.
- Work "around" the body or joints to change muscle groups.

Movement Suggestions

Basic move

- Scissors/jax in the diagonal plane.

Low intensity

- Enlarge the range of motion or surface area.
- Move "around" the body or joints.
- Increase speed.
- Change working positions.

Higher intensity

- Travel.
- Use an interval format. (Create intervals by changing working position and speed.)

A Music Note ♫

Music that has a motivating, steady, strong beat helps participants push beyond feeling comfortable to overload for training benefits. Longer songs and medleys work well for continuous training sets. Music that has natural volume or tempo changes is great for interval work!

Muscular Endurance and Strength Training

This section includes sample objectives, suggested movements, and music recommendations for muscular endurance and strength training.

Muscular Endurance Objective Checklist

- Isolate target muscles and perform repetitions at the target level to near fatigue. Resistance levels are determined by working against buoyancy, speed, surface area, leverage, the inertia of currents, and the effects of action/reaction.
- Have participants determine their level of intensity, and work there.

- Cue participants to use stabilizers (trunk and hands) to balance the body in water.
- Cue participants to use synergistic (coordinated arm or leg) movements to keep the body warm and assist with balance.
- Sequence exercises to alternate working joints.
- Cue participants to actively rest with targeted range-of-motion exercises.
- Monitor exercise intensity by having participants use perceived exertion and listen to their bodies.

Muscular Endurance Movement Suggestions

Change the exercise intensity for moving muscles by increasing or decreasing surface area, force, or speed; increasing buoyancy for downward action; increasing gravity and impact by decreasing buoyancy; or using water-filled weighted equipment for overhead work.

Change the exercise intensity for stabilizing muscles by changing working positions and depth, working single levers, or increasing the intensity of moves.

Muscle group—Triceps

LOW INTENSITY

- Submerge a joint (such as the elbow) and stabilize your stance with a lunge or jog.
- Practice a pattern of movement such as elbow extension (palms supine or prone).
- Wear gloves and slice the hands through the water. Add power on the extension and recover on the flexion.
- Add speed, but always slow down before changing to the next intensity.
- Change the surface area of the gloves (fist, open hand).

HIGHER INTENSITY

- Add speed, but always slow down before changing to the next intensity.
- Travel backward in shallow water. Power down and lift the body upward in transitional and deep water.

Total 8–15 repetitions for each exercise.

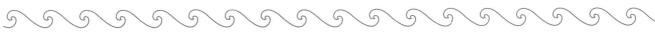

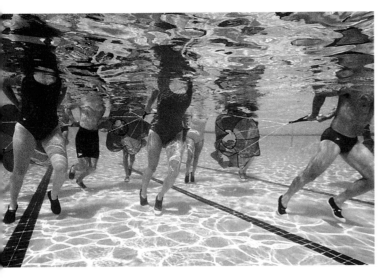

Muscular Strength Objective

It's difficult to achieve a sufficient overload for strength training without using equipment. Try using fitness paddles and chutes in shallow water. Strength training objectives may be met if surface area and buoyancy are increased and participants work at a sufficient speed.

Muscular Strength Movement Suggestions

Muscle group—Triceps

EQUIPMENT
- Power buoys/fitness paddles

LOW INTENSITY
- Submerge a joint (such as the elbow) and stabilize your stance.
- Practice a pattern of movement such as elbow extension.
- Hold buoys and slice the hands through the water. Add power on the extension, jog, and recover on the flexion.
- Add speed, but always slow down before changing to the next intensity.
- Change the surface area of the buoys.

HIGHER INTENSITY
- Add speed, but always slow down before changing to the next intensity.
- Travel backward in shallow water. Push the body upward in transitional and deep water.

Total 8–15 repetitions.

A Music Note

During muscular conditioning sets, use background music (instrumental, classical) rather than music with a strong tempo (beat) so participants can work at their own pace. Have participants work shorter sets to allow for rest.

Flexibility Training

In this part we look at sample objectives, suggested movements, and music recommendations for flexibility training.

Objective Checklist

- Cue participants to use the target muscle groups.
- Change the exercise intensity by adjusting buoyancy and resistance (gravity, manual resistance).
- Keep participants warm by alternating flexibility exercises with low-intensity cardiorespiratory sets. Perform flexibility exercises for both the upper and lower body.

Movement Suggestions

Muscles—Hamstrings, abductors/adductors

SHALLOW WATER—LOW INTENSITY
- Walk or otherwise travel forward, sideways, diagonally, or backward.
- Enlarge the walk by extending the legs or the stride length.

SHALLOW WATER—HIGHER INTENSITY
- Leap or otherwise travel forward or sideways.

DEEP WATER—LOW INTENSITY
- Do a suspended seated hamstring stretch, straddle the legs, and point the toes up and down.

DEEP WATER—HIGHER INTENSITY
- With a partner, do a suspended hamstring stretch and straddle the legs with a tilt side to side.

TRANSITIONAL WATER—LOW INTENSITY
- Hop lightly on one leg, do a hamstring stretch, stand tall, rotate a leg to the side, and point the toes forward.

TRANSITIONAL WATER—HIGHER INTENSITY
- Hop, stretch, and travel backward. Leap sideways and land tall.

A Music Note

Let the pool temperature determine the tempo of your music. If it's warm, use a slow and relaxing sound; if it's cool, play something that will keep participants moving all the way to the locker room.

Functional ADL

Water-specific exercises designed to target improvement of functional ADL on the land are to be performed in shallow water. This allows us to use gravity as part of the work in order to carry over the effects of these water exercises to specific tasks on land. Here are sample objectives, suggested movements, and music recommendations for functional ADL conditioning.

Objective Checklist

- Choose exercises that closely simulate identified functional activities. Examples might be gait and balance training, reaching and dynamic postural work, walking up or down stairs, or carrying groceries or children.
- Determine which muscles are to be stretched and which are to be strengthened, design the pattern, and practice the skills. Use cues for both the stabilizing muscles and the moving muscles. Work through the appropriate intensity progression for each skill.

Movement Suggestions

See part IV for functional ADL training exercises.

A Music Note

The older population who wants to achieve these objectives may prefer the music of their generation. Use the music to make the participants want to move and work through the water's resistance. Music with lyrics can make it hard to give verbal cues, so use instrumental music when you are teaching new exercises or skills.

Health, Activity, and Fun

Finally, some of your activities should just promote physical activity and fun. Here are some sample objectives, suggested movements, and music recommendations for these activities.

Objective Checklist

- Movements are done safely and effectively, but involve lots of laughter and fun.
- Make sure everyone has a smile.
- Be playful!

Movement Suggestions

- Do some choreography primarily for Fun, for example, customizing the Macarena or the Achy Breaky for the water! (see the Instructor videos).
- Twist to the song "Twist and Shout." Keep shoulders, hips, knees, and feet in alignment, moving together. Perform it from a stationary position, or travel sideways or backward.

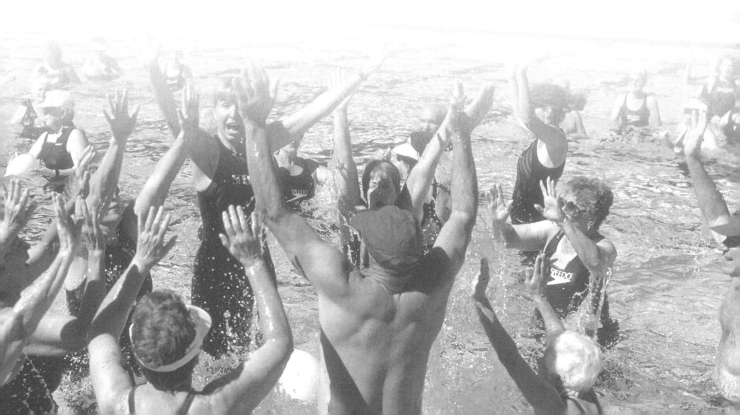

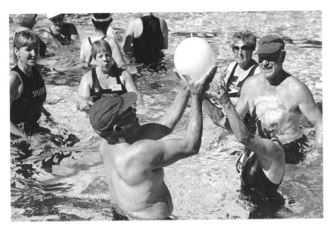

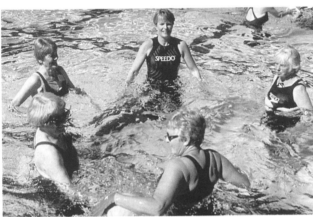

- Try different class formation patterns, such as circles, line dancing, the "Hokie Pokie," square dancing, lines that cross, or zigzagging down the pool and then running a straight line through (the Snake).
- Use movements from games, such as tag, jump rope, sports moves, hopscotch, or freeze frame.

A Music Note

Fun movements are often created from the lyrics of the music that is selected.

Warm-Down and Stretch (2–5 Minutes) (All depths)

The warm-down is essential at the end of a workout to promote a gradual reduction in cardiorespiratory function while balancing body warmth. Postexercise stretching is done to improve the range of motion of specific joints. As participants work out less intensely, the cooling effect of water increases, causing them to rapidly lose body heat. If the water is cold, keep participants from becoming chilled by immediately transitioning to active stretching or by having them exit the pool. Encourage them to stretch at home or after a shower in the workout room.

Here are some suggested warm-down movements and ideas for accompanying music.

Movement Suggestions

DECREASING INTENSITY

- Do an easy kick or jog.
- Perform an enlarged walk forward, backward, and sideways.

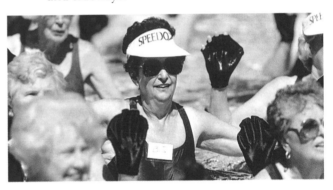

- Try walking and then freezing in order to work on balance and range of motion for the ankles.
- Do a stationary jog with an upper-body range-of-motion active stretch.
- Try an upper-body scull (to stay warm) with lower-body stretches.
- Jog (to stay warm) while performing range-of-motion actions with the wrist, fingers, and neck.

ACTIVE EXIT

- Do a light, loose jog.
- Try leaping or falling sideways or backward gently, allowing buoyancy to support the movement.

A Music Note

Make the warm-down music short, fun, and "humable," so participants end the workout on a happy note. After class, play music to make the walk to the shower room and beyond enjoyable (play it soft enough that it doesn't compete with talking). Make their day!

Putting It All Together

To see how you might combine the parts of the workout and various types of training, look at the sample classes in figures 10.2, 10.3, and 10.4. A class is described for each of the three water depths: shallow, transitional, and deep. The acronym **S.W.E.A.T.** is used in these figures to indicate the intensity variables involved: Surface area and Speed, Working positions, Enlarge movements, work Around the body, and Travel.

Figure 10.2 *Sample shallow water class*

Shallow Water Workout

This sample demonstrates how to blend the workout essentials with a variety of training options to create a workout with purpose and clear objectives. Your job is to encourage your participants with positive, responsive, and corrective coaching. Put some of your favorite music together and use this sample for your next class format, or start mixing and matching your own!

Set and objective	Basic move or muscle	Intensity variables (Movement variations)
Set 1: Buoyancy warm-up	Stationary jog/kick	S.W. (neutral) E.A.
Set 2: Cardiorespiratory (CR)	Travel/walk/jog Assist/resist scull	E.A.T.
Set 3: Cardiorespiratory	Jog/kick	S.W.E.A.T.
Set 4: Muscular endurance (ME)	Biceps	S.W. (submerge joint while in neutral working position) E.T.

Set 5: CR	Walking/jumping	S.W.E.A.T.
Set 6: ME/ Functional (balance) Adduction/abduction	Hip adduction/ abduction Walk/jog/freeze frame	S.E.A.T.
Set 7: CR	Scissors	S.W.E.A.T.
Set 8: ME	Triceps/pectorals	S.W.E.A.T. (submerge joint while in neutral working position)
Set 9: CR (Traveling/upper-body surface area changes)	Jogging	S.E.A.T.
Set 10: ME	Rhomboids, trapezoids Biceps (small range)	S.W.E.T. (submerge joint while in neutral working position)

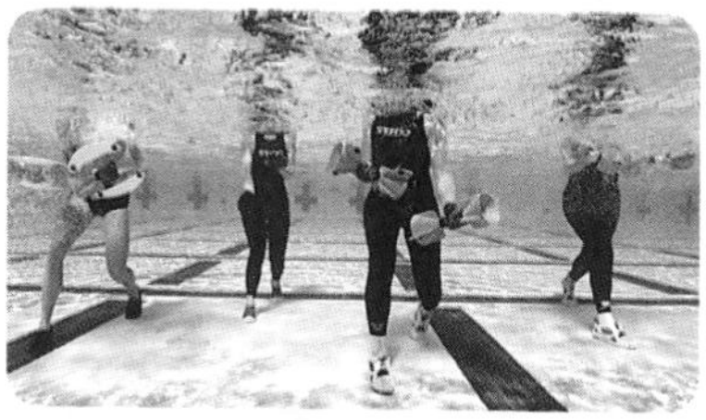

Transition into a whirlpool formation. Use a 30-second musical cue.

Set 11: Functional (balance) and Fun	Jog/whirlpool	S.W.E.T.
Set 12: Range of motion/ Warm-down	Jog/walk	S.E.A.T.
Set 13: Warm-down/stretch	Active stretching	S.W.E.A.T.
Set 14: Exit pool warm	Anything fun!	----

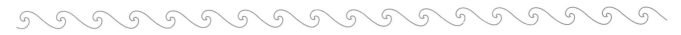

Figure 10.3 *Sample transitional water class*

Transitional Water Workout

Equipment needed: Webbed gloves, buoyancy belts, aquatic steps, resistance bands

Set and objective	Basic move or muscle	Intensity variables (Movement variations)
Set 1: Buoyancy warm-up (shallow water)	Jog, kick, rock	S.W.E.A.
Set 2: Cardiorespiratory warm-up (shallow water)	Jog, kick, scissors	S.W.E.A.T.
Transition to the transitional water level	Jog/bicycle	S.E.T.
Set 3: Cardiorespiratory (CR)	Modified scissors Jog (Use hover jog—push off into suspension, then jog as long as possible before falling back to the bottom.)	S.W.E.A.T.
Set 4: Muscular endurance (ME)	Upper back/pectorals (stand tall, jump back to suspended seated position)	S.E.T.
Set 5: ME	Triceps (suspended modified scissors jump)	S.E.T.
Set 6: CR/Interval (use aquatic step)	Scissors	S.W.E.A.
Transition to shallow water.	Bicycle/jog	
Set 7: Range of motion/stretch	Jump/leap/falling backward, sideways hamstring/quadriceps stretch	E.A.T.

Figure 10.4 *Sample deep water class*

Deep Water Workout

Deep water workout formats are based on the fitness goals of the program,
the equipment used for bouyancy support, and the pool depth.

Pre-class: Equipment orientation and safety skills review (2 minutes)

Set 1: Skills warm-up: **A.B.Y.S.S.S.**
(1 minute)

A. = Adjust to buoyancy (change the belt or adjust buoyancy after "hanging").

B. = Breathe against the pressure. Practice at least six full breaths.

Y. = Yield to the new freedom to extend the legs downward and use the full range of motion.

S. = Scull for balance and to assist travel.

S. = Synergize—work the same arm and leg, then use opposing arm and leg (scissors move). Feel the balance difference.

S. = Safety skills practice (recover to vertical from supine and prone falls).

Set and objective	Basic move or muscle	Intensity variables (Movement variations)
Set 2: Buoyancy warm-up	Stationary jog/kick	S.W.E.A.
Set 3: Cardiovascular warm-up	Bicycle	S.W.E.A.T.
Set 4: Muscular endurance/ trunk stabilizers	Tilting (enhance by using resistance bands for fun and ROM feedback)	S.E.A.
Set 5: Cardiovascular (CR)	Jog	S.W.E.A.T.

Work or rest interval: Perform a CR high intensity or active rest interval for one minute. For high intensity, do scissors with the legs only and slice hands through the water while wearing mitts. The legs must drive the intensity. For active rest, do easy jogs, supine or vertical. For an interval workout, insert an interval between each CR set.

Set 6: CR/intervals	Scissors, bicycle	S.W.E.A.T.
Set 7: ME	Kick/quadriceps/hamstrings	S.W.E.A.T.
Set 8: ME	Adductors/abductors	S.W.E.T.
Set 9: ME	Pectorals/rhomboids/trapezoid	S.E.T.
Transition to shallow water	Bicycle to shallow/rock in shallow	S.E.T.
Set 10: Range of motion/stretch (remove flotation belts)	Quads/hamstrings/hip flexors, pectorals/rhomboids, adductors/ abductors, neck, triceps, deltoids	W. (neutral) E.T.

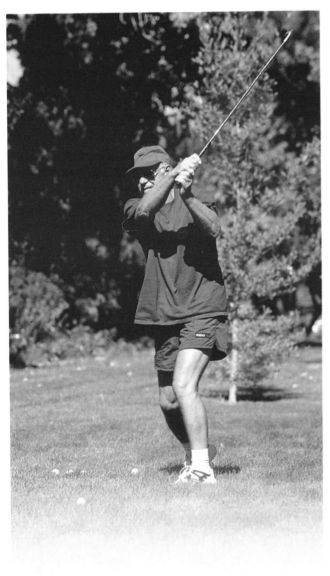

Music and Movements

Music seems to be a natural accompaniment to movement. Scientific findings also have shown that it can affect exercisers in various ways:

- Music, being nonverbal, can travel through the auditory cortex to the limbic system, the midbrain network that governs most of our emotional experiences as well as basic metabolic responses.

- Music may activate the flow of stored memory material across the corpus callosum, connecting the left and right sides of the brain, and helping the two work in harmony.

- Music stimulates production of endorphins, the natural opiates secreted by the hypothalamus that provide a feeling of involvement and dull the perception of pain and stress while working out.

Your choice of music should communicate the quality of the accompanying movements, be entertaining, and motivate participants to maintain the desired intensity. However, due to the high resistance and buoyancy of water, participants cannot always move to the beat as they do on land. Since water exaggerates individual differences such as body composition, skill, movement speed, and timing, we don't recommend counting off "steps" in choreography.

Before you use music with a strong beat, consider these questions:

- Does your beat vary? A class in which the music maintained 125 beats per minute throughout the entire workout would soon become boring. Offer a varied tempo for variety and to motivate different intensities of movement.

- Does the beat motivate the movement? Using a slow tempo when you want to get your group moving will never work. Choose a tempo that matches the type of movement you want to achieve.

- Does the beat compromise the movement? Individual differences in skill, body composition, and fitness level are just a few of the reasons why everyone moves through the water differently. If the external beat dictates the speed, not everyone will be able to keep up with that beat, and the size and quality of the movement is compromised.

To summarize, when you design your classes, begin with an inspection of the pool and get an idea of the possibilities for exercise design based on space, water depth, and equipment available. Keep in mind the objectives of the workout and the fitness level of your participants, then set the mood with some music that will enhance the experience and make it a success for you and your participants. Ask participants what they would like to target for training, and be sure to include some sets addressing their objectives. For example, if George wants to get better at playing golf, include some range-of-motion work for golf in your workout, and let George know this is for him!

Each pool and class and day will be different. Stay alert to respond to the needs of the group or the conditions in the environment, and make sure that participants are safe and successful! Be flexible.

Allow the internal beat to motivate the movement, not force everyone to move at the same time. This gives participants permission to feel the music and move with the "feeling," regulating their own intensity and pace. Attend to the qualities of music such as pulse, continuity, flow, expansion, and points of energy or relaxation. Choose music artistically in order to create a composition that involves participants in the sensuality of water and captures a spirit of adventure. When you design a travel set through water, choose music that is "going somewhere" to motivate pushing heavy water out of the way! Music that communicates feelings such as power, force, lightness, looseness, or buoyancy can help communicate movement quality and involve participants in their personal workout expressions.

Deciding Whether to Use Music

Evaluate your situation when you consider whether to use music in your water fitness class. Pool acoustics, the quality of the sound system, and the availability of money and time may all play a part in your decisions.

The acoustics in a pool environment are usually poor. The whirlpool, the waterslide, lap swimmers, and children's swimming lessons may create enough background sounds to turn the best music into noise. In this type of situation, playing music may not be an option.

The quality of the sound system also can make a difference in whether the music can be heard. Systems can range from a portable cassette player to a built-in system (the budget of the facility usually dictates the system that is used). Current compact stereo systems are portable enough to put on a movable cart, and many offer dual cassette players, a CD player, high-speed dubbing, and a microphone jack for a headset microphone. Make sure that the outlet for your sound system is grounded. The humid pool environment can be hard on electronic equipment, so your sound system should be stored in a humidity-free storage area.

Keep in mind that using music in your water fitness classes can be expensive and time consuming. While you can purchase premade music tapes offered through a variety of companies, selecting and purchasing the right music tape is no easy task. It takes time, a budget, and an ear sensitive to the kinds of music that can work.

Turning off the tape player and tuning into the "music" of the water also has its advantages in a water fitness class. Given the challenges of the pool environment, silence may be the only option for some facilities. Silent segments in your workout tape can be used to teach new skills, to create a "gear down" time in an interval set, or to just allow participants to tune into their bodies and hear the sounds of the water.

Choosing Which Music to Use

Ask yourself these evaluation questions to help you select music:

- Do you *like* it? Answering this question may require you to play the song a few times, but if you don't care for the song, it won't be one that will motivate you once the class has begun.

- Is it *appropriate* for the participants or for the movement objectives?

- How does it make you *feel*—energized, relaxed, powerful?

- What is the *style*—country, swing, jazz, mambo?

Be sure to take into account your participants' musical preferences and choose music that is motivational to them. If you have a multigenerational group, offering a variety of music styles and tempos can

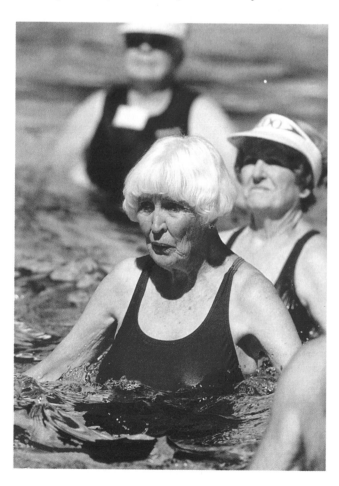

make it enjoyable for them to work out together. Also consider whether the music you want to use is vocal or instrumental. Each has its own pros and cons.

Vocal music selections can stimulate psychological and emotional responses in your class participants. A sing-along can help regulate intensity for a moderate-paced workout. Lyrics also can create the theme for a workout set. For example, "Take Me Out to the Ballgame" can help set the mood for a playful sport set. However, many older adults have trouble hearing, and lyrics may make it more difficult for them to hear your directions. You also must be sensitive to the content of the lyrics, eliminating those that might be offensive or intimidating to your participants.

Instrumental music offers a broad range of choices such as classical, Big Band, jazz, international rhythms, and even sound effects. These selections are good choices when you are teaching skills and want your voice to be the primary focus.

Music and Class Formatting

Music is an important tool for class formatting. Changing the tempo, style, and mood of the music can define the beginning of a new set.

Use one workout tape and let it play continuously, with no interruptions. Cue changes in mood or activity by using tapes that include fade-ins and fade-outs or by turning the volume up or down, but keep the music flowing. Changing the music each time the objective of the exercise changes alerts participants to the new objective. Create meaning by tying the music choices to the purpose of each component:

- Warm-up music should be uplifting and stimulating, something that makes participants want to move.
- Cardiovascular training may use music that is strong, steady, and smooth.
- Muscular conditioning music should promote a feeling of power and strength with a bigger sound.
- Transition music or sounds such as bubbling water can keep the class flowing and the participants warm and involved through equipment changes, water breaks, and teaching moments.
- Warm-down music should be upbeat to ensure participants are warm for the walk to the showers.

Your enthusiasm and teaching are the foundation to your workout, but the addition of music can make it become "magic."

Bibliography

Sanders, M., and N. Rippee. 1994. Speedo aquatic fitness system, instructor training manual. London, UK: Speedo International.

Sanders, M.E. 1991. Aqua music. *IDEA Today,* 9(4): 24–25.

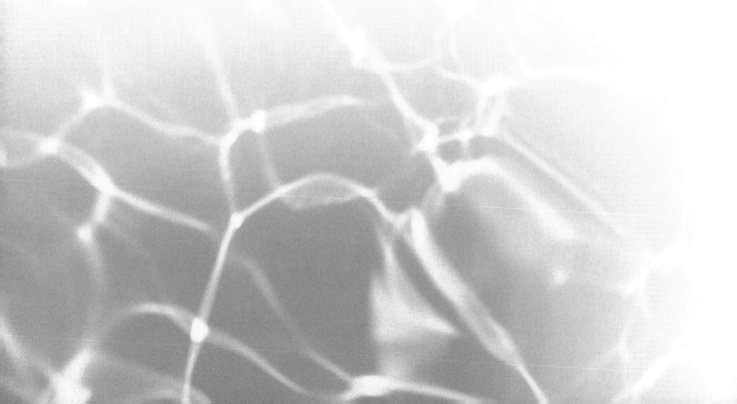

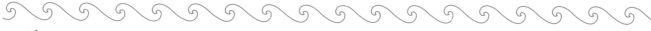

 Instructor Training Workout Videos

Introduction to the Waterfit Aquatic Fitness System, Shallow Water:
One shallow water workout.

Specificity of Training and Deep Water Program:
Two workouts, one in deep water and the other using all three depths of water.

The Aquatic Step Program:
One shallow water circuit type workout using the step (may also be performed without the step). You may substitute traveling for the step overload.

Tidal Waves:
One shallow water workout with fun choreography.

Golden Waves Program, Functional Water Training for Health:
One shallow water workout, targeting ADL.

Golden Waves, Video II:
Over 50 exercise progressions targeting functional activities to add to your shallow water program.

One With Nature™:
A complete mind/body workout based on learning from the beauty of the ocean creatures.

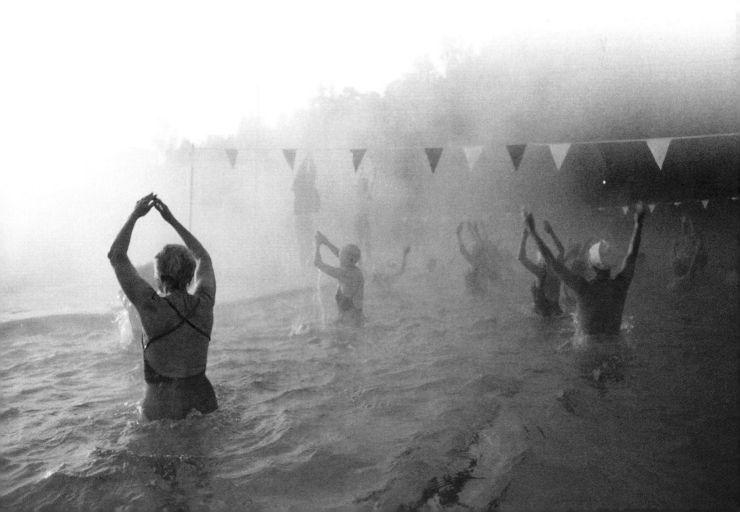

11

Teaching Responsively

MARY E. SANDERS AND DEBBIE MILES-DUTTON

Objectives:

- To choose a teaching method for water fitness that works
- To learn how to be a responsive teacher, including developing a verbal and visual cueing system and using equipment
- To provide a checklist for running a successful class
- To identify what instructors need to do to take care of themselves

B eing a responsive instructor means responding to the workout environment, the participants' needs, and your own needs. Since water is a much different exercise environment than land, you will have to think about how to adjust your teaching methods for water and choose ones that work best with your class and situation. You'll do best if you can teach participants the water fitness skills they need to regulate their own exercise intensity, so you can coach rather than instruct all the time. Verbal and visual cues are an important part of instruction, and you may need to use equipment to get the best workout possible. We've provided a checklist you can use in planning for your water fitness classes, and we also include some tips on taking care of yourself as well as your participants.

Finally, a note before we begin: You need to know the basic water safety skills in order to keep your participants safe during water fitness training. Review the materials from your YMCA Lifeguard or Aquatic Safety Assistant training as necessary.

Choosing a Teaching Method

It is much different to teach exercise in water than it is on land. You need to consider those differences and how best to deal with them when you teach. This section explains some of the differences, then gives you four possible methods.

Land vs. Water Teaching Techniques

On land we can participate fully in the workout, using mirrors and a microphone to assist with demonstration and explanation of the moves. When we participate and teach from the water, only the portion of our bodies not submerged is visible. Participants have more difficulty seeing movements, and pool acoustics may make audio cues impossible to hear. You or your assistant need to demonstrate some movements on the deck without participating directly in the workout. In this case, clear instruction, safety, and motivation outweigh the importance of a personal workout.

Deck teaching is more physically difficult than teaching in the water. Take special care when teaching from the deck to demonstrate safely while still cueing water-specific moves at appropriate water speeds. If the moves look like those in a land aerobics class, they probably are not water specific. You may not be able to mimic all water movements on deck, so use other methods such as in-water demonstration to help participants learn the skills.

Equipment such as a teaching stool (a waist-high bar stool or chair for standing support), well-cushioned nonslip shoes, and a water-resistant microphone can help make teaching water moves from the deck safer. Microphones are now available that go into the water with you! You also can provide corrective feedback from your view from the deck; however, the best view is achieved by wearing a mask or goggles underwater. That's the place from which you can truly evaluate participants' alignment and technique; you can't teach from there, but visit periodically.

If you do teach in the water, you'll rely primarily on verbal cues to describe the move and some demonstration, along with guided, supervised practice of the skills. To make learning as easy as possible, turn off the music and focus on your verbal instructions.

Ideally, you can combine both deck and water teaching to protect yourself and to participate in the fun of working out. Also, the more the participants know, the easier it is to teach from the water. Learn water-specific teaching skills to add to your current teaching skills on land.

Since exercising in water is so different from exercising on land, you should view exercises as skills that need to be mastered so participants can be successful in achieving results. People must learn how to swim before they can swim for fitness; the same is true for water fitness workouts. Teaching participants how to move efficiently for work and rest helps them achieve training results within their own levels. In order to communicate these skills, you need to choose a method or combination of methods that ensures safe and effective results.

Weighing the Options

Let's examine four methods and find those that make your classes safe, effective, and fun:

- Teaching from the deck
- Teaching in the water
- Teaching from the deck and in the water
- Demonstrating in the water or with a video

Watch Session 5 in *The Specificity of Training and Deep Water Program*, Session 4 in *The Aquatic Step Program*, and the Teaching Session in *The Golden Waves II* videos to observe demonstrations of these teaching methods.

Method 1: Teaching From the Deck

Teaching from the deck has the following advantages:

- It's easy to see participants and provide feedback.
- You can provide quick visual cues, thus stressing your voice less.
- You can observe participants and pace the workout according to their fitness levels.
- You may find that new participants learn the skills more quickly with both visual and verbal teaching.

The disadvantages are that it is difficult to mimic water moves on land safely and effectively and that high air temperature and slippery surfaces can be dangerous.

When you teach from the deck, demonstrate a move, then use visual cueing to have participants continue the movement while you coach them without performing the move yourself. Give participants

feedback and motivation, and use visual cues to show them how to manipulate their bodies to change the intensity of the move as it progresses. Occasionally cue close to the water's surface to help participants maintain good neck and head alignment. After participants have learned the intensity progression, they can be encouraged to look at each other as they work while keeping their necks in neutral alignment. If they have to keep their eyes glued on you, their necks may stay hyperextended throughout the workout. Remember to teach safely.

Here are some tips for teaching from the deck:

- Always wear shoes with traction and impact protection.
- Adhere to land training guidelines for safety.

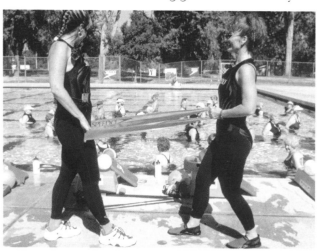

- Keep all movement low impact.
- Coach, lead, and cue, but don't do the entire workout on the deck!
- Check participants' head alignment; step away from the pool if the participants in the front line have to hyperextend their necks to see you.
- By mirroring individual participants, you can feel their intensity levels, share their workout experience, and give them support. For example, you can say to the class

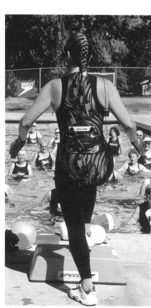

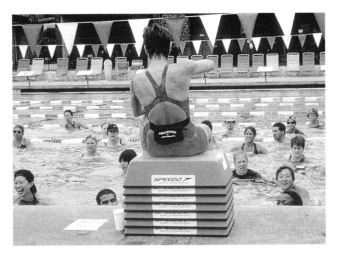

"I'm with Molly now." Everyone has permission to work at his or her own pace.

- Use a training mat if available to reduce impact.
- Use aids such as a chair for balance and for mimicking suspended moves.
- Wear clothing that is professional, but that will keep you comfortable by providing protection outdoors or allowing heat to escape indoors.
- Don't yell! Use a microphone if possible.

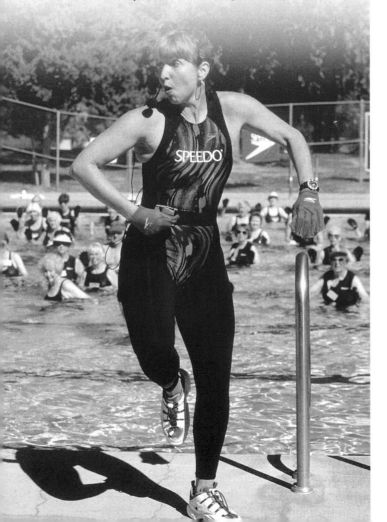

Method 2: Teaching From the Water

Another method you may enjoy is teaching from the water. As your participants can't see the parts of your body that are submerged, you'll have to verbally describe the exercises.

Advantages of teaching from the water include these:

- You share the workout environment with the participants.
- You can do hands-on teaching, assisting people to learn to trust buoyancy and providing one-on-one corrective feedback.

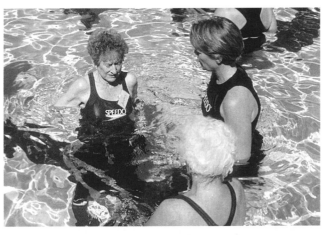

- You can assist participants with pool entry.

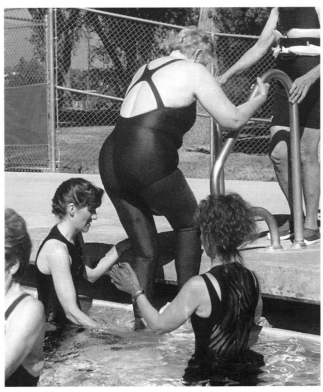

- It's safer and more fun for you.
- It may be very motivating for participants as you work out together.

However, it also has the following disadvantages:

- It's difficult for you or your participants to see your lower body.
- You must verbally describe the exercises and it may be difficult for participants to hear and quickly understand the descriptions.
- New participants may have a difficult time keeping up with seasoned participants who already understand the skills.

The following are some tips for teaching from the water:

- Wear shoes that provide good in-water traction.
- Keep your verbal cues concise and audible.

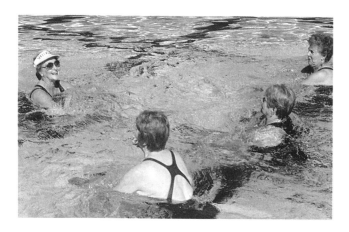

- Perform visual cueing signals high enough above the water that everyone can see and understand them.
- Wear colored tights and position yourself so you can move through the class providing feedback.
- Ask participants to describe where they feel the muscles working so you can check for proper exercise execution (it's difficult for you to see participants in the water, too).

As the participants become more skilled, this method becomes more effective and will probably be more fun for you.

Method 3: Teaching From the Deck and From the Water

Many instructors combine in-water teaching with on-deck demonstrations. It is a good balance for instructor comfort, safety, and fun.

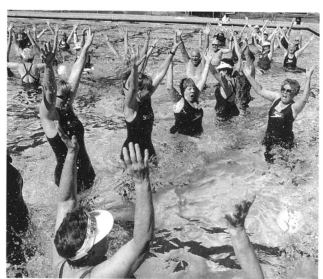

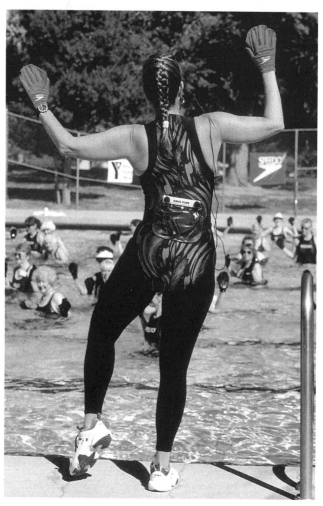

These are some tips for using a combination method:

- Wear shoes that provide impact protection and have good traction when wet.
- Be sure to use safe entrances and exits during transitions.
- If your back is turned, be sure the lifeguard is alert.
- Before you begin your transition, cue participants to continue the move, so they don't stop working!

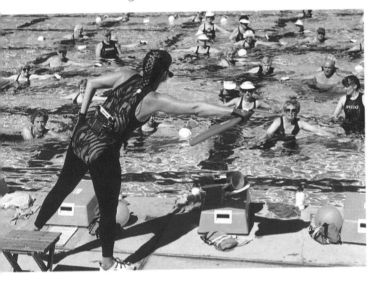

- Give yourself time to adjust to gravity before you begin your deck demonstrations, and also give yourself time to adjust to buoyancy when you re-enter the pool.

Plan in advance the deck moves you'll demonstrate, but be flexible enough to ask participants during class, "Do you understand the move?"

- For suspended kickboard work, include both deck and in-water demonstrations, as the position is possible only in water. Have participants practice this position before performing the set.
- If you have new participants, you may need to demonstrate on the deck more than you teach in the water until they master the basic skills and understand your cues.
- Ask participants if they understand the movement as you lead in the water.
- Wear clothing that provides comfort in or out of the water when wet and presents a professional appearance without requiring a lot of readjustment during transitions.

Method 4: Demonstrating in the Water or With a Video

Help participants learn new exercises using one of these two methods:

- To demonstrate in the water, have participants stand on the edge of the pool to watch. A corner is the best position. You or a skilled participant can then get into the pool and demonstrate the move as it's explained.
- To demonstrate on video, have participants watch the section of the video that illustrates the new exercise. Repeat the section enough times so they understand. State the objective of the exercise and any suggested modifications if needed.

Either way, participants see a visual image, so when the move is cued they understand how it's actually performed in water. Ask if they have any questions before they begin performing the movement.

Responsive Teaching

No matter which method or combination of methods you choose, you must learn how to respond to your participants, how to be there to coach them, teach them, and guide them through skill development. The word *responsive* means giving a response, reply, or feedback. By providing positive, specific, corrective, and motivational feedback during class, participants will develop skills so they can take charge of their own workouts.

The key is to teach water fitness not as random movements, but as self-paced, skilled exercises that participants can adjust through a progression by making small changes in factors such as force applied, speed, or size of movement. Applying these variations to an exercise that is performed correctly (properly coordinated using good body alignment) allows participants to take charge of their own bodies. Since water is resistive, coaching participants through progressions, and letting them find the speed or size for a movement that works, allows them to target the right level of resistance for them.

Let's start out with an example of teaching responsively, then look at the use of verbal and visual cues and equipment.

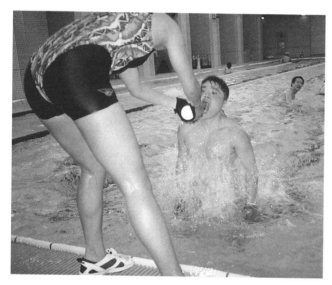

Example of Teaching Responsively

The following is an example of how to teach participants a progression that they can apply to an exercise. You can gently coach them to perform each exercise properly and find their own levels of intensity.

To start, you do not use music, as participants are just learning the skills. Without music, participants can concentrate on learning, feedback, and corrections. Once participants understand the skills and have achieved good performance, you can add music for fun and motivation.

Begin with a warm-up, focusing on basic skills for balance and safety such as recovering to a stand, sculling, and keeping good posture (see chapter 8). Allow participants to adjust to buoyancy and practice moving their joints through a range of motion, feeling the buoyancy and the resistance of the water. Have them feel the weight of the water and ask them to trust buoyancy. Cue their breathing. Teach them the 4 S's they can use to lower intensity, if necessary:

1. *Slow* down.
2. Make the move *Smaller*.
3. *Stabilize* and check balance and posture.
4. *Substitute* a modified move if needed.

Then use the following teaching progression:
- Demonstrate the basic move, thermal movements, and stabilization skills (such as flat sculling and jogging).
- Show participants how to keep proper alignment using the ready position (described in chapter 8). Check and correct them as necessary.

- Tell participants the objective for each exercise, such as cardiorespiratory training or improving the ability to climb stairs.
- Point out to participants the primary muscles that are involved in each exercise, and have them practice the pattern of movement:
  - ➤ Have participants adjust the size of the move as necessary, and check participants' functional range of motion.
  - ➤ Cue participants to use proper posture and biomechanics.
  - ➤ Cue participants in how to breathe during the exercise.
  - ➤ Check and correct them as necessary.
- Gradually increase resistance overload by applying the **S.W.E.A.T.** formula.

During class, do the following:
- Observe participants and respond as needed. If you have a large class, you may want to have participants wear colored name tags. The colors can be keyed to specific special needs (for example, pink may mean to cue for a knee condition), and the tags make it easier for you to address participants by name.
- Remind participants to adjust exercise intensity using the 4 S's. Encourage participants to work at their own pace.
- Check that participants use proper biomechanics and correct them as needed.
- Encourage and celebrate their efforts!
- Ask if they are warm while they are working. If not, tell them how to get warmer.
- Provide personal, positive, and specific feedback.
- Remind participants to monitor their exercise intensity (rate of perceived exertion or talk test).

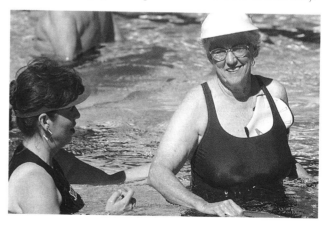

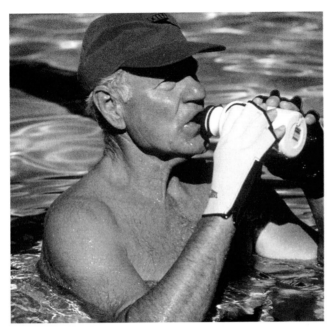

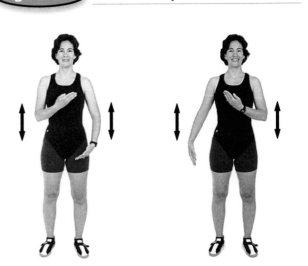

Figure 11.1 *Visual cues for water exercise*

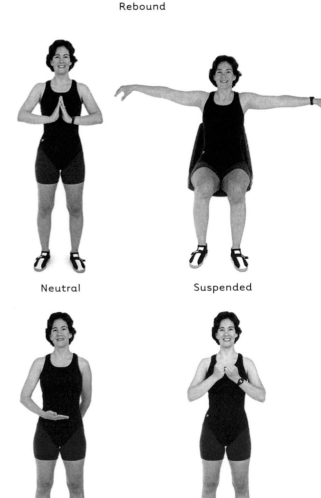

Rebound

Neutral

Suspended

Ready position/
Neutral posture

New move

- Give participants water breaks.
- Vary the exercise and continue the set, or reduce intensity and begin a new move.

Choose a safe teaching style that works for you and your group. Educating participants and developing their skills will empower them to take charge of their own workouts. You then can enjoy being their coach rather than teaching skills.

Verbal and Visual Cues

The purpose of visual cueing is to minimize the use of voice commands, especially if you don't use a microphone. Visual cues provide participants with quick information on movement variations and help them "read" your body language. The repeated use of a combination of consistent verbal and visual cues will help participants become familiar with both the terms and visual commands. After they've mastered the meanings of the visual commands, you can use the visual cues without verbal cues to protect your voice, especially when music is being played or competing noise makes hearing difficult.

Teach the cues a few at a time and watch how well participants learn to respond to visual cues. Remember to cue early so participants have time to see, hear, and make the transitions, as water slows their movements. Figure 11.1 shows some visual cues you can use.

 Video Reference:

The Golden Waves Leadership Program, Session 10, Responsive Teaching Tips.

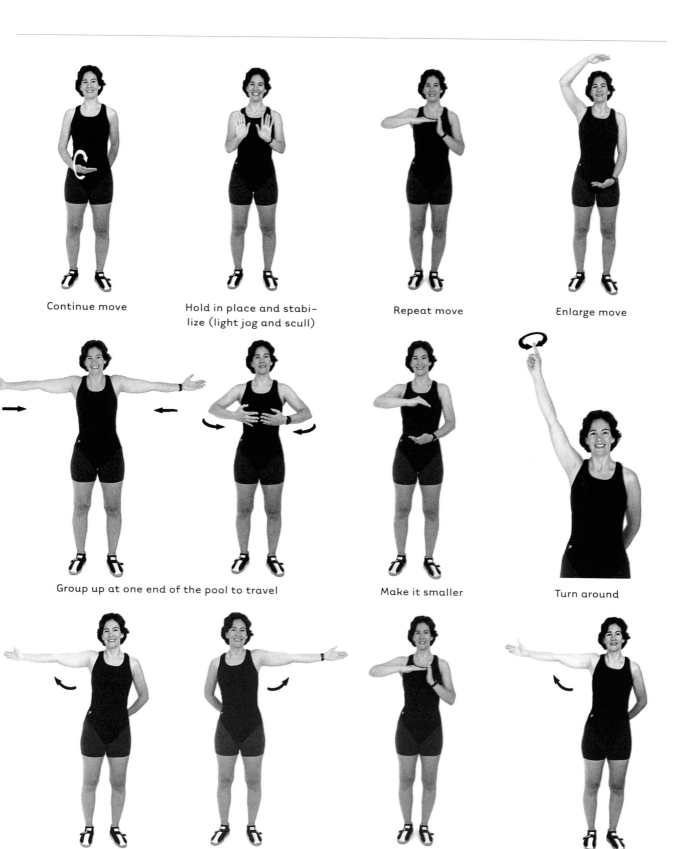

Continue move

Hold in place and stabi-
lize (light jog and scull)

Repeat move

Enlarge move

Group up at one end of the pool to travel

Make it smaller

Turn around

Travel (cue direction with point)

Repeat on other side (touch side and point)

(Continued)

Figure 11.1 *Visual cues for water exercise (continued)*

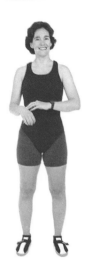

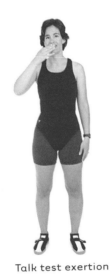

Talk test exertion

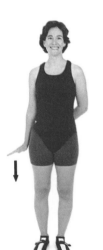

Slow down

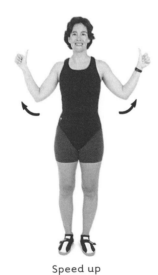

Speed up

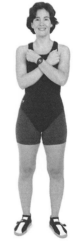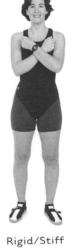

Rigid/Stiff

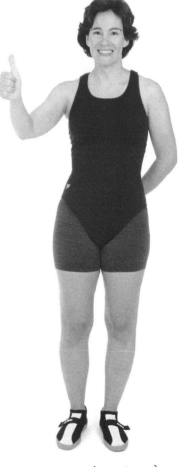

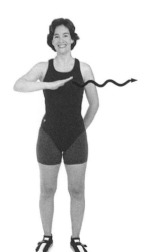

Soft/Flexous

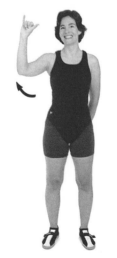

Light, loose, and buoyant
(hang loose, thumb and
pinkie finger up)

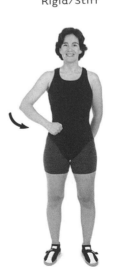

Power and force (move
fist across body)

Good Job! (thumbs up)

Adding Equipment

You can add basic equipment such as webbed gloves to your program. The primary purpose of the gloves is to increase the surface area of the hand. This increased surface area uses the property of action/reaction; as you push down on the glove, the upper body is assisted upward. Participants can lean on the enlarged surface area like a table top for support. They also can use the gloves to maintain better postural position, adjust to leg movements, and push the water to assist with change of direction. They need to be taught how to change the positions of the gloves to adjust intensity during resistance work.

Any time you add a piece of equipment to your workout, you must consider it to be a new program. Everything will feel different and require new skills. Participants will need to be taught how to use the equipment, understand its purpose and how it works, and know how to use it safely. Every piece of equipment should provide participants with the opportunity to work in a progression, allowing them to target the levels that are right for them.

Some equipment compromises balance, so teach the specific safety skills for each piece of equipment to ensure a safe and comfortable experience for participants. Check that participants use proper body alignment while using the equipment and know how to control buoyancy if it's being added. Make sure the overload or buoyancy support is appropriate for participants' body types and fitness levels. Teach participants effective resting positions or release procedures, and watch that participants use the equipment safely.

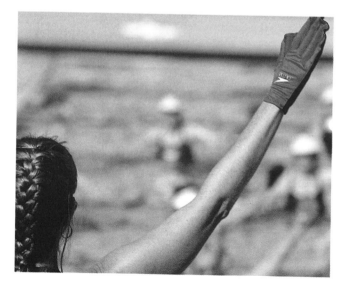

Checklist for a Smooth Class

Here are the steps to follow to ensure your water fitness class goes smoothly.

BEFORE CLASS

- Design your workouts to be site specific, taking into account pool depth, temperature, pool size, class size, and deck space available. Use all your available space.
- Plan for classes to have a ratio of no more than 25 participants to each instructor.
- Cue tapes beforehand for smooth transitions.
- Test your microphone for volume and fresh batteries (waterproof microphones are available).
- Set up your equipment and teaching aids, but otherwise clear the deck.
- Greet your participants and get to know them. Use health history questionnaires. Buddy up new participants with seasoned participants.
- Always have a "Plan B" ready in case the pool cannot be used. An effective program design includes at least one class that can keep your participants on track with their fitness program without getting wet. "Plan B" land classes could include stretching, resistance band work, or simply an informative lecture on nutrition, stress relief, or the benefits of exercise.

DURING CLASS

- On the deck or in the water, teach where you are effective according to the needs of the class. Greet the class right to left and front to back. Move around; everyone is important and each group is different.
- Get in and out of the pool safely and demonstrate moves the best you can from the deck safely. Wear water shoes and keep movements low impact and safe.
- Teach participants how to recover to a stand in shallow water or to use the resting position in deep water for their own personal safety. Check their ability to perform these skills.
- Have participants wear water shoes for traction and to protect their feet, both during the workout and in the shower room.
- Tell participants that wearing tights, leotards, and special water-fitness gear can provide them with increased warmth and support for vertical exercise in water. Share information on shopping outlets for this special gear with participants.

- Encourage participants to pace themselves, and be sensitive to different body types. Twenty people working out together are having twenty different experiences. Challenge and moderate through effective coaching.

- Your body language and cueing should reflect the actual water pace. Cue your participants using consistent body language and verbal/visual cues that make sense to them.

- Educate participants constantly so they learn the skills necessary to take responsibility for their own work and rest. Every participant should understand the basic principles of hydrodynamics so he or she can take command of his or her own workout. Share current and accurate exercise and nutritional information with participants. Teach them and they become your teachers!

- Protect and pace yourself according to your own fitness level. Use your body to teach basic moves, then coach participants through progressions with short demonstrations or verbal/visual cues. It's their workout, not yours.

- Motivate participants with positive feedback. Remind them to go at their own pace, and congratulate them when they do!

AFTER CLASS

- Have fun with your group and end class by giving them information on the next class, handing out health information, or encouraging them to cross train on land. Thank them, for they are your greatest teachers!

- Share with other instructors and learn all you can about health, fitness, and water exercise so water fitness can grow. We have a long way to go, and it's going to take teamwork!

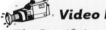 **Video References:**

The Specificity of Training and Deep Water Program, Session 5

The Aquatic Step Program, Session 4

The Golden Waves II Advanced Progressions, Teaching Session

Water Fitness Instructor Survival

Water is a forgiving environment for our participants, but if we teach incorrectly, the participants' healthy program may create unhealthy results for us. While we're busy motivating participants in and out of the water in all possible conditions, we often overlook our own physical and mental fitness. The following are some of the challenges we face as instructors and some tips to prevent or recover from them:

 Teaching unsafely on deck or on deck and in water can produce injuries to your feet, shins, knees, and low back. *Wear well-cushioned, nonslip, supportive shoes (the styles that go in and out of the pool are the best). Work on a mat and limit your moves to low-impact demonstration exercises. Remember, you are not performing, you are teaching skills. Use stools or chairs to assist with your demonstrations and to provide a resting place. Teach skills using visual and verbal cues.*

 Environmental risks may include sun exposure, temperature and humidity extremes, and chlorine or other chemicals. All of these can be hazardous with overexposure. *Wear sunscreen, sunglasses, and a hat (and a T-shirt, if desired) to minimize sun exposure dangers. Layer on apparel that encourages either heat loss in hot conditions or heat retention in cool situations. Shower before entering the water so the skin absorbs nontreated water, minimizing the absorption of chlorine. Then shower in clear water after immersion and apply a petroleum jelly-based lotion while your body is still wet. Drink water to help thermoregulation in any temperature, and be sure the facility has good ventilation. If you detect a strong chemical smell, check immediately with the pool manager. Refer to* Teaching Swimming Fundamentals, *p. 168–169 for more information.*

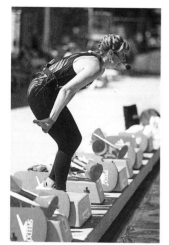

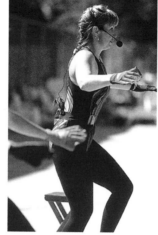

To be a good instructor, you must be flexible and knowledgeable. By observing and responding to the big picture (the facility, participants, distractions, challenges), you provide a fun and safe environment for your class. By being aware of factors such as the pool facility and fitting them to the participant's needs, you should be able to make every class a success. Every situation, day, and class is different, so use these tips to help you respond no matter what happens that day!

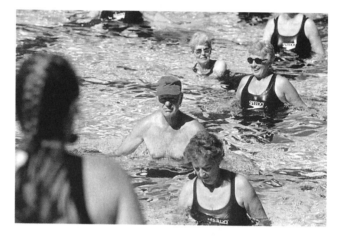

 Nonimpact and overuse injuries can result from yelling, working out in or out of the water while teaching too many classes, or working out too hard. The shoulders, neck, and low back may fatigue due to body position. *Use a microphone. Turn off the music so you can cue without competition. Teach skills in the water in small groups so you don't have to yell to be heard. Limit your own personal workout intensity and the number of classes you teach, and take a break from exercises to coach. Upper-body and low-back fatigue are usually caused by leaning forward toward participants during deck teaching. Check your stance, stand tall and centered (don't lean forward). Instead of teaching near the deck's edge, stand back a little to encourage a more neutral neck and low-back position.*

 If you are injured or ill. *Take care of the condition, and rest to ensure recovery. Check the medical conditions section of this book for some specific suggestions for injury.*

 If you are "burned out" or feel like you can't face another class with enthusiasm. *Take a break, attend someone else's class, do something else, buy a new water exercise video for ideas, attend a conference, or ask your supervisor to help you get recharged. Don't just keep showing up! Participants do not need just a "warm body" to coach them to a great life; they need someone who's professional, enthusiastic, and ready to share himself or herself in the process. The greatest gift you can give your participants is you as a healthy role model.*

Bibliography

Durrett, A. 1996. Are you set to get wet? *IDEA Today* 14(3): 30–35.

Miles-Dutton, D. 1996. Water fitness for beginners. *IDEA Today* 14(8): 29–31.

Miles-Dutton, D. 1994. Teaching with a splash. IDEA World Fitness Convention Presentation.

Miles-Dutton, D. 1994. Deck tips and teaching tricks. IDEA World Fitness Convention Presentation.

Sanders, M., and N. Rippee. 1994. Speedo aquatic fitness system, instructor training manual. London: Speedo International.

Sanders, M., and C. Maloney-Hills. 1998. Aquatic exercise for better living on land. *ACSM's Health & Fitness Journal* 2(3): 16–23.

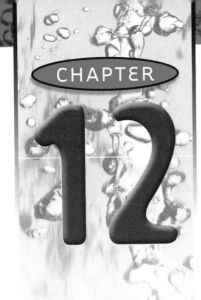

CHAPTER 12

Progressing Your Programs: Equipment and Advanced Formats

MARY E. SANDERS AND TATIANA KOLOVOU

Objectives:

◎ To determine why equipment is added to water fitness classes

◎ To identify equipment categories

◎ To review a number of evaluation questions that can help instructors properly choose and use equipment for specific exercises, sets, and programs

◎ To identify some methods and ideas for progressing sets, workouts, and programs

When you create a good basic water fitness program and it becomes successful, your next challenge will be to expand the available program choices to keep continuing participants' interest and to raise their exercise intensity for further fitness gains. Both can be accomplished by the proper use of water exercise equipment and variations in sets, workouts, and program development.

Equipment

Equipment can increase the quality and safety of a water fitness program while offering participants an opportunity to progress their training by increasing exercise intensity. To use equipment properly, you need to understand the purpose of each piece of equipment and to design movements with that equipment based on the properties of water and exercise science. You need to evaluate the function and safety of each exercise with equipment before you use it in class.

Using equipment can do the following:

- Add variety to the class.
- Increase (or decrease) the intensity of the workout.
- Provide buoyancy support.
- Add resistance to movements to create greater work while training.
- Give participants the opportunity to progress their exercise.

Equipment changes the way water acts against the body in a number of ways, making classes more interesting. The shape and size of the equipment can change how water flows over the body, either impeding movement by increasing surface area (increasing resistance) or assisting movement by streamlining it (decreasing resistance). Additionally, equipment that floats can add buoyancy to the arms, legs, or entire body. Full-body buoyancy support allows participants to work out in a suspended position for as long as they want and to rest as needed, which is especially important in deep water. In transitional depth, full-body buoyancy support allows participants to work for extended periods of time in a suspended position and can increase the drag resistance during shallow water moves modified for transitional depth (using the pool bottom for rebounding). Full-body buoyancy gear worn in shallow water provides support for vertical balance and decreases lower-body impact. Buoyancy equipment that is held or worn on the arms and/or legs impedes downward movements, requiring the user to work harder.

Other types of equipment can be used to target a variety of training objectives by changing how water's properties act on the body. Aquatic steps used in shallow water increase the effect of gravity and decrease the effects of buoyancy against the body. Without equipment, buoyancy minimizes most of the eccentric overload. Tethers or elastic resistance bands can be added to provide resistance that includes both

Parts of this chapter adapted with permission of IDEA, The Health and Fitness Source. (800) 999-IDEA or (619) 535-8979. See page x for complete source information.

concentric and eccentric contractions while using the water to minimize impact and provide support during the exercises.

Equipment should be added to a program to meet certain training or safety objectives for each individual. This means that different participants in a group exercise class may perform the same exercise with different pieces of equipment based on their fitness level and/or safety objectives. For example, one participant may choose to wear a flotation belt during a shallow water class and to use webbed gloves for the upper-body conditioning set. Another participant may choose to not wear a belt and work the upper body using fitness paddles, which provide a larger surface area that creates a higher-intensity workout during the same set of exercises. Both participants are using the same type of equipment (surface area), but due to the different sizes of the equipment, the overload varies.

It's important to know how to match the type of equipment (and how it affects the body) with the objectives. For example, the same upper-body exercise in which buoyant dumbbells are used may overload different muscle groups if fitness paddles are used, and it may not be targeting the desired objective. *The main reasons for using equipment are to enhance training and to provide a safe working environment.* Now let's turn to the types of equipment available and how to choose which equipment to purchase and use for each training objective.

Equipment Types

Different types of equipment help to target different objectives effectively. Let's examine the two main types: water-specific equipment and land/water integration equipment.

Water-Specific Equipment

Water-specific equipment falls into two categories: equipment that increases surface area and equipment that is buoyant.

Surface Area Equipment

Surface area equipment increases the surface area to be worked, increasing drag without providing any buoyancy. Devices vary in size, can have flat or shaped surfaces, and can be handheld or worn. The amount of overload generated depends on the size of the device and the drag resistance it creates during movement. The equipment can increase the intensity of the work (or overload) by making a movement less streamlined. As the surface areas of our arms and legs are usually too small to provide an adequate overload for

strength training, equipment is essential to progress training for muscular conditioning. However, it's also important to check that the shape or size of the equipment does not interfere with good body mechanics and proper body alignment.

Here are some examples of surface area equipment:

- Webbed gloves
- Nonbuoyant dumbbells
- Fitness paddles
- Swim fins
- Water parachutes

Each has specific ways it can be used in training.

- **Webbed gloves.** Webbed gloves provide a "table top" surface for better support of the upper body during sculling motions. As participants press downward, the gloves give extra lift upward for stabilization and vertical support.

  Gloves also can be used to provide variable on-demand resistance for the upper body, enhancing muscular conditioning by allowing participants to adjust the amount of surface area being moved through the water. While gloves may create too much upper-body overload, they can be removed easily anytime during the workout.

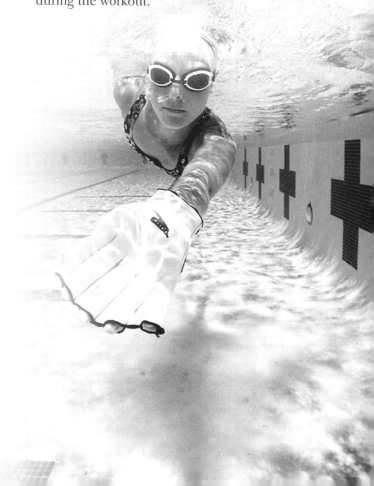

In addition, gloves help to contribute to general cardiorespiratory conditioning by assisting with faster movements through the water. Participants can use the gloves to push and pull the body through the water faster or to help with balance during changes in direction. When it is added to the effort of the lower body, the extra armwork may contribute to higher-intensity training and enhance calorie expenditure for each session.

Finally, by using the gloves' surface area for upper-body support, participants can extend through their maximal ranges of motion for the lower body. The extra surface area can help to stretch the fingers as the hands are pushed through the water.

- **Nonbuoyant dumbbells or fitness paddles.** Handheld surface area dumbbells may offer upper-body support when held on the surface. When the dumbbells are large enough to provide a "table top" support, participants can lean on them during range-of-motion exercises to enhance work.

Dumbbells or paddles provide resistance in any direction and are the most versatile equipment for targeting muscle groups. Various sizes and shapes can be moved in any plane through the water to create overload. On land, participants choose various weights or machine settings for overload. In water, they must learn which piece of equipment creates the optimal overload for them and apply the right speed to feel some muscle fatigue within 8 to 15 repetitions. Check that the size of the device does not compromise body alignment.

When the equipment impedes movement of the legs by creating more drag, the effort of the legs can be increased, which in turn increases cardiorespiratory intensity.

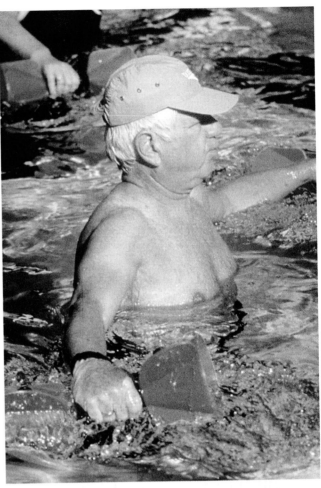

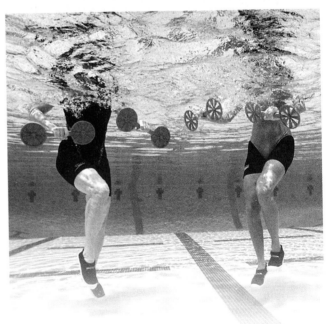

- **Swim fins.** Fins provide muscular overload during leg extension and flexion, significantly working the lower body, especially during large kicking movements. This lower-body work can contribute to effective cardiorespiratory as well as muscular training.

- **Water parachutes.** Parachutes provide very large unstreamlined surfaces that can be pulled by a handle for upper body and trunk muscular work or attached to a sports belt (nonbuoyant) for additional drag resistance during running or walking. The parachute provides effective high-intensity concentric and eccentric contraction work, as the participant slowly resists extension while dragging the parachute. As the parachute is soft and moves around the body, participants can easily maintain proper body alignment.

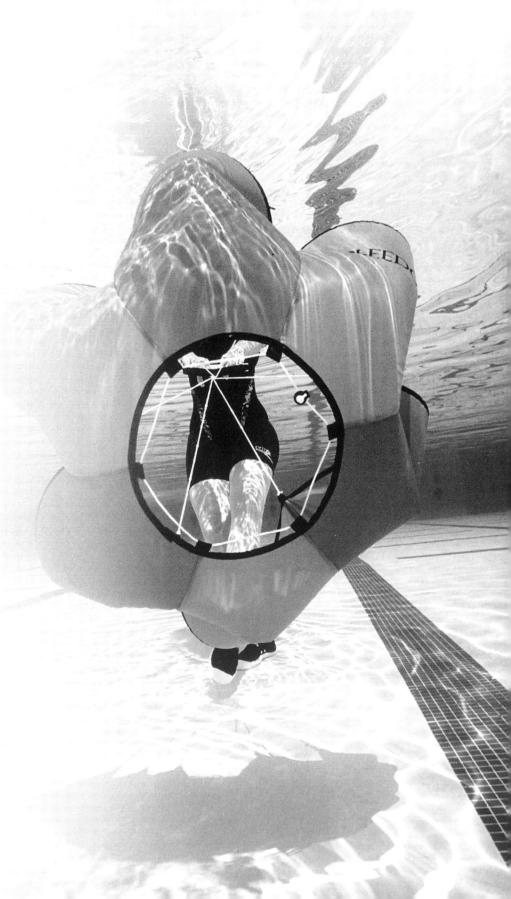

Buoyancy Equipment

Buoyancy equipment floats enough to provide flotation support for an arm or leg or the entire body. The purpose of buoyancy equipment is to increase the buoyancy of the limb or body, providing resistance to downward movements against buoyancy's upward force. The amount of buoyancy overload varies with each type of equipment and the individual's body composition. We do not recommend you use milk jugs or other containers as exercise equipment at any time. They do not allow participants to maintain proper joint alignment and are unreliable for support.

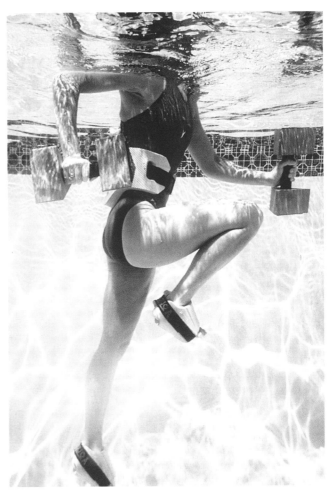

These are some examples of buoyancy equipment:

- Whole-body devices, such as belts (foam or inflatable)

- Arm and leg devices, such as dumbbells (foam or air-filled) or cuffs (foam or air-filled, attached to the ankles or upper arms)

- Free-floating devices, such as noodles, logs, or kickboards

The following are some ways this equipment can be used.

- **Whole-body devices.** Belts attached to the body (waist) provide full-body support for any depth, and they are especially important for deep water. Without buoyancy gear in deep water, participants must work to keep their heads above water by performing advanced skills, such as eggbeater kicks or sculling. This can be appropriate for some participants, but it is exhausting for most. Also, in a balanced deep water strength training program, some movements require the power phase to be upward, toward the surface. For example, during a biceps curl the hand is pulled upward, propelling the participant downward (action/reaction). Buoyancy gear keeps the participant from going underwater. Thus, deep water exercises should include buoyancy support for the entire body to allow participants to relax during the workout and to ensure muscles can be worked in a balanced way.

Flotation belts can be used in transitional and shallow water as well as deep water to extend the length of time that participants can stay in a suspended working position and to provide extra balance and support. Also, surface drag from the bulky shape of the belt may con-

tribute to overload during rebound movements, further increasing intensity.

Whole-body devices support participants so they can exercise suspended in the water, allowing a freedom of movement and an ability to maximize range of motion that may not be possible on land. They also provide participants with stabilization, balance, and lift. For example, in shallow water a participant can remove the belt and place it under a leg to assist in stretching the hamstrings upward.

- **Arm and leg devices.** Some buoyancy equipment is handheld or is attached to the upper arms or ankles to provide resistance to downward movements. This works in opposition to gravity and is especially useful for muscular training. The amount of resistance a buoyancy device provides depends on its density and volume (size). Small foam dumbbells may offer lower levels of resistance, while larger

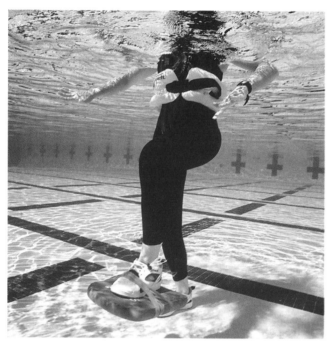

foam devices or air-filled dumbbells can provide higher resistance.

Participants can easily release handheld devices if they lose their balance, and these devices are effective at any depth. However, undue stress may be placed on participants' shoulders if these devices are the only equipment used for full-body support during a deep water class. Have participants wear flotation belts to minimize shoulder stress and support the body. Buoyant cuffs attached to the ankles are more difficult for participants to manage and require more advanced skills for safe use, but the cuffs can provide fun and challenge for more advanced participants. Be sure to follow the manufacturers' program guidelines for use of the cuffs to ensure your participants' safety.

Participants can hold buoyant dumbbells at the surface for stabilization and support. Be sure the dumbbells are buoyant enough to support the participants.

Handheld gear can increase support so participants can work the lower body more effectively. Additional energy expenditure may result from pushing or pulling the devices through the water.

Finally, buoyant devices can assist the arms or legs upward to enhance the range of motion. The body should be aligned properly during these movements, and to prevent overstretching

you should check that the buoyancy of the devices is not more than participants can control.

- **Free-floating devices.** Kickboards, noodles, and logs are not attached to the body and can be used for both full-body and limb support. They can be held at the surface for support and balance. As this equipment is handheld and can slip away, advise weak swimmers or participants who are insecure in the water to wear a flotation belt for support, even in shallow water.

Noodles or water logs provide buoyancy support that can be used in any depth of water. Working positions can be changed by moving the long foam cylinder around the body or by sitting on it. Participants can work their cardiorespiratory systems by performing any of the basic moves in any depth. Kickboards can be used for kicking on the back, side, or front.

Participants can sit on kickboards, noodles, or logs for lower-body muscular work and can push or pull the devices through the water for upper-body muscular work. Equipment also

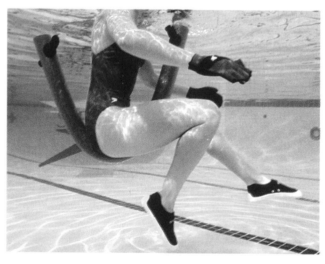

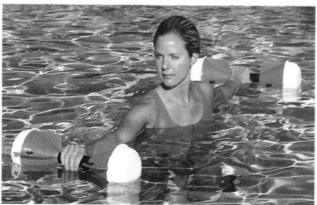

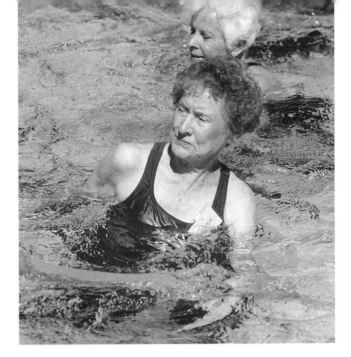

can be placed under the arms or legs to assist with upward directed stretches.

Land/Water Integration Equipment

This category includes pieces of equipment that are either the same as or similar to those used on land, such as resistance bands or aquatic steps. Most provide an opportunity to bridge from land to water training by permitting modification of land exercises for the water.

These are examples of land/water integration equipment:

- Aquatic steps
- Tethers
- Resistance bands
- Balls (air-filled, weighted, and foam)

Here are some uses for these devices.

- **Aquatic steps.** Used on the bottom of the pool, a step designed for in-water use only provides added leverage for vertical propulsion and a platform that minimizes the effects of buoyancy, thereby increasing the effects of gravity and overloading the lower body. Balancing on top of the step is harder than standing on the pool floor, adding difficulty to balance exercises. Basic moves for muscular and cardiorespiratory conditioning can include simple up-and-down movements or dynamic propulsion jump training exercises. Also, the platform provides

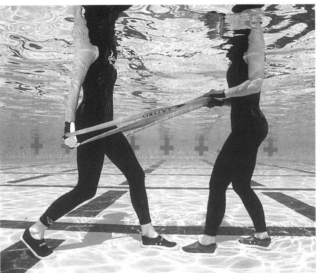

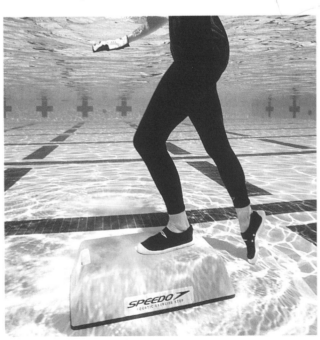

something to lean on so participants can use their own body weight to enhance stretches.

- **Resistance bands.** Resistance bands (or tubing) are available in various levels of elasticity. Once cut to five-foot lengths, they have a wide variety of uses. They can be used for performing both concentric and eccentric muscular work, and cardiorespiratory work can be added to upper-body strengthening by having participants jog through the water during the muscular sets. The bands can be used for support, can be leashed to an object to provide resistance for trunk strengthening, and can provide range-of-motion feedback as they are moved through the water during flexibility sets. Participants can gauge how far they are reaching by watching the shape and size of the patterns they make with the bands.

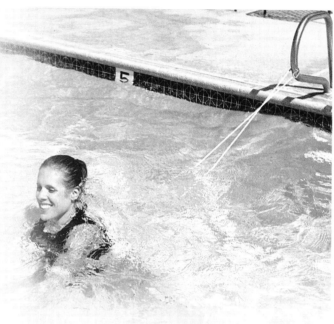

Weighted balls, such as medicine balls or water-filled "thumper" balls, also can be used to improve lifting, lowering, and passing strength. In the water, normally this overhead range of motion is impossible to overload without weighted equipment. Weighted balls offer this opportunity.

Foam balls are available in many sizes and densities for complex drills that combine catching, throwing, and walking, or jogging for training in agility, coordination, balance, and endurance. Smaller foam balls can be used for grip-and-release drills to increase finger, hand, and wrist strength, mobility, and flexibility.

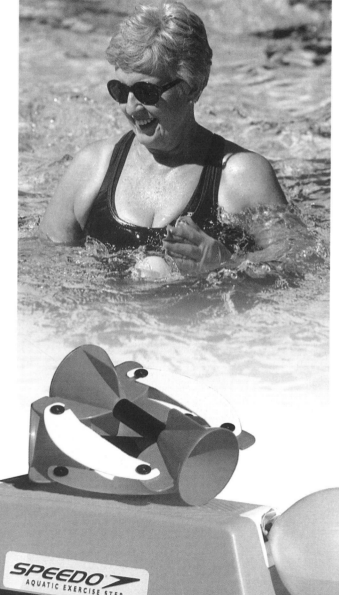

- **Tethers.** A tether is resistance tubing that is designed to be attached in a number of ways to provide multiple exercise options. Tethers can be used by individuals or partners for muscular and cardiorespiratory endurance work, for balance drills, and for tether-together exercises (two people pulling away from each other). Tether systems should be water resistant (have no metal) and should be designed to attach to a belt bilaterally, one on each side of the body for balance. A sliding attachment on the belt can be used for individual tether exercises (the tether attached to the wall) or to drag a water parachute. Sports drills can be created by attaching a tether to the pool wall to increase resistance against the body, especially the trunk, for running, kicking, and lateral movements.

- **Balls.** Air-filled balls or water polo balls add variety to exercise. They provide stability training for the shoulder area when used in overhead motions and torso strengthening when used in passing motions.

Equipment Combinations

Some equipment has a combination of properties that affect overload and skills. For example, kickboards provide both buoyancy and surface area resistance. Equipment can also be combined for training variety. Participants can wear flotation belts while using aquatic steps during intervals that alternate high-intensity rebound work on the steps with suspended work performed above the steps! Be sure to evaluate how these combinations will affect exercise in each water depth.

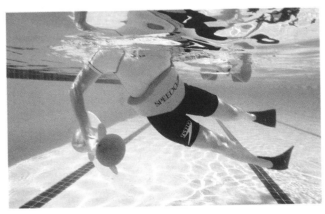

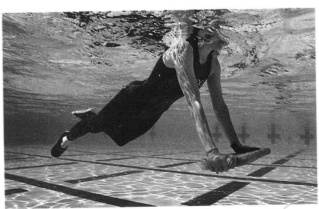

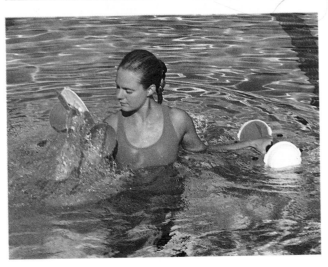

Progressing a Program With Equipment Applications

As participants improve their fitness levels, they will need more challenging exercises to continue the training effect. The **S.W.E.A.T.** formula and the basic equipment, along with water depth and exercise design variations, can challenge most participants for quite a while. However, stronger participants and those who need to overload more will need to be challenged with additional equipment, just as the weights are progressively increased in the weight room. Not only does the equipment challenge individual muscles, but each piece of equipment requires participants to learn and develop unique stabilization and performance skills. Each piece of equipment presents its own program!

Before you add equipment to an exercise, ask yourself the following questions as a guide:

- What is the purpose of the equipment?
- What are the fitness benefits of using the equipment?
- What is the cost of the equipment, and is it worth it compared to the benefits?

Purpose of Equipment

Equipment can provide buoyancy, amplify resistance, increase surface area, increase or decrease gravity, or any combination of these. If your pool has deep water, you will need some type of buoyancy equipment if you are going to fill the pool with participants who are working out effectively and safely! Table 12.1 shows various pieces of equipment and the workout objectives that they can be used to meet. Table 12.2 indicates, for the same pieces of equipment, the depths of water in which they can be used.

Fitness Benefits

When you consider purchasing equipment, think about what that equipment does and how it does it. Determine which properties of water it utilizes. Ask yourself if individual participants can use it to create their own progressive overload, and think about what skills you will need to teach them so they can use the equipment properly.

Consider the safety aspects of using the equipment. Can participants use this equipment and still maintain body alignment? Will you need to teach them special safety skills?

Table 12.1 Workout Objectives and Equipment Use

Equipment type	Cardiovascular	Muscle strength-muscle endurance	Flexibility	Sports functional training
Webbed gloves	X	X	X	X
Ankle fins	X-overload	X	0	X
Large surface area dumbbells	X-overload	X	0	X
Swim fins	X-increase speed	X-lower body	0	X-sports
Kickboards	X	X	X	X-sports
Fitness paddles	X-overload	X	0	X
Small surface area dumbbells	X-overload	X	0	X
Power buoys system	X	X	X	X
Water parachutes	X	X	X	X
Buoyancy belts	X	X	X	X
Buoyancy ankle cuffs	X	X	X	X
Buoyancy dumbbells	0	X	X	X
Water noodles/logs	X	X	X	X
Aquatic steps	X	X	X	X
Resistance bands	0	X	X	X
Water polo balls	X	0	X	X
Sponges/foam balls	0	X	0	X
Tether system	X	X	0	X
Sloggers (large foot sandals)	X	X	0	X

X = recommended   0 = not recommended

Table 12.2 Pool Specifications and Equipment Use

Equipment type	Shallow water depth *Navel to nipple*	Traditional water depth *Nipple to shoulders—feet in contact with pool bottom*	Deep water *Shoulders submerged and body suspended*
Webbed gloves	X	X	X
Ankle fins	X	X	0
Large surface area dumbbells	X	X	X-with flotation belt
Swim fins	0	X	X-with flotation belt
Kickboards	X	X	X-without flotation belt
Fitness paddles	X	X	X-with flotation belt
Small surface area dumbbells	X	X	X-with flotation belt
Power buoys system	X	X	X-with flotation belt
Water parachutes	X	X-with flotation belt	X-with flotation belt and swim fins
Buoyancy belts	X	X	X
Buoyancy ankle cuffs	X	X	X-with flotation belt
Buoyancy dumbbells	X	X	X-with or without flotation belt
Water noodles/logs	X	X	X-without flotation belt
Aquatic steps	X	X-flotation belt recommended	0
Resistance bands	X	X	X-with flotation belt
Water polo balls	X	X	X
Sponges/foam balls	X	X	X
Tether system	X	X	X-with flotation belt
Sloggers (large foot sandals)	0	X-with flotation belt	X-with flotation belt

X = recommended   0 = not recommended

Cost of Equipment and Its Worth

In some cases, you know you will need equipment. If you have only deep water, you will have to have equipment for support. If you want to expand your program, you may want equipment for variety and to meet different participant objectives. However, which equipment you buy and in what order is a matter of preference based on your market, facility, storage space, and budget.

Ask yourself some of the following questions as you assess whether you should purchase equipment:

- Will this equipment provide safe and progressive work?
- Will this equipment help my participants meet their objectives?
- Can it be used for a number of intensity levels? Can it be used in a number of ways?
- Is the equipment safe, durable, and comfortable to use?
- Will the cost of the equipment fit in my budget?

Table 12.3 Exercise Type and Intensity Potential for Equipment

Intensity	Type of Exercise			
Low	**Cardio**	**Muscular**	**Flexibility**	**Functional ADL**
↓	Gloves	Gloves	Gloves (finger)	Gloves
	Belts	Bands/fitness paddles	Belt/bands	Belts
	Steps	Power buoys	Steps	Fitness paddles
	Fins	Steps		Power buoys
High		Fins		Steps

Table 12.4 Equipment Cost*

Equipment type	Under $20 per participant	$20–$30 per participant	Over $30 per participant
Webbed gloves	X		
Ankle fins		X	
Large surface area dumbbells	X		
Swim fins	X		
Kickboards	X		
Fitness paddles	X		
Small surface area dumbbells	X		
Power buoys system			X
Water parachutes			X
Buoyancy belts, foam		X	
Buoyancy belts, inflatable	X		
Buoyancy ankle cuffs			X
Buoyancy barbells	X		
Water noodles/logs	X		
Aquatic steps			X
Resistance bands	X		
Water polo balls		X	
Sponges/foam balls	X		
Tether system		X	
Sloggers (large foot sandals)			X

*NOTE: Estimates are for 1998 costs

- Can the equipment be shared? For example, fitness paddles come in pairs, but each participant may use only one paddle.
- Do we have sufficient storage space for the equipment? Can we keep the equipment out of the sun and away from mildew?

Some pieces of equipment are better suited for individual use, such as inflatable belts that must be blown up or webbed gloves. These items are relatively cheap, and once participants own them, they can use them to work out anytime and anywhere.

One way to look at costs is to compare the expense of obtaining equipment with the number of ways it can be used and the amount of intensity it can add to water fitness workouts. Table 12.3 shows the types of workout and intensity levels for which they can be used.

Table 12.4 shows price ranges for each of the pieces of equipment listed in tables 12.1 and 12.2.

Advanced Formats: Sets, Workouts, and Programs

Another way to progress your program besides adding equipment is by using variations to progress a set or a workout, or developing advanced programs.

Progressing a Set

Here are some suggestions for progressing a set for each type of training:

- **Cardiorespiratory training.** One idea is to use intervals to individualize sets. Another is to teach participants how to use equipment and allow them to choose individual overloads. For example, some participants may benefit from using a step during a set, while others may need to go without.
- **Muscular endurance/strength training.** Try encouraging participants to select the equipment type that provides the appropriate overload. Some participants may need to exercise with only webbed gloves, while others may need to add fitness paddles to overload for muscular strength training. You also might allow time for participants to perform the proper number of repetitions and sets. If some participants need more time for their exercises, cue the others to perform an independent cardio set, such as jogging the length of the pool, while the rest complete the work.

- **Combination cardiorespiratory and muscular endurance/strength training.** Include exercises in the set that focus some of the time on muscular work and the rest of the time on cardiorespiratory work. Organize "Tag Exercises" in which one person performs muscular exercises (using overload equipment such as fitness paddles) while the other does a run (or swim) down the pool and back, and then they switch activities. One set of paddles works for two participants!
- **Flexibility and range-of-motion training.** Design partner- and equipment-assisted exercises that can increase the challenge.
- **Functional ADL and sports training.** Include combinations for ADL training that progress challenge. Medicine balls (weighted balls), passed between partners while they walk, stop, and change directions, overload many areas during exercises that may be riskier to load on land. These combinations may improve responses to activities on land such as lifting an object, turning, and walking. For athletes, encourage them to work high-intensity exercises for a longer duration to increase the volume of work performed without increasing potential risk.

Use these questions to evaluate a set for effective progression:

- What is the set objective?
- What depth(s), space, and equipment are required for the group?
- Does the set format (travel, stationary, interval, etc.) meet the objective?
- How will depth changes affect intensity, safety, skills, and achievement of the objective?
- Does the set challenge individual participants through progression? How?
- What responsive teaching skills need to be applied to meet individual objectives?
- Can the set be formatted better or differently?

Progressing a Workout

To progress workouts, you must be in tune with your participants' objectives and skill levels. During group exercise in which participants can "drop in," the challenge becomes the greatest. You probably will have a combination of both skilled and unskilled participants, each needing very different attention. The easiest way to progress workouts is to limit the class to only those registered for a certain time frame, but if it's not possible, you may have to cue participants differently based on their skills.

Another challenge occurs when the pool is small, it has three depths, and the class is large. In order to fill the pool, using all available space, you must cue three different exercise variations. The all-depths workout shown in figure 12.1 is advanced for both the instructor and the participants. Beginners can work in the shallow water, while participants in the transitional and deep water will need to have a baseline skill level to be successful at this workout. With water classes growing and limited pool space, you may have to be able to lead and manage this type of advanced format. If possible, team teach it with another instructor, one of you teaching participants in shallow and transitional water, and the other leading those in the deep water (refer to the *Specificity of Training and Deep Water Program* video for a demonstration).

Progressing a Program

As the popularity of and participation in your water programs increase, people will look to you to expand the program for them as they continue exercising.

Two ways that you can progress your program are through instructional design and progressive program design. You also can decide to offer water fitness as part of post-rehabilitation for those with injuries or chronic medical conditions. If you are a personal trainer, you should consider using water fitness as part of your work with clients.

Instructional Design

Design your programs to target participants in a number of ways, giving them a choice of their own schedules, fitness and health objectives, and preferences. Offer group exercise classes as both drop-in programs and closed registration classes (to allow more effective skills progression). All group exercise instructors need to be skilled at teaching a variety of levels under a wide variety of conditions.

Create cluster groups that target people who share similar conditions, such as classes for the low back, pre- and postnatal classes, and weight management classes. Your facility also may want to offer a kids' water fitness program that bridges to swimming skills, especially for those who need to learn how to enjoy the water and feel safe in the pool.

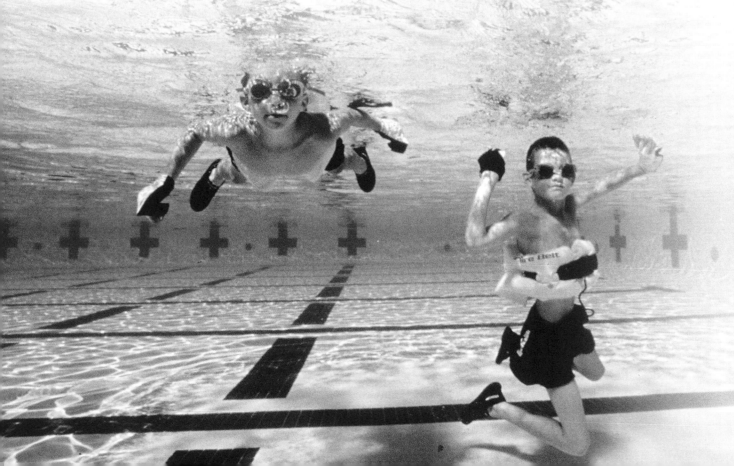

Figure 12.1 *Sample all-depth water fitness workout*

Teaching to the entire pool may require three different variations in movement to optimize training. Be sure you're effective at cueing each depth individually before trying to lead a class in three different depths! You can also use these guidelines and move one group from depth to depth, with all participants wearing flotation belts. Move them after each set. The primary objective is to fill the entire pool with participants and provide them with the proper moves for each depth of water.

The basic progression for all depths is this:

1. Begin with a basic movement (jogging, kicking, etc.) and stabilize.
2. Vary the intensity by using the **S.W.E.A.T.** formula.

EXERCISE CONSIDERATIONS FOR SHALLOW WATER (NAVEL TO NIPPLE DEPTH, FEET AS CENTER OF BALANCE)

- Research suggests that traveling through navel-deep water seems to provide optimal cardiorespiratory endurance work, resulting in an opportunity to maximize the percentage of $\dot{V}O_2$max.

- Since shallow water is the most similar to land, it may provide a more stable environment for people who are new to the water.

- Workouts do not require buoyancy equipment. We recommend that participants wear shoes for protection and traction and wear webbed gloves for enhanced balance.

- A wide variety of exercises can be designed using the hips as a stable center of balance, the same as with land-based exercise. Participants have the opportunity to use the feet as the base of support and also use the chest as the **center of buoyancy** by performing movements suspended with feet off the floor, mimicking deep water.

- Shallow water provides some gravity as overload for the lower body.

- Working positions for intensity regulation in shallow water are rebound, neutral, and suspended.

EXERCISE CONSIDERATIONS FOR TRANSITIONAL WATER (NIPPLE TO NECK, LUNGS SUBMERGED, FEET TOUCH THE BOTTOM, CENTER OF BALANCE BETWEEN THE CHEST AND HIPS)

- Both shallow and deep water exercises can be modified for this depth. Participants can perform deep water exercises using buoyancy gear.

- Due to the amplification of the properties of water surrounding the body, especially buoyancy, you'll need to provide more time for the legs to move and create work.

- Cue sculling that provides lift to allow the legs more time to work through a full range of motion. Sculling also can balance moves so participants can focus on working the legs while keeping the head above water at all times.

- Try to land all moves in an extended position (tall) to keep the head above water, and cue the hands to assist with stabilization and "landing."

- Monitor the height of kicks, cueing to limit range of motion to comfortable ranges. Buoyancy assists the limbs upward more dramatically in transitional water than in shallow water. In shallow water, participants can lean back to protect their backs during hip flexion, but in transitional water this position may cause a loss of balance and control.

- Have participants use gloves to pull upward toward the surface, assisting with pulling the hips down for centering over the feet.

- For most people, travel usually doesn't contribute to cardiorespiratory work by increasing resistance against the body. Buoyancy may be too difficult to

(continued)

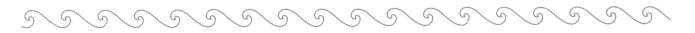

Figure 12.1 *Sample all-depth water fitness workout (continued)*

overcome and may negate the speed necessary to optimize resistance. However, travel at this depth may be effective for upper-body muscular endurance work, since the arms are necessary for movement.

- Exercise design should include vertical propulsion and long lever moves for intensity overload for both cardiorespiratory and muscle conditioning.

- Transitional water also can be treated as deep water when buoyancy equipment is used.

- Working positions for intensity regulation in transitional water are rebound (landing tall), neutral, and suspended.

SOME EXERCISE CONSIDERATIONS FOR DEEP WATER (OVER NECK DEPTH, FEET NOT TOUCHING BOTTOM, CENTER OF BALANCE AT CHEST)

- We recommend buoyancy equipment to maintain proper alignment, target muscle balance, allow rest/recovery during the session, and provide a stable base of support for speed, surface area, and lever variations.

- At this depth, submersion to the neck obscures body movements. Position yourself so you can see the movements for coaching and skills development.

- Of the three depths, deep water most highly amplifies the properties of water and individual body differences. Participants need to master the basic skills for stabilization and be allowed to work movements through the progressions at their own pace, including taking self-directed rest periods as needed.

- Every piece of equipment requires its own exercise design based on how its application affects the body, especially with regard to buoyancy gear, which may challenge a person's center of balance. Personal safety and balance skills

should be taught for each type of equipment used.

- Working positions for intensity regulation in deep water are "Power Pops" for vertical propulsion; the body positions of vertical, seated, and horizontal; and arm positions on the surface, submerged, and overhead (to decrease body buoyancy).

Resources:	Speedo Aquatic Fitness System, Instructor Training Course Videos: *Art and Science of Wave Aerobics, Specificity of Training and Deep Water Program*
Music:	*Music With a Splash, I and II Muscle Mixes: Signature Tape, Gin Miller Rocks*
Equipment:	Gloves on all participants; flotation belts on the deep water group only if the groups do not change depths; belts on all participants if they change depths during the workout

FORMAT TIPS

- All participants can optimize use of the depth if you cue them all to a basic move, then cue modifications.

- When teaching three depths at a time, cue in this order: shallow, transitional, then deep (participants in deep water move the slowest and require the most time).

- If you are moving groups from one depth to another, all participants should wear belts all the time.

- During travel sets, stop periodically and work the exercise in whatever depth they end up in!

- If you only have enough flotation belts for some of the participants, have them exchange equipment so everyone gets to go into deep water.

Set 1

1. In His Kiss — Warm up, enlarge, move around the body, stabilize, scull, balance

2. Dangerzone — **Cardio:** All depths: Jogging
Deep: Bike

3. Opposites Attract — **Cardio:** Shallow/Trans: Rock, Kick, Jumping
Deep: Tilting, Kick, Power Pops

4. Forever Man — **Cardio:** All Depths: Jax/Scissors

5. Medley: — Muscular conditioning:
Don't Leave Me — **1.** Jax (abduction)
Make You Want Me — **2.** Rhomboid/lats
Fire and Steel — **3.** Scissors for gluteals/hamstrings
Wipe Out — **4.** Triceps

Set 2

6. Hanky Panky — Warm up for depth

7. Conga — **Cardio:** All depths: Jogging
Deep: Jog/Bike

8. Alright — **Cardio:** Shallow/Trans: Rock, Kick, Jumping
Deep: Tilting, Kick, Power Pops

9. Dancing in the Streets — **Cardio:** All Depths: Jax/Scissors

10. Medley: — Muscular conditioning
Rhythms of Hope — **1.** Jax (abduction)
Jump — **2.** Rhomboids/lats
Stealing My Time — **3.** Scissors for gluteals/hamstrings
Hollywood Nights — **4.** Triceps

Set 3

11. Love Shack — Warm up, enlarge, move around the body, stabilize, scull, balance

12. Great Balls of Fire — **Cardio:** All depths: Jogging + clapping hands and pulling arms back
Deep: Bike

13. Nowhere to Run — **Cardio:** Shallow/Trans: Rock, Kick, Jumping
Deep: Tilting, Kick, Power Pops

14. Brown Sugar — **Cardio:** All Depths: Jax/Scissors

15. Medley: — Muscular conditioning
Reaching for the Best — **1.** Jax (abduction)
William Tell — **2.** Rhomboid/lats
Shout — **3.** Triceps
So Strong — **4.** Scissors for gluteals/hamstrings

For all depths, range-of-motion work for the upper body and lower major muscle groups. Participants in transitional water move to shallow. All presenters come close on deck to finish.

Play a fun song as they exit, and use moves such as Snake! or Jacuzzi!

Small group formats provide interactive time for those with shared interests, allow instructors to interact with participants on a more personal basis, and may create a more private environment for people who need special attention. If you work with cluster groups, you should be qualified to teach in the special areas that you are assigned. You also should be prepared for more personal interaction, which may include performing fitness assessments, reading and responding to participant journals (diaries of personal responses to exercise), and communicating with health care providers for those with health conditions.

Personal training presents a challenge for you to be responsive to the individual needs of a single participant. You should be ready to take responsibility for guiding the participant to a positive outcome that in most cases needs to be measured using fitness assessments and also may need to be monitored by the participant's health care provider.

Other personal training opportunities may exist with athletes who need post-rehabilitation work or who simply are seeking to supplement their land training with water training. Working with their physical therapists or their coaches is a must to ensure positive results.

Participants who want to bridge land-to-water training, learn new skills to enhance their training program, or introduce themselves to working out in the water and maybe even swimming can benefit from working one on one with a personal trainer. The trainer can respond to their specific objectives with an effective, well-designed program.

For more on this topic, see the section "Personal Training" later in this chapter. Part Four provides training information for working with specialty groups and participants with medical considerations.

Progressive Program Design

Having a wide variety of programs gives participants choices, whether they are members of group exercise or personal training classes.

Skills and drills classes offer participants the opportunity to develop, work, and practice their skills. These popular classes are usually taught without music so instructors can provide effective feedback for skill development.

Advanced classes are necessary so participants from skills and drills classes can eventually move into more advanced workouts, such as the all-depths workout in figure 12.1, or athletic training. Classes such as these should be limited to participants who are highly skilled so intensity and skills can be more challenging.

The mind/body approach to class design has an inward focus and includes exercises that are "breath centered." The program should be "process oriented" and most probably will be conducted at a lower intensity than mainstream fitness programs. Cues need to focus on "mindful movements" that integrate the body's movements with breathing and the feelings of energy flowing through the body. This type of class requires special training and cueing to invoke the inward focus participants need to discover their own mindful approach to health.

In land and water bridging classes participants are encouraged to do land exercise as well as their water program. A good resource for simple, supplementary exercises, especially for women, is the book *Strong Women Stay Strong* by Miriam E. Nelson. You can recommend that participants purchase the book and work on their own, or you can hold a dry land class to teach them exercises that they can perform on days when they cannot get to the pool or as additional work.

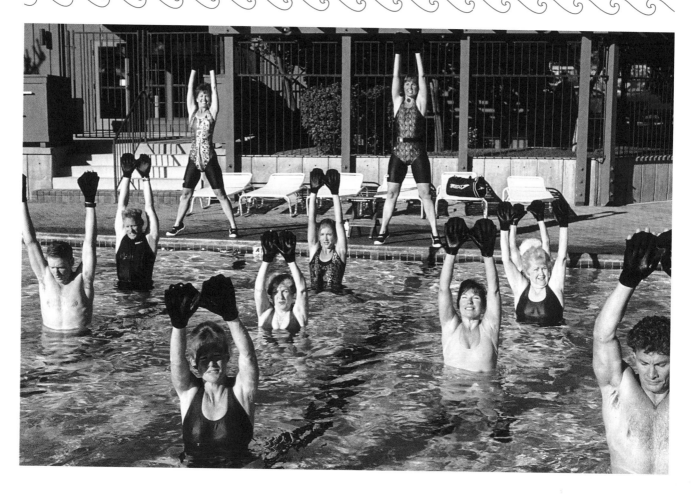

Water Fitness During Recovery From Injuries

"My knees ache during step class so I'd like to try water exercise instead."

"I have a stress fracture in my foot, and my doctor told me I could exercise in the water."

As a water exercise instructor or personal trainer, are you prepared to meet the specific needs of these participants? If not, you're missing a golden opportunity to add more participants to your classes and meet their needs.

Water exercise is becoming increasingly popular for individuals recovering from injuries. In fact, with recent changes in the health care system, it's likely that individuals with stress fractures, chronic knee pain, and other injuries will be mainstreamed into your water program. Rich Ruoti, founder of the American Physical Therapy Association Aquatic Therapy Section, believes that insurance changes with health care reform will result in less direct physical therapy care. This means more people may be participating in water exercise after rehabilitation.

To ensure that these individuals enjoy water exercise and don't aggravate their injuries, both you and your participants must nurture working relationships with their medical providers. Easier said than done? Not if you follow some general guidelines for working successfully with the medical community.

Physicians and physical therapists are more likely to recommend your program to their patients if they believe you are knowledgeable and offer safe, effective exercises. Personally visit local medical providers to promote your program. Dress professionally for the appointment and keep your visit brief. You will want to do the following:

1. Provide evidence of staff credentials, class protocol, and emergency procedures.

2. Show off your facility. Take a promotional brochure or videotape of the facility.

3. Explain specific exercises and equipment used in your classes. Use diagrams of moves and take samples of equipment, or show a promotional videotape demonstrating exercises and equipment.

4. Solicit specific recommendations from the physician or physical therapist about exercise protocol and equipment.

Fostering communication between your participants and their medical providers will help to make mainstreaming participants easier and more effective. Participants who discuss their exercise programs with their medical providers will have a better understanding of what to do in the water.

As an instructor, you can supply participants with a list of questions to promote discussion between them and their medical providers, including the following:

- What is my injury?

- Do you feel it is safe for me to exercise in the water?

- Does the water need to be a certain temperature? (For example, arthritis sufferers perform better in warmer water.)

- How much weight can I place on my injury while in the water? (Forty to fifty percent weight bearing indicates that waist-deep water is appropriate; ten percent weight bearing calls for neck-deep water; zero percent weight bearing means deep water with flotation devices.)

- Are there certain exercises/moves I should not do in the water?

- Are there specific exercises you want me to do in the water?

- Can I increase my joint range of motion if the injured area is pain free? (For example, individuals with an anterior cruciate ligament [knee] sprain should not perform full-knee extensions, even if they are pain free.)

- Should I restrict my exercise intensity while in the water? (For example, participants with myofascial pain generally must perform at low intensity.) If so, can I increase the intensity if I am pain free?

- Are there certain pieces of buoyancy equipment, such as dumbbells, that I should not use?

- If I experience pain, stiffness, or swelling during water exercise, should I stop, decrease my intensity, or keep going? (In instances in which participants are working to increase joint range of motion, they can reasonably expect some discomfort. These individuals would probably be instructed to continue water exercise without restrictions.)

Participants should obtain this information from their physician or physical therapist and return it to you prior to participating in your program.

You can use a health screening form such as the PAR-Q (recommended by the American College of Sports Medicine) to determine participants who are at risk. In addition, you can ask participants to complete a more detailed health history form. A form such as this must be kept confidential and should be given to anyone whose responses to the health screening form indicate potential risk factors that may preclude participation in water exercise. Follow your YMCA's policy on assessing participants prior to exercise.

Whether you communicate with medical providers through a personal visit or information from a participant information form, it is important that you make contact. Water exercise is becoming increasingly popular as a form of physical therapy. After being released from their medical providers, many participants will want to continue exercising in the water. It offers a safe exercise environment, providing less stress to the joints than land exercise. Water resistance also is an excellent way for individuals with musculoskeletal problems to increase strength and improve their overall health and fitness. With the American College of Sports Medicine and Centers for Disease Control's new recommendations emphasizing improved health through safe and moderate workouts, water exercise is sure to be a mainstay!

Refer to Part Four for information on working in this area of health.

Personal Training

The demand for trained fitness professionals to serve personal training clients is growing. Clients who have special needs can benefit from a trainer who is educated in both land and water exercise programs. An increasing number of health care providers are referring clients to personal trainers to bridge the gap between therapy treatments performed by licensed therapists and post-rehabilitation fitness/wellness programs. "Apparently healthy" clients can be trained one on one using the skills already discussed in this book, while in Part Four we will address some of the specific skills needed to work with special populations.

According to personal trainer Douglas Brooks (1997), "individual, personal commitment and service are the essence of personal training" (p.11). One size fits all definitely does not apply to the individual needs of clients. Personal trainers should provide individualized programs that clients will be motivated enough to continue for a lifetime of personal health. To be able to understand clients' needs and to respond effectively, personal trainers must have strong communication skills. As clients need to find value in the programs being offered to them by the trainer, trainers need to know how to meet the training objectives of their clients while keeping clients motivated.

Trainers commonly use periodic fitness assessments to track the progress of their clients and to evaluate their program's effectiveness. For clients from special populations, these assessments are an important component of their health care program, measuring post-rehabilitation or functional gains that will lead to more independence.

Kathie Davis, executive director of IDEA, The Health and Fitness Source, reports (1999) that IDEA members say "in addition to the skills to design appropriate exercise programs for their clients, trainers need the ability to answer clients' questions on a variety of issues and know how to handle business challenges" (p.7). Clients may require diverse health programs that include areas of expertise outside the personal trainer's scope of practice or training. For example, clients may need coaching for nutrition, motivation, psychological problems, medical conditions, or lifestyle problems. Besides being able to understand and respond to a client's needs within his or her area of expertise, a personal trainer must also know how and when to refer clients to other professionals who can help clients meet their wellness objectives.

Personal trainers also need to be educated in the business and legal aspects of fitness, including forms of businesses, insurance coverage, billing practices, contractual agreements, and balancing of personal and professional workloads. While it can be very rewarding to see clients succeed, trainers who work with many different clients must be skilled at balancing their own lives with their clients' needs if personal training is to work for both clients and trainer.

For more information, look at the YMCA's personal training program for personal trainers.

Bibliography

Brooks, D. 1997. *Program design for personal trainers: Bridging theory into application.* Champaign, IL: Human Kinetics.

Davis, K. 1999. Your need to know. *IDEA Personal Trainer Magazine* 10(6): 7.

LaForge, R. 1996. The science and application of mind-body fitness. Presentation at YMCA of the USA Healthy People Conference, October 10–13, Orlando, FL.

Nelson, M. 1997. *Strong women stay young.* New York: Bantam Books.

Sanders, M. and N. Rippee. 1994. *Speedo aquatic fitness system, instructor training manual.* London: Speedo International.

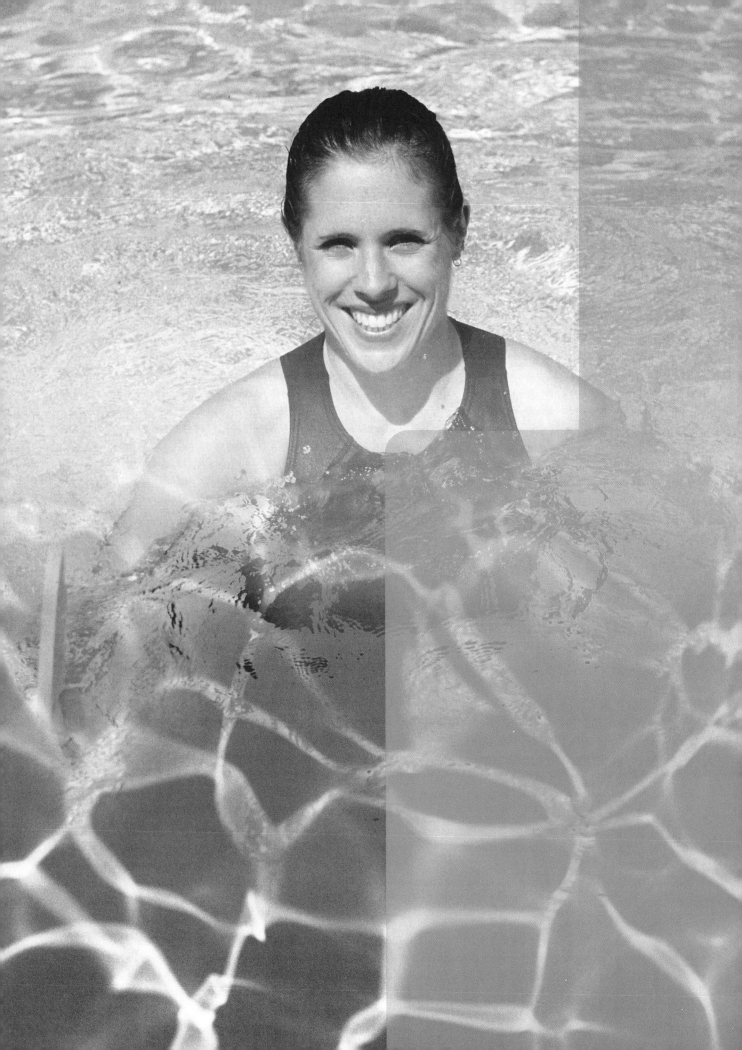

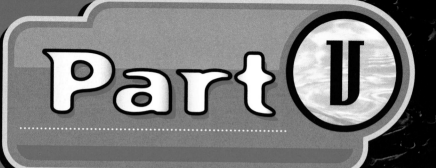

Part V

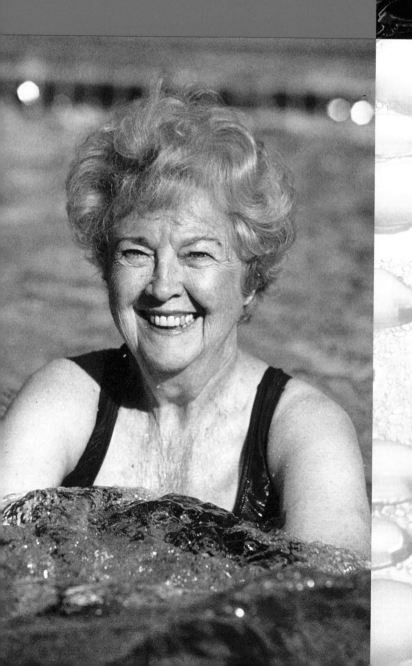

Responsive Programs
for Participants With
Individual Challenges

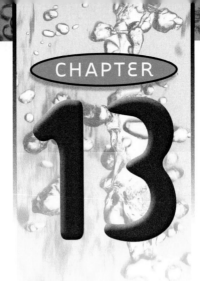

CHAPTER

13

Functional Training for Healthy Living on Land

MARY E. SANDERS AND CATHY MALONEY-HILLS

Objectives:

- To describe the various aquatic exercise programs available to YMCA members and the types of exercise training activities offered in each program

- To define the terms *functional ADL* and *functional exercises* and to describe the purpose of assessing function for water exercise participants

- To describe the YMCA's Golden Waves™ program for functional ADL fitness

- To describe sample exercise progressions and a workout format for a functional ADL fitness program

The YMCA Water Fitness Program is designed to satisfy a wide range of individual needs. As membership and participation in YMCAs grow, we need to provide programs that best meet the abilities and interests of each member and participant. In the past, many Ys offered only a small number of water exercise classes that did not address special conditions presented by many of the participants. With the introduction of YMCA Water Fitness, YMCAs will be able to serve the wide range of needs of individuals across the country. YMCA Water Fitness is progressive, challenging the interests and abilities of all participants.

The goal of YMCA Water Fitness is to help participants improve their health and functioning in their daily lives. A variety of programs should be offered in order to challenge the broad spectrum of individual

health and fitness levels common today. The different levels of participation include post-rehabilitation, functional and physical fitness programs, as well as sports-specific training. All instructors, participants, and health care providers involved should have a clear understanding of each of these programs. The following descriptions may help with appropriate placement of participants in each program and with identifying professionals' roles in these programs:

- **Rehabilitation.** Rehabilitation can be defined as restoration or enhancement of functional ability following disease, illness, or injury (Stedman, 1976, p. 1217). Goals of rehabilitation can include improving strength, range of motion, cardiorespiratory endurance, muscular endurance, coordination, balance, flexibility, and communication skills. Achieving these goals enables individuals to perform activities of daily living (ADL) safely and with the greatest independence possible. ADL include transfers (moving in or out of the bed, toilet, bath, chair, car, floor), dressing, bathing, cooking, cleaning, carrying, lifting, doing yard work, and all activities performed in the home or outside environment. Rehabilitation is provided by a licensed health care provider such as a physical, occupational, recreation, or speech therapist.

- **Post-Rehabilitation/Therapy.** Clients who have been discharged from treatment by their health care providers can be cleared to participate in community-based exercise programs.

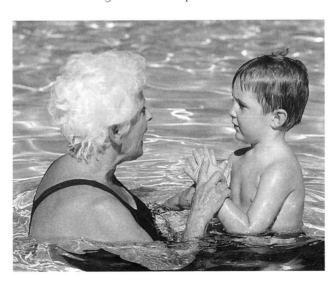

Close communication between the health care provider and fitness professional is essential to provide appropriate placement, specific goals, guidelines, and modifications for the former patient's safe participation in the exercise program. Progression to more challenging programs occurs after the goals are reached. Primary objectives for these individuals would include increasing range of motion, muscular strength and endurance, and cardiovascular-respiratory endurance, and improving balance and the efficiency of ADL.

- **Functional Fitness.** The emphasis in functional fitness is to improve the quality of life for spirit, mind, and body. It targets improvement in ADL with specific objectives in mind. Outcomes related to the objectives can be measured and documented, such as decreased blood pressure, body fat, or cholesterol or increased bone density, strength, range of

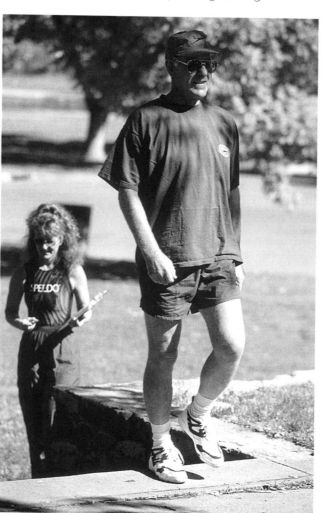

motion, endurance, or functional abilities. Functional gains can include something as simple as the ability to walk up a flight of stairs without stopping. Functionally designed exercises can help participants minimize the limiting effects of aging and help them maximize their independence. Measurements are taken to document the improvements that participants have achieved and the specificity of the training they receive. Participation can help prevent loss of bone and muscle mass, improve cardiovascular-vascular health, avoid or delay surgery, and decrease the use of medication (with the physician's guidance). Individuals can manage chronic problems such as arthritis, hypertension, asthma, or back pain more effectively.

- **Physical Fitness.** Physical fitness is a state characterized by an ability to perform daily activities with vigor. It also decreases the risk of developing diseases or medical conditions associated with inactivity (Pate et al., 1995). Fitness programs are geared to healthy, motivated individuals who want little supervision and are able to work out on their own. The primary emphasis is on the improvement of cardiorespiratory endurance, body composition, muscular endurance, and flexibility. Fitness programs may also provide training for specific sports.

A large number of YMCAs have collaborated with local hospitals or clinics in providing rehabilitation by licensed health care providers on-site at the Y. This is a growing trend that enables the general public to have easy access to all aspects of health and fitness enhancement. Providing all components of rehabilitation and fitness at the Y also increases awareness and communication between health care providers and fitness professionals. This optimizes the progression of participants through all appropriate levels from rehabilitation to fitness and sports-specific training.

The purpose of this chapter is to describe the type of program needed for a water fitness ADL training program. We provide brief descriptions of a sample program, sample workouts, and class format. A good ADL training program has appropriate screening, program placement, goal setting, reassessment, and communication with health care providers when necessary. This ensures that participants can progress safely through the various training levels to their goal of enjoying complete independence and health.

Table 13.1 *Suggested Program Placements*

Intensity (low)   *(high)*

	AFYAP training	AFYAP plus	Functional fitness	Physical fitness	Elite athletic
	Low int. ex. ROM Mulitdir. walking Balance act.	Same as AFYAP plus higher CV workout	ADL Musc. strength and endurance ROM CV Balance act.	Musc. strength and endurance CV Body comp. Rec. and life enh. act.	Sport-specific training CV Body comp. Musc. strength and endurance
Post-rehabilitation training	+	+	+	+	+
Ready to be fit	+	+	+	+	
Healthy population with no special conditions			+	+	+
Athletes				+	+

KEY

Multidir. walking = Multidirectional walking

Low int. ex. = Low intensity exercise

ROM = Range of motion

Balance act. = Balance activities

CV = Cardiovascular training

AFYAP = Arthritis Foundation YMCA Arthritis Program

ADL = Activities of daily living

Musc. strength and endurance = Muscular strength and endurance

Body comp. = Body composition

Rec. and life enh. act. = Recreation and life enhancement activities

Table 13.1 shows suggested program placements for various populations, ranging from post-rehabilitation/ therapy to elite athletes. It also includes the types of exercise training and activities performed in each program. The + represents the potential starting level for each group, with placement determined from PAR-Q and fitness assessment results. Trained instructors assist participants in developing specific goals and objectives that can be measured and evaluated. This motivates participants and builds their self-management skills. Participants should move up to the next level, establishing new long-term goals and short-term objectives, when they have reached the goals of the current program.

Functional ADL Fitness

When fitness professionals know the definitions and examples of functional activities and exercises, they can use them appropriately in fitness activities. Functional activities, or ADL, are those tasks an individual performs in order to care for himself or herself, be mobile in the environment, and care for all daily needs. The list of tasks can be limitless, depending on the individual's activity level and independence within or outside of his or her home environment. A great variance in functional activities can exist, especially with older adults, depending on their health, lifestyle, occupational status, and activity level (Lewis, 1985).

Functional exercise can therefore be defined as those exercises designed to most closely simulate the individual's identified functional activities. The most fundamental principle taught to physical education teachers is that *learning is specific to the task* (Lewis, 1985). Performing active range-of-motion exercises and walking will improve range of motion and walking. Improving one's ability to vacuum a rug requires exercises that incorporate walking and multidirectional lunging (with correct body mechanics, of course), balance activities, and pushing and pulling against resistance. To set goals, instructors must define the individual's current functional abilities, set goals for improvement, and then reassess progress in order to set future goals. Even when it is impossible to evaluate and set goals on an individual basis, most older adults would improve their efficiency in performing functional activities through practice.

A number of studies support the idea that water training, when properly designed, can improve land tasks, whether it's running a marathon or climbing up and down stairs. (See "Functional Exercise" in chapter 6 for details of these studies.) The water is the perfect environment in which to do this because it provides variable, multidirectional resistance; greater safety than land (especially for balance activities); and the benefits of not loading the joints. However, simulating land tasks in the water requires that the instructor correctly apply the properties of water to the simulations. He or she must have a thorough understanding of how buoyancy and resistance can be varied to most effectively mimic land activity.

Listening to conversations among older adults, one can hear comments such as "Things just aren't the way they used to be" or "I'm finding it harder to _____ every day." As a result of the changes to the mind and body that occur with aging, older adults find many functional activities become more challenging. Some common functional difficulties include getting out of bed or a chair, walking up or down stairs (especially on buses), pushing a shopping cart, walking fast, making directional changes, reaching, recovering balance, carrying groceries, or picking up items from the floor. Picking up and holding a grandchild can be a physical challenge.

Difficulty with functional ADL is usually associated with older adults, but a recent study dispels this belief. Preliminary findings from a study of 10,000 women aged 40 to 55 (Gold, 1998) show that 20 percent have trouble with simple functional activities such as walking a block or up a flight of stairs and carrying groceries. Obesity and sedentary lifestyles have begun to take their toll on a much younger population. This study demonstrates the importance of functional assessments and training for populations of all ages (Gold, 1998).

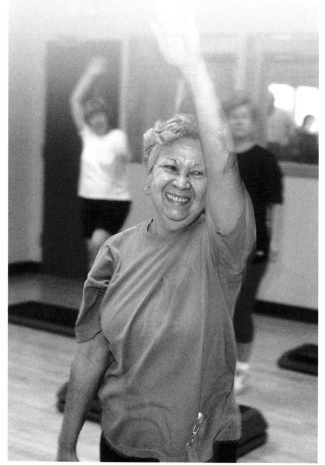

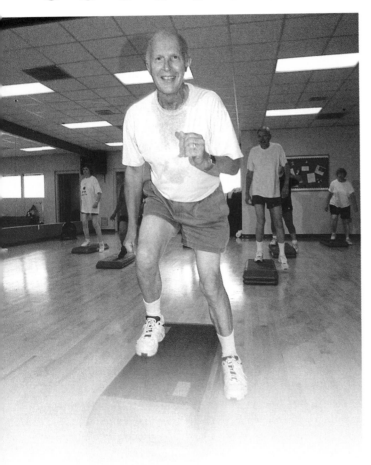

A number of tests are available to evaluate functional abilities, with some examining all aspects of function including communication, eating, hygiene, and personal care and home management. A simple assessment of function appropriate for individuals participating in a community-based group exercise program has been provided (see chapter 16). It measures basic functional activities for older adults who are independent in home and community activities. All or part of this evaluation potentially can be used to assess individual performance.

Functional assessments are typically not done until an individual has an impairment that requires it. Information gained from evaluating functional abilities in seemingly self-sufficient older adults, combined with some basic safety guidelines for home and community, could prevent future falls and accidents. This would be a tremendous service to provide to our rapidly growing older adult population.

This section has clearly defined functional ADL and functional exercise, emphasized their importance in all fitness training, and provided tools to evaluate functional activities. Now let's look at an ADL training program already in use at YMCAs.

Golden Waves ™ as a Sample Functional ADL Program

Functionally targeted ADL programs are not limited to older adults. Other adults who have any type of limitation or who may be unable to perform tasks to achieve their optimal quality of life can be encouraged to add tasks specific to their life objectives. Whether a participant wants to improve at playing golf or at getting into and out of a chair, exercises can be designed to address the goal. In this section, we'll investigate a basic ADL program that targets common ADL such as lifting groceries, walking quickly, balancing, reaching, gripping, and moving from a sit to a stand more efficiently.

The Golden Waves ™ Functional Water Training for Health Program began as a research study, funded in part by a grant from the Sanford Center for Aging, University of Nevada, Reno. The program continues now as a YMCA program. During the study, program adherence was 94 percent, and after two years, over 50 percent of the original subjects still participated in the program as members of the local YMCA. The program is conducted in shallow water at water temperatures of approximately 27 to 29 degrees C (81 to 84 degrees F). Program format consists of 60-minute sessions, with the first 15 minutes for undirected pool activity. This time is used for individual special coaching by an instructor if necessary, but primarily it's the group's time for social interaction, gentle walking and talking to warm up and catch up! Waterproof name tags ensure personal interaction. The final 45 minutes are directed by instructors (1 instructor to every 10 participants). Class meets three days a week. A sample weekly training progression is shown in table 13.2.

As participants become more skilled, workouts include additional progressions and faster transitions, with less time spent on skill development and more time on performance. The instructor-to-participant ratio may change, with fewer instructors needed.

Table 13.2 *Weekly Training Progression*

Day	Learning objective	Instructor intervention
Monday	New skills learning, directed participant practice. Usually music is not used.	Deck instruction plus one-on-one instruction as needed in pool.
Wednesday	Skills review and progressive drills practice for individualized overload and modifications. Music is used intermittently.	Deck instruction plus cluster group work with pool instructors.
Friday	Application of skills and progressions into a continuous workout sequence using music.	Deck instruction. In-water instructors cue, motivate, and give general feedback.

The exercises are designed primarily to target improved functional capacity for activity on land. Careful consideration is taken to use the properties of water effectively in maximizing resistance for strengthening the quadriceps, hamstrings, gluteal muscles, trunk stabilizers, and upper-body muscles. A thermal component is included so participants can stay warm. Most of the exercises are performed while traveling through the water and all are done without wall support. Some participants wear inflatable flotation belts to assist with balance. The belt can be inflated partially or fully, depending on the amount of support necessary (and for which part of the body it's needed), and can be adjusted on the spot. Participants who need more support are encouraged to use a buoyancy dumbbell or in some cases a ski pole with a tennis ball on the tip. Wall support is advised only as a last resort to encourage participants to "trust" buoyancy for support as they work beyond their gravity-based center of balance. They are encouraged to make errors in movement in order to learn balance correction and minimize fear of falling in the water. Functional movement patterns are performed in the pool to target agility, stair climbing, standing from a sitting position, balance, speed walking, stride length, and error corrections during many movement patterns.

Participants are carefully coached to go at their own pace and modify each exercise as needed. (Movement modifications for participants' individual needs are discussed in chapter 14.) Instructors help participants learn to regulate and modify their own exercises and teach participants the skills to monitor their own intensity. Perceived exertion and occasionally heart rate monitors are used to monitor intensity. Participants are taught the 4 S's (see chapters 9 and 11) and they are reinforced during every class. The 15-minute class period before instruction begins gives instructors time to work with special participants, designing appropriate modifications in response to individual needs. After participants learn these, they are empowered to take responsibility for their own intensity and modifications. All of the participants suffer from at least one chronic condition (usually arthritis or hypertension) and/or post-rehabilitation conditions.

Participants are encouraged to keep journals, which are collected regularly for review and comment by the instructors. By learning about the participants, instructors can design classes responsively so that the program can be based on individual experiences and needs. Health care providers monitoring a medical condition appreciate the dated documentation written by their patients themselves. Additionally, instructors create a newsletter for participants that has educational tips to reinforce learning. It includes the purpose of the exercises, the major muscle groups worked, the training objectives, the intensity progressions, definitions of terms used in class, and topics related to general health.

Figure 13.1 is an example of a handout developed to teach participants the names of the major muscle groups and how they function during daily tasks.

Figure 13.1 *Sample muscle identification handout*

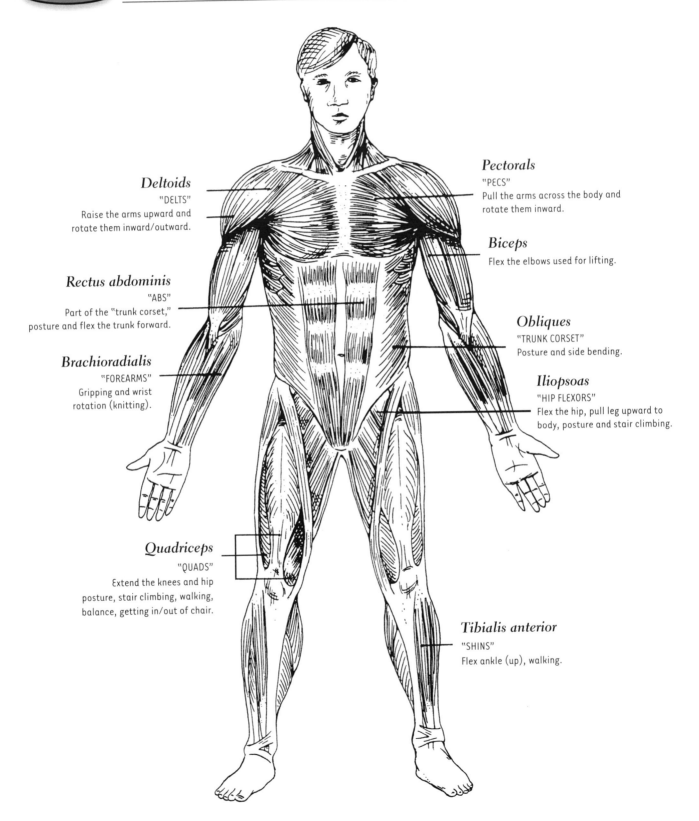

Deltoids
"DELTS"
Raise the arms upward and
rotate them inward/outward.

Rectus abdominis
"ABS"
Part of the "trunk corset,"
posture and flex the trunk forward.

Brachioradialis
"FOREARMS"
Gripping and wrist
rotation (knitting).

Quadriceps
"QUADS"
Extend the knees and hip
posture, stair climbing, walking,
balance, getting in/out of chair.

Pectorals
"PECS"
Pull the arms across the body and
rotate them inward.

Biceps
Flex the elbows used for lifting.

Obliques
"TRUNK CORSET"
Posture and side bending.

Iliopsoas
"HIP FLEXORS"
Flex the hip, pull leg upward to
body, posture and stair climbing.

Tibialis anterior
"SHINS"
Flex ankle (up), walking.

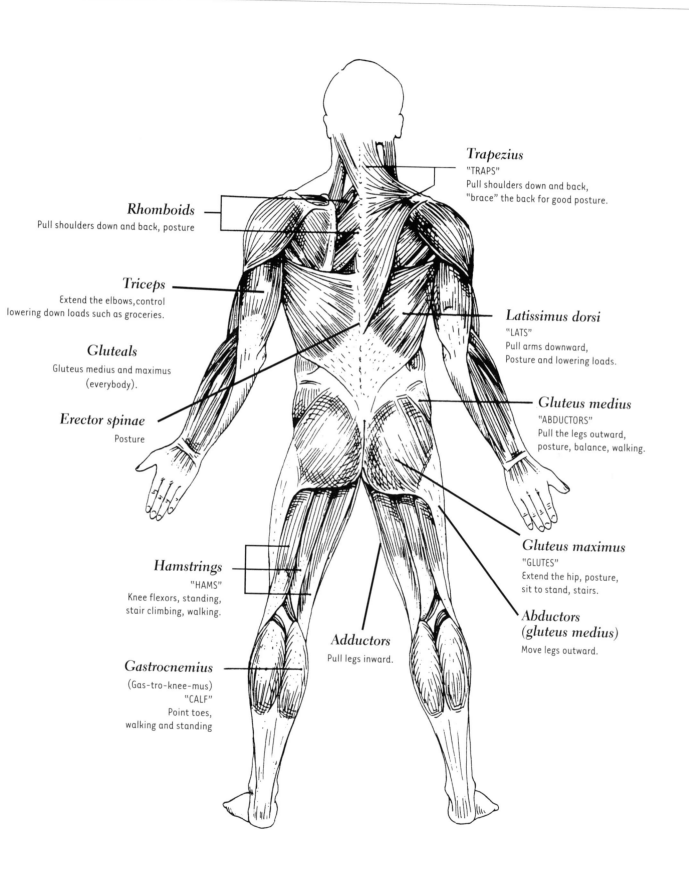

Trapezius
"TRAPS"
Pull shoulders down and back,
"brace" the back for good posture.

Rhomboids
Pull shoulders down and back, posture

Triceps
Extend the elbows, control
lowering down loads such as groceries.

Latissimus dorsi
"LATS"
Pull arms downward,
Posture and lowering loads.

Gluteals
Gluteus medius and maximus
(everybody).

Erector spinae
Posture

Gluteus medius
"ABDUCTORS"
Pull the legs outward,
posture, balance, walking.

Gluteus maximus
"GLUTES"
Extend the hip, posture,
sit to stand, stairs.

Hamstrings
"HAMS"
Knee flexors, standing,
stair climbing, walking.

**Abductors
(gluteus medius)**
Move legs outward.

Adductors
Pull legs inward.

Gastrocnemius
(Gas-tro-knee-mus)
"CALF"
Point toes,
walking and standing

Sample Golden Waves™ Exercise Progressions

Appendix B shows some sample exercise progressions from Golden Waves™. We recommend that participants complete a screening form and a health history questionnaire before they participate in your program. Begin each session with a thorough thermal warm-up that includes water adjustment, stabilization skills (sculling), neutral posture and gaze stabilization practice, modified recovery to a stand (lift feet slightly, small movements, more vertical position), range of motion with cues for functional range, and suggested modifications (see chapter 15). Review the responsive teaching progression in chapter 11. Let your participants know the workout objective and get going!

Encourage participants to work the progression until they find the level that provides enough overload for work but is not so high that they feel uncomfortable. If they experience any pain or limitations in range of motion, they should modify the move or replace it with a similar move that feels comfortable. Motivate participants to try to work up the progression, and review the 4 S's so they can easily lower intensity for comfort and control.

The exercises in the ADL section of appendix C are provided to functionally challenge participants in aquatics fitness classes. They are by no means the only exercises to do, for the best exercises are those based on what participants demonstrate or mention as their functional difficulties. The limits are set only by the instructor's creativity. The responses of participants will be very enthusiastic, and the rewards will be very noticeable in six to eight weeks!

Sample Workout Format

When you design a functional ADL workout, follow the same guidelines as you would for a basic workout (presented in chapters 9 and 10), but give special consideration to creating exercise progressions that keep participants warm when working out in cool water (below 84 degrees F.). Consider the skill and fitness levels of the participants, the class objectives, and any special medical modifications that may be needed. If you create interval workouts, participants have built-in times to rest, so when you alternate a muscular endurance set with a cardiorespiratory endurance set, participants may be able to pace themselves more easily. Teach progressions so participants can find the level that's right for them.

Figure 13.2 shows some sample lesson plans for a functional ADL workout. For additional exercise progressions and workouts, watch the following two videos, *The Golden Waves™ Functional Water Training Program for Health* and *The Golden Waves™ Functional Water Training II Advanced Progressions*, and read *The Golden Waves™ Aging Adults Leadership Course*.

Figure 13.1 *Sample functional ADL workout lesson plans*

Class 1

*One instructor on deck, two in the water;
45 min on deck, 15 min in pool*

1. Give participants an orientation to the program. Ask them to fill out health history and screening forms, then talk to each participant individually about his or her interests and needs related to the program. Show participants the *Golden Waves™ Functional Water Training Program for Health* video.

2. Demonstrate how to pack a workout bag: towel, water shoes, lotion, hair gel, webbed gloves, swimsuit, cosmetics, plastic bag for wet items. Place water bottles at poolside.

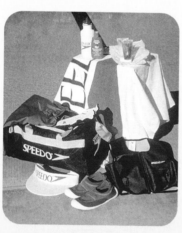

3. Introduce participants to the workout environment. Explain the sign-in sheets and your method of taking attendance. Give participants a tour of the pool working areas, pointing out the shallow and deep water and the locker room. Provide them with precautions and safety tips for the pool, deck, and locker room. Demonstrate how to safely get into and out of the pool.

4. Have participants practice getting into the pool. Have spotters at the ladders or stairs.

Once they have gotten into the water, they should splash water under their arms. If they are using webbed gloves, they should put them on and practice using them, feeling the water's support. (They should never put them on before entering the water.) Show them how they can use the gloves as rudders for balance. They should find their proper water depth, check their posture, and practice getting into correct posture against the wall. Have them practice sculling, both flat and with fingers down or up to assist with travel forward and backward. Show them how to take the ready position (see chapter 8).

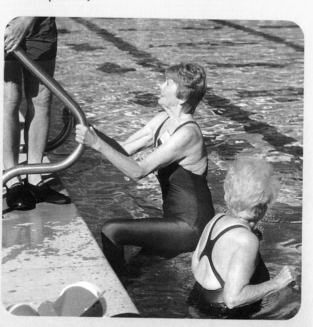

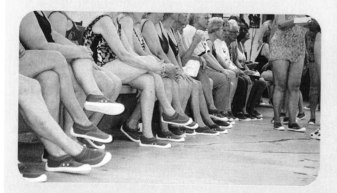

(continued)

Figure 13.1 *Sample functional ADL workout lesson plans (continued)*

5. Do some workout activities (stationary movements only, if necessary). Have them practice sculling, both for stabilization and travel (if possible). Have them jog for a lap or circle around, then take the ready position. They can walk or jog in a number of ways: working legs around the body; traveling, then stopping and stabilizing; moving forward, sideways, or backward. If participants cannot travel, have them work in place, jogging or performing crosswise patterns. Finally, have them practice gentle range-of-motion work.

6. Have participants exit the pool, with spotters in place.

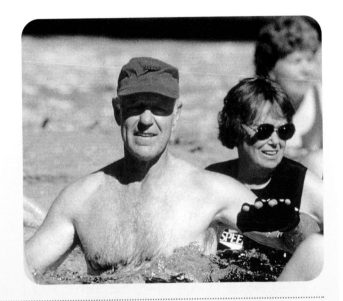

Class 2
15 min on deck, 30 min in pool

1. Prepare for entry. Check the sign-in sheets and put the water bottles at poolside. Have participants enter the pool. If needed, have two spotters in the pool to assist participants in entering and exiting the pool.

2. Have participants perform skills development activities. Find the correct depth for participants and then have them practice sculling and walking. Teach them how to

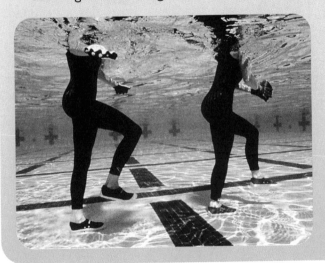

recover to a stand. Have them warm up by sculling and marching in place, then walk or jog working the legs around the body. Review proper body alignment, and teach them the ready position and the "I surrender" position for upper-body posture. (The "I surrender" position is with arms at the sides, elbows bent and palms forward. Arms are lifted to shoulder level, then lowered back down.) Finally, teach them the cues for "new move" and "enlarge the move."

3. Have participants practice marching in place or jogging through the 4 S's. Use the "Joint Energy" movements (walk/jog and range of motion) from *The Golden Waves Functional Water Training Program for Health.* Follow this sequence:

- Jog sideways, hold. Perform range-of-motion movements for the shoulders.

- Jog sideways, hold. Perform range-of-motion movements for the elbows.

- Jog sideways, hold. Perform range-of-motion movements for the hip.

- Jog, hold, repeat hip range-of-motion movements on the other side.
- Jog, hold, perform range-of-motion movements for the knee.
- Jog, hold, repeat on the other knee.
- Jog, hold, relax the hands by swishing them back and forth in the water.

This can be done to the song "Rum and Coca-Cola."

4. Have participants perform the walking and "Freeze Frame" progression (see *The Golden Waves™ Program* video or appendix B). It can be done to the song "Bop."
5. Lead participants through a warm-down. Have participants do a shoulder stretch, a giant walk for hip flexors, a pectoral stretch in which they drag the arms behind, neck tilts (tilt head gently side to side, lift chin up and forward), and an Indian sit (squat with one leg crossed) for the gluteals. Tell participants to exit from the pool.

Classes 3 and 4

60 min: 15 min of self-directed walking and 45 min of instructor-directed progressions

1. Have participants warm up using coordinated skills: jogging and kicking or rocking.
2. Use the following exercises from *The Golden Waves™ Program* video (and appendixes B and C):

- "Joint Energy" for joint range-of-motion and light cardiorespiratory work

- "Freeze Frame" for balance and walking
- "Play Ball" for gripping and light cardiorespiratory work
- "Clock Squats" for lower-body strength, balance, and coordination

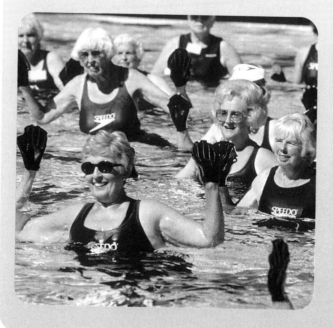
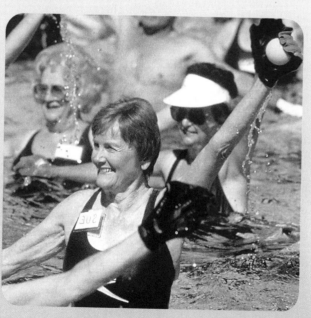

(continued)

Figure 13.1 *Sample functional ADL workout lesson plans (continued)*

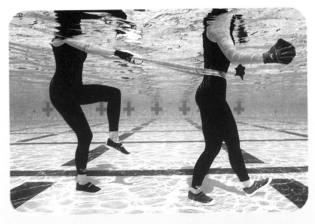
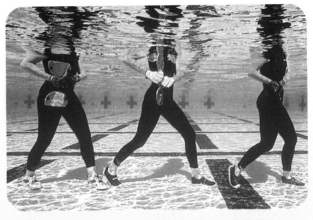
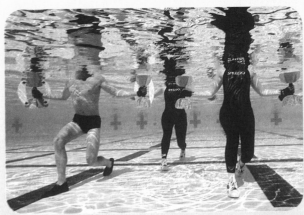
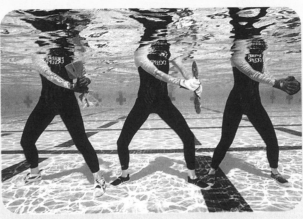

- "Leash Me" for balance correction and increasing stride length for the person walking and cardiorespiratory training and thermal work for the person who tugs on the resistance band
- Upper-body resistance work wearing webbed gloves, targeting the upper back
- Pretending to vacuum, working the trunk and upper body

3. Have participants warm down with active stretches: "Back Rub for Range of Motion," dynamic stretching using the water's buoyancy (fluid stretches), falls backward, neck and shoulder stretching, hamstring and quadriceps stretching, pectoral stretching, and back releases.

Bibliography

Bushman, B., M. Flynn, F. Andres, C. Lambert, M. Taylor, and W. Braun. 1997. Effect of 4 weeks of deep water run training on running performance. *Medicine and Science in Sports and Exercise* 29(5): 694–699.

Gold, E. 1998. Interview by author. University of California, Medical School, Davis, The study of women across the nation (SWAN).

Landgridge, J., and D. Phillips. 1988. Group hydrotherapy exercises for chronic back pain sufferers. *Physiotherapy* 74(6): 269–273.

Lewis, C. 1985. *Aging, the health care challenge: An interdisciplinary approach to assessment and rehabilitation management of the elderly.* Philadelphia: F.A. Davis.

Lewis, C., and K. Knortz. 1993. *Orthopedic assessment and treatment of the geriatric patient.* St. Louis: Mosby Yearbook.

Michaud, T., D. Brennan, et al. 1995. Aquarunning and gains in cardiorespiratory fitness. *Medicine and Science in Sports and Exercise* 9(2): 78–84.

Pate, R., M. Pratt, S. Blair, W. Haskell, C. Macera, C. Bouchard, D. Buchner, W. Ettinger, G. Heath, A. King, A. Kriska, A. Leon, B. Marcus, J. Morris, R. Paffenbarger, K. Patrick, M. Pollock, J. Rippe, J. Sallis, and J. Wilmore. 1995. Physical activity and public health: A recommendation from the Centers for Disease Control and Prevention and the American College of Sports Medicine. *JAMA* 273(5): 402–407.

Sanders, M., N. Constantino, and N. Rippee. 1997. A comparison of results of functional water training on field and laboratory measures in older women. *Medicine and Science in Sports and Exercise* 29(5): Abstract 630.

Sanders, M., and C. Maloney-Hills. 1998. Aquatic exercise for better living on land. *ACSM's Health and Fitness Journal* 2(3):16–23.

Sanders, M., and N. Rippee. 1993. *Speedo aquatic fitness system, instructor training manual.* London: Speedo International.

Siegel, A.J., M.J. Warhol, and E. Lang. 1986. Muscle injury and repair in ultra long distance runners. In *Sports Medicine for the Master Athlete*, eds. J.R. Sutton and R.M. Brock, pp. 35–43. Indianapolis, IN: Benchmark Press.

Simmons, V., and P. Hansen. 1996. Effectiveness of water exercise on postural mobility in the well elderly: An experimental study on balance enhancement. *Journal of Gerontology: Medical Sciences* 51A: 5 M233–M238.

Smit, T., and R. Harrison. 1991. Hydrotherapy and chronic lower back pain: A pilot study. *Australian Journal of Physiotherapy* 37(4): 229–234.

Spirduso, W. 1996. *Physical dimensions of aging.* Champaign, IL: Human Kinetics.

Stedman, T.L. 1976. *Stedman's medical dictionary* (23rd ed.) Baltimore: Williams and Wilkins.

Suomi, R., and S. Lindaur. 1997. Effectiveness of Arthritis Foundation program on strength and range of motion in women with arthritis. *Journal of Aging and Physical Activity* 5: 341–351.

Templeton, M.S., D. L. Booth, and W.D. O'Kelly. 1996. Effects of aquatic therapy on joint flexibility and functional ability in subjects with rheumatic disease. *Journal of Orthopaedic and Sports Physical Therapy* 23(6): 376–381.

14

Exercise Considerations for Older Adults

CATHY MALONEY-HILLS AND MARY E. SANDERS

WITH ADAPTED EXCERPTS FROM *ACTIVE OLDER ADULTS IN THE YMCA:
A RESOURCE MANUAL BY ANN HOOKE AND MARY ZOLLER**

Objectives:

◎ **To describe common physical changes due to aging**

◎ **To describe the benefits of exercise for older adults, particularly water exercise**

◎ **To explain exercise modifications related to physical changes due to aging**

◎ **To review the principles of specificity of training and overload as applied to exercise for older adults**

◎ **To look at the components of fitness programs for older adults that develop cardiorespiratory fitness, flexibility, muscular strength and endurance, and ability to perform activities of daily living (ADL)**

◎ **To discuss the need for health screening and assessment for older adults in exercise programs**

◎ **To provide safety and injury prevention tips for working with older adults**

Older adults entering water fitness classes today are quite different from those who entered classes 10 to 20 years ago. Unlike earlier class participants, the baby boomers who are now turning 50 are aware of the importance of exercise and healthy diet and lifestyle habits to staying healthy and active. In addition, new medications and advances in medical technology have decreased the risk and incidence of lifestyle-related diseases. The result is that many of the older adults who are exercising today are healthier and less frail than earlier exercise participants. The 1998 IDEA Fitness Programs Trend Report (IDEA, 1998) states that the number of older adults (people aged 56 and older) participating in fitness programs rose 23 percent from 1997 to 1998. Water exercise classes are now offered in 46 percent of all exercise facilities (and in 63 percent of all YMCAs). The attitudes and characteristics of the aging population are in the process of changing, and the result of that change is an increased demand for water fitness programs today.

Water fitness training design for older adults must take into account the many physical changes aging brings. However, exercise can help to alleviate many of the problems caused by those changes, as long as the exercise has been appropriately modified to accommodate older adults' reduced physical abilities. Using some of the same principles as land exercise but using water's qualities to enhance the effects of

exercise, you can create water exercise programs that target older adults' cardiorespiratory fitness, flexibility, and muscular strength and endurance, plus improve their ability to perform ADL (activities of daily living). You'll need to do some health screening and assessment before beginning your program, and following guidelines on safety and injury prevention will protect your older adult participants from harm.

Physical Changes Due to Aging

Aging is a part of life. Nothing will prevent it, but certain things can be done to postpone it. Maintaining a healthy lifestyle, having healthy relationships with others, and keeping a positive attitude have been shown to slow down some of the effects of aging. Feeling younger is correlated with good health; higher levels of income, education, and activity; a more positive outlook; and high self-esteem.

There is no magical age at which someone officially becomes "old." Though for purposes of this manual we have selected 55 as the minimum age for participation in an older adult program, each of us ages differently and views becoming older from a slightly different perspective.

Regardless of our perceptions, certain changes take place in all people as they move past middle age. For any given individual, a few changes may be very marked, whereas other changes may be essentially insignificant from a functional standpoint. However, we as YMCA staff and leaders must accept that in any given group of older adults, most of the changes listed in this section will be manifested in one individual or another. Similarly, the related common chronic diseases of the aged, usually associated in one way or another with lifestyle habits, age-related changes, or both, will be represented, such as heart disease, arthritis, or diabetes.

As we design programs for older adults, we must recognize that they range in age from 55 to over 90. That is a span of more than 35 years. In general, the 55- to 75-year-old age group is able to do most of the same things they've always done; the 75- to 85-year-old age group experiences some limitations and has begun to look at things differently; and the 85-and-over group is the one that tends to be in poor health with marked limitations.

Within any age range of older adults there is enormous variation from one individual to the next in the degree of any particular change. Take, for example, a married couple, both of whom are aged 72. The husband may be hard of hearing but able to move easily, whereas the wife may have perfect hearing but be limited in her mobility because of age-related joint deterioration.

Any particular change can have, in the long run, a positive or negative outcome, depending on the individual's coping ability and the understanding and support he or she receives from other people. YMCA staff and leaders can have an enormous impact in facilitating a positive outcome to the inevitable changes. Program modification based on the characteristics of any given group of individuals is essential.

Some physical changes seem to originate from normal age-related processes, some from lifestyle habits, and some from disease processes. Although disease processes are not normal, unhealthy lifestyles unquestionably contribute to the development of many diseases. The changes are presented in seven categories; sensory, mental, body size and appearance, mobility and response time, cardiorespiratory system, musculoskeletal system, and lower digestive and urinary systems (Astrand and Rodahl, 1986; Birrer, 1989; Shephard, 1978).

Sensory

Sensory perception—vision, hearing, taste, smell, and touch—does change with age, but the nature and degree of change vary greatly among individuals.

- **Vision.** Vision changes may involve a decrease in acuity (sharpness of perception), a decrease in the size of the visual field, an increase in sensitivity to bright or glaring light, a slowing of dark adaptation, and increasing difficulty in judging the speed of moving objects. Thirteen percent of Americans over age 65 have some form of visual impairment, with 8 percent having a severe impairment. Many older adults are unaware of the changes in their vision, and up to 25 percent may be using incorrect lens prescriptions.

- **Hearing.** Hearing changes may involve a decrease in acuity; a sensitivity to loud noise, causing pain; and a decrease in sound discrimination of significant sound from background noise. Nearly one in four persons (23 percent) between the ages of 65 and 74 has a hearing impairment. The risk of having problems with hearing continues to increase with age from one in three for individuals aged 75 to 84 to one in two for people aged 85 and over.

- **Taste and smell.** Taste and smell acuity may decline. The decline is often limited to specific tastes or smells. For example, the sensitivity to sweet and salty flavors declines faster than the sensitivity to bitter or sour flavors.

- **Touch.** Touch sensitivity involves pain, pressure, and temperature sensors. An individual may experience age-related declines in one or more of these.

Mental

Older adults normally remain mentally alert until very, very late in life unless disease processes intervene. This alertness is maintained if lifestyle choices encourage active involvement with life.

Memory loss plagues most adults, but older adults fear it as a sign of impending incapacity and total dependence on others. Yet there is little decline in long-term memory (recollections of events occurring several years ago) and short-term memory (the first few seconds following an event). It is intermediate memory, the retention of information for minutes to months, that may decline. Lifestyle, physical health, and emotional health all seem to affect this intermediate memory.

People are able to learn new and complex material at any age. However, older adults do need extra time to integrate new ideas. This may be because older adults learn by reflection, making connections between their past experiences and new information, and they have large stores of prior knowledge. Older adults also often have to unlearn old material before they can incorporate new information.

As a result, although older adults enjoy learning, they like to set the pace. They do not learn well when conditions demand speed or are competitive or stressful. They have little tolerance for threatening situations but respond well to a safe, accepting environment. Also keep in mind that the sensory changes and day-to-day energy level fluctuations related to aging can affect older adults' ability to learn.

Older adults prefer learning information that is relevant and meaningful to them. They do well with hands-on experiential learning, and they also enjoy participation in planning and evaluating training objectives.

Body Size and Appearance

The appearance of the body reveals some of the visible signs of aging.

- Body height decreases, with the loss of height taking place in the spine. This contributes to the frequent complaint from older adults about midsection spreading.

- Body weight may increase somewhat during midlife, followed by a gradual decrease starting during the 60s. Marked weight changes from young adulthood are not normal.

- Normal body composition changes include a decrease in lean body mass due to the decrease in muscle mass. A related increase occurs in percentage of body fat. As an individual ages, more body fat is stored beneath the skin as opposed to within deep body sites.

- Abdominal and chest girth normally increase and limb girth normally decreases. These changes are due mostly to the decrease in muscle mass and the increase in body fat.

- Hair becomes thinner and often changes color.

- Skin loses its elasticity, becoming drier and wrinkled.

Mobility and Response Time

Our position in space and our movements are controlled by the brain's intricate coordination of sensory information and muscular response. By the time a person reaches extreme old age, he or she can experience an enormous loss in the number and sensitivity of nerve cells. There is also a decrease in the production of regulatory hormones and nerve transmission substances. Yet miraculously, the system continues to function.

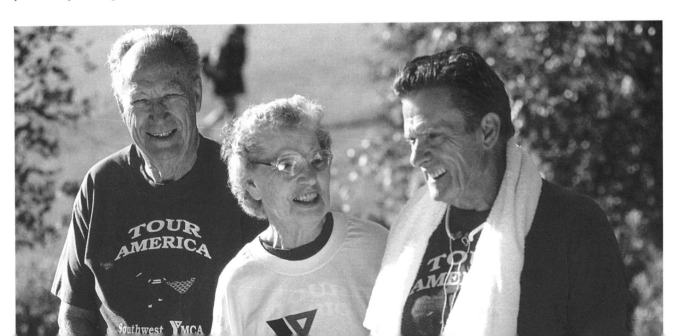

One of the most important age-related changes that staff and older adult participants must recognize and accept is the slowing of response time (Ostrow, 1984). Total response time involves reaction time (reception of sensory input from internal or external cues) and movement time (muscular response). If, in addition, the sensory information is complicated or requires a high degree of coordinated response, the reaction time can be markedly slower than usual. The actual muscle contraction time will also be slower. For older adults to function comfortably and successfully, they need to be given extra time to react and respond to a situation. Older adults do not enjoy being rushed or forced to complete tasks within a timed period.

Balance and coordination are complex functions that also require coordination between nerves and muscles. Many older adults assume that poor balance and lack of coordination are inherent characteristics of aging. It is true that they may experience a modest decline in these functions, but the decline is readily slowed with use.

Spatial awareness is an important function in controlling the body as it moves through space. Most people don't even stop to think about the sensors and reflexes that prevent us from bumping into each other, from falling over, or from tripping over sidewalk irregularities. The number and acuity of each of these sensors decline with age and, unfortunately, injuries related to these changes increase.

Cardiorespiratory System

The cardiorespiratory system includes the heart, lungs, blood, and blood vessels. The efficiency of this system is strongly affected by genetic, lifestyle, and disease factors. In any case, some changes are inevitable.

- The maximal attainable heart rate declines with age. The resting heart rate normally does not change significantly. The result is a reduced heart rate reserve available for vigorous activity.
- The volume of blood pumped by the heart each minute decreases, reducing the older adult's possible workload capacity.
- Both the systolic and diastolic blood pressure increase with age due to the loss of elasticity of blood vessel walls and to the narrowing of the vessel openings caused by fatty deposits. The fatty deposits are related to the normal increase with age in blood cholesterol.
- Blood vessels rupture more easily, causing bruising.

- Blood vessel valves (in the veins) become less efficient, which contributes to fluid retention and swelling. Sitting for long periods will often cause uncomfortable swelling in the feet and legs.
- Regulatory systems controlling blood flow redistribution, breathing depth and rate, and blood pressure adjustments become less efficient. It takes an older adult longer than a younger person to change gears to a higher or lower level of activity. It also takes longer for the blood pressure in an older adult to adjust to body position changes from reclining to sitting or standing.
- Regulatory systems that control responses to both cold and heat are less efficient. In addition, the ability to sweat to cool the body and the ability to shiver to warm the body are reduced.
- Regulatory systems controlling immune responses are less efficient. By old age, illness occurs more frequently and recovery takes longer.
- The vital capacity of the lungs decreases. Vital capacity is the total volume of air that can be forcibly expired following a maximal inspiration. Respiratory efficiency, both the mechanics of breathing and the exchange of gases at cell boundaries, is decreased.

Musculoskeletal System

The older adult's most visible body changes are those that affect the musculoskeletal system. This system is composed of bones, muscles with their attaching tendons, joint-binding ligaments, and joint-cushioning cartilage. This is also the system to which the statement "use it or lose it" most strongly applies.

- Bone density decreases, with a resulting increase in susceptibility to fractures, particularly at the wrist, hip, and cervical and lumbar spine.
- Muscle strength decreases due to a decrease in the number and volume of muscle fibers. The degree of this decrease is strongly affected by use. However, it is important to remember that older adults experience a normal decrease in maximum power output, in the number of fast-twitch muscle fibers, and in muscle bulk.
- The strength of particular muscle groups, such as the back, seems to decline faster than that of other muscle groups.

- There also seems to be an increase in muscle cramping of the hands, feet, calf muscles, hamstrings, quadriceps, and lumbar spine. The exact cause of this increased cramping is not known, but inactivity, poor flexibility, and inadequate potassium in the diet are considered to be contributing factors.

#4
- Muscle flexibility decreases. Muscle tearing is more common, causing muscle soreness in mild cases and major disabling injury in more severe cases.

- The tendons are also more prone to strains, tears, and ruptures during sudden, unaccustomed bursts of activity.

- Cartilage (such as disks in the spine) becomes less elastic, less able to cushion the compressive forces involved in movement. Sharp or jarring movements are more likely to cause pain or injury.

#5
- Joint mobility decreases for a variety of reasons. The production of lubricating synovial fluid declines, resulting in stiffness. Blood circulation to and around the joints becomes less efficient. Calcification deposits may occur and impede movement. Joint surfaces become furrowed and irregular. Joints also become noisier! The clicking and popping sounds an older adult may experience are harmless unless there is associated pain. Joint range of motion is significantly affected by individual use patterns.

Lower Digestive and Urinary Systems

Changes in the lower digestive and urinary system do create embarrassing situations for older adults. The decline in kidney efficiency may result in fluid retention. There is an unrelated decrease in thirst sensation. Deliberate added water intake will ease the kidney dysfunction and fluid retention problems. Therefore, the older adult needs to empty the bladder more frequently. Bowel problems, both constipation and looseness, are more common than in younger adults. Research suggests that diet, exercise, and lifestyle changes may improve these common problems.

Benefits of Exercise

Although everyone can benefit from exercise, perhaps no other segment of the population benefits as greatly from regular, consistent exercise as older adults. For older adults, exercise not only reduces or eliminates

such common physical problems as stiff joints, aching backs, and reduced energy levels, but it also improves the quality of life. They will find ADL easier and the physical demands of their preferred recreational activities enjoyable. Active older adults remain functionally independent longer than inactive seniors and continue to make valuable contributions, which is rewarding both to them and to their communities (Smith & Serfass, 1981).

Let's look at the specific benefits exercise brings to the following areas:

- Sensory and psychomotor
- Psychological
- Body composition
- Cardiorespiratory system
- Muscular system
- Skeletal system
- Internal organs

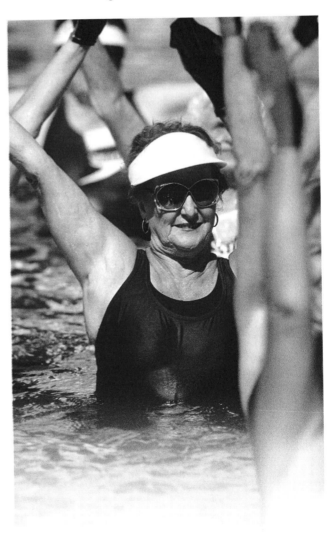

Sensory and Psychomotor Benefits

Exercise has positive affects on the sensory organs' functions of sight, skin sensitivity, position awareness, and balance and on the psychomotor function, the interaction among the brain, the nerves, and the muscles:

- Tones the eye muscles.
- Stimulates the sense of touch.
- Stimulates the senses associated with body position awareness.
- Helps maintain one's sense of balance.
- Helps maintain nerve-muscle reaction speed.

Psychological Benefits

Research also demonstrates that exercise has positive affects on brain function, memory, and emotional health:

- Aids in efficient brain function.
- Helps slow memory loss and may even improve one's memory.
- Reduces emotional stress and anxiety.
- Increases one's sense of well-being and ability to relax.
- Improves one's self-image.

Body Composition Benefits

Exercise affects the body fat and muscle mass components of body composition in the following positive ways:

- Aids in the reduction of body fat.
- Aids in maintaining or increasing muscle mass.
- Slows the age-related decline in basal metabolic rate, the minimum energy required to maintain life processes (retaining muscle mass is directly associated with maintaining a higher basal metabolic rate).

Cardiorespiratory Benefits

Exercise benefits the heart, lungs, and circulatory system in the following ways:

- Increases the efficiency of the heart.
- Improves lung capacity and breathing efficiency.
- Aids the circulation of oxygen and nutrients throughout the body.
- May slow the development of arteriosclerosis.

- May lower or normalize blood pressure.
- Aids the maintenance of healthy blood chemistry by increasing high-density lipoprotein (HDL) levels and increasing insulin sensitivity and glucose tolerance (for diabetics this means better use of insulin and regulation of blood sugar).

Muscular System Benefits

Exercise improves muscle health in the following ways:

- Helps reduce the loss of muscle mass.
- Improves muscle strength and endurance.
- Improves muscle flexibility.
- Reduces the risk of injury and facilitates healing, if orthopedic injury occurs.
- Strengthens ligaments and muscles, which aids in maintaining one's balance.
- Helps reduce muscle tremors.

Skeletal System Benefits

Exercise improves the strength of bones and the flexibility of joints in these ways:

- Slows the degeneration of joints and increases their range of motion.
- Increases the efficiency of skeletal support through increased muscle strength and endurance.
- Increases bone density, which reduces the incidence of broken bones caused by osteoporosis (i.e., loss of bone mass), particularly in the hip, the spine, and the wrist.
- Increases the flow of synovial fluid to the joints.

Benefits to Internal Organs

Exercise also benefits the internal organs in these ways:

- Stimulates and regulates digestion and elimination.
- May slow the decline in hormone, enzyme, and neurotransmitter production.

The Unique Benefits of Water Programs for Older Adults

Another advantage of water exercise is that the buoyancy of water helps to minimize the risk of falling.

Water exercise has always been a favorite form of activity with older adults, and it is particularly beneficial for them. Given the normal changes that take place as people age, water activities can easily be modified by the participant to accommodate individual challenges. In addition, close communication and cooperation between staff of land and water programs ensures that cross-training classes (exercising on both land and in water) can provide a balanced program for healthy living on land. Water fitness classes should be listed with the land fitness programs, and land-based older adult fitness classes, such as walking, Tai Chi, and resistance training, should be listed as part of the comprehensive fitness program. In this way, the Y's ability to meet the needs of older adults is strengthened as the participants themselves go through the changes in their lives.

As mentioned, we recommend that participants exercise both on the land and in the pool to maintain independence and health. There are some unique benefits of water programs that may not be experienced on the land that are important to consider when talking to your participants and designing all your fitness programs.

For example, people who suffer from pain of limitations during range-of-motion work can benefit greatly from warm water exercise, where the joints and body are supported by buoyancy. Water's resistance can aid in strengthening weak muscles and provide an opportunity to train the healthy limbs aggressively while training injured or limited areas of the body with reduced intensity.

Another advantage of water exercise is that the buoyancy of water helps to minimize the risk of falling. It provides a safe environment in which participants can reach farther safely and improve their balance and recovery skills.

Water's buoyancy also provides participants with an opportunity to adjust the level of impact, especially on sensitive joints and those that are weight bearing. Impact levels in the pool must be considered with regard to a person's body composition (the percent of body fat) in relation to water depth:

- **Low- or no-impact exercises** in the pool place minimal or no stress on the back, hip, knee, or ankle joints. They are usually performed in nipple-deep or deep water (with a buoyancy device for support). They do not include jumping or rebound moves, but should be performed in neutral or suspended working positions. These exercises may require more coordinated upper-body movements to stabilize the body. In deep water, participants need more advanced skills to be able to maintain neutral spine or joint position and good body alignment. Armwork in deep water may increase aerobic intensity for participants, so be sure they pace themselves.

- **Medium-impact exercises** in the pool place less stress on the back, hip, knee, and ankle joints than do high-impact exercises. Medium-impact exercises include activities such as walking or jogging in navel- to nipple-deep water, although impact levels depend on the body composition of the participants. Participants with high body fat float more easily and experience less impact than more muscular or lean participants in the same water depth. Have participants adjust the intensity. Medium-impact exercises may include moves such as kicking, jumping jax, or any other move performed in light rebound or neutral working positions.

- **Higher-impact exercises** in the pool are characterized by movements that work against gravity more by rebounding off the pool floor in navel-depth water or by rebounding off a step. These higher-impact exercises may not be appropriate for some older adults; however, with training and in the proper water depth, participants may be able to work the moves without contraindication. Water cushions landings and softens the effect of gravity on landings, but for some participants, bending their knees on landings may still be too much. Higher-impact exercises are characterized by jumping, hopping, and rebounding moves in navel- to nipple-depth water or off the top of a step. They may be performed at lower speeds or with the aid of a flotation device in shallow water to allow participants to perform propulsive moves while the extra buoyancy softens the landings. These exercises require different balance skills and should be taught using coordinated arm movements for control. Webbed gloves are especially helpful in providing extra balance for the upper body.

The hydrostatic pressure of water provides resistance to any movement in any direction, allowing participants to improve muscular endurance during any movement, even if the movement is limited. Participants can modify moves to adjust to individual limitations without losing a training effect.

Some older adults suffer from a limited capacity to breathe normally. By simply immersing the lungs underwater during breathing exercises, participants can help improve lung ventilation ability on the land (Kurabayashi et al., 1997).

Water exercise is beneficial for participants who may have poor body images. They can "hide" their bodies in the water and move without feeling "watched."

Finally, water exercise provides the chance for everyone to go at his or her own pace, so the level of intensity can be self-regulated, personalizing each exercise, each set, and each session. And water exercise skills can be performed for a lifetime!

Exercise Modifications for Older Adults

Because older adults experience normal, age-related physical changes that become increasingly marked over time, fitness programs, in order to be safe, effective, and enjoyable, must be designed to accommodate these changes. The design takes into account the functional ability of a particular group and of each individual within that group.

In addition to normal, age-related changes, the incidence of chronic disease and disability increases in the older adult population (Birrer, 1989). At any given time, 5 percent of those over 65 are in acute, intermediate, or long-term care facilities. The remaining 95 percent live at home (Piscopo, 1985). Yet, as people age, the limitations of common chronic diseases and disabilities progress to more noticeably disabling stages. Though these limitations often require some modification of their lifestyle, most older adults remain functional.

Not long ago these people would often say that they could not participate in exercise because they had one or more common chronic conditions. Today they often say they must exercise because they have these conditions. Exercise can play a significant role in preventing or reducing the incidence of various conditions and their negative effects. Older adults with some degree of limitation will always be present in older adult fitness classes. Learn the limitations of individual class members and provide appropriate exercise modifications to allow them to achieve success.

Participants with more marked limitations should be directed to appropriate special programs—YMCA Healthy Back Program, general postcardiac exercise classes, or Arthritis Foundation YMCA Aquatic Program—or to local health care professionals.

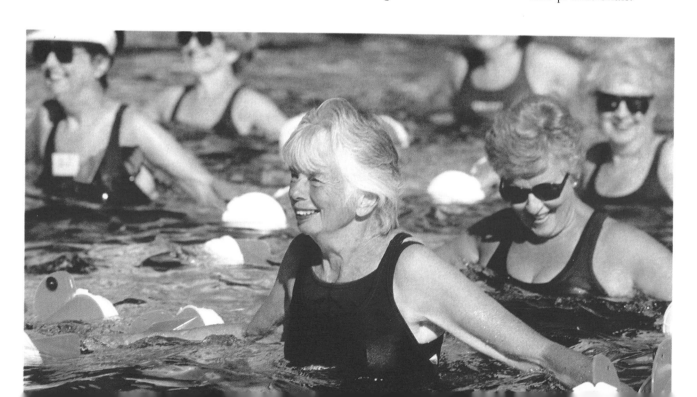

In this section, we'll now discuss exercise modifications related to changes in the following areas:

- Sensory abilities
- Psychomotor abilities
- Body composition
- Cardiorespiratory system
- Musculoskeletal system
- Conditions due to sedentary lifestyles
- Psychological and social conditions

Modifications Related to Sensory Changes

To accommodate the sensory changes affecting hearing and spatial awareness, several modifications must be incorporated into exercise programs.

Auditory

Because many older adults have hearing problems, you should rely more on visual cues than on verbal ones: The eye is quicker than the ear. Often a verbal cue can be replaced by pointing or simply moving clearly. Let your body do the talking by moving with boldness, clarity, and energy. Eliminate confusing, irrelevant movements such as toe tapping and finger snapping unless such movements are the exercise focus. When you use verbal cues, reduce them to the bare essentials and speak clearly. Use a wireless microphone when teaching poolside to help those with hearing problems to hear better.

Though the use of music for motivation is important in older adult fitness classes, some modifications must be made in its use. First, keep the volume down. Loud music is often physically painful to older ears. The volume should be low enough so that you can give verbal cues in a normal tone of voice and still be heard easily over the music. Also, instrumental music is less confusing than vocal music. Second, if participants are wearing hearing aids, exercises that bring the arms close to the ears (overhead arm stretching) create an unpleasant whistling sound. Instruct participants to move their arms just in front of or just behind their ears while maintaining good shoulder and spinal alignment.

You may choose not to use music in your water exercise programs. In these programs, participants often have more difficulties hearing you because water splashing creates a lot of distracting background noise. Also, many older adults do not wear hearing aids in the water and the acoustics in pool areas are poor. For these reasons, your participants' ability to hear your instructions and perform the exercises

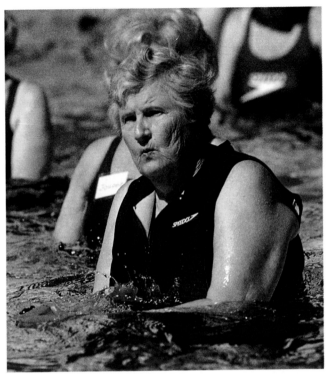

safely and correctly may be compromised if you play music.

Spatial Awareness

The decline in balance and spatial awareness creates unusual problems (Ostrow, 1984). Older adults are prone to tripping, backing into objects, and bumping into each other. Always allow extra space between participants in older adult fitness classes. Use positive cues such as "move backward carefully" and monitor the participants' positions often!

Moving laterally or backward is very challenging for older adults, even in the safer environment of the pool. Remind the participants to maintain proper body alignment, especially neutral spinal position, during all traveling activities in the water.

A great advantage of water exercise is the ability to make errors in balance and self-correct without fear of falling onto a hard surface. The pool is the ideal environment in which to challenge balance and practice preventing falls. We recommend that all water exercises be performed away from the pool wall unless participants' ability to balance is so compromised that holding onto the wall is necessary for safety. Exercises performed while holding onto the side of the pool prevent the participants from experiencing safe challenges to balance that can prepare them for similar challenges on land. Also, the sustained muscle contraction that results from holding onto the side of the pool can increase stress and strain on the fragile joints of the neck and may lead to shoulder pain or dysfunction (especially in older adults).

Modifications Related to Psychomotor Changes

Psychomotor changes are less obvious to older adults and are therefore the underlying cause of many accidents (Ostrow, 1984). Here are some suggestions for how to accommodate these changes:

- The speed of movement is slower in the water and requires greater effort than movement on land. Therefore, you may have to motivate participants when you want them to increase the speed of their movements through the water.

- When teaching a new activity, allow participants time to visualize each movement and sense its wholeness—its sequence from beginning to end. This is particularly important at the beginning of class and for new participants.

- Increase the amount of space around new participants and put them around the perimeter of the group. This allows water currents to subside before reaching these participants, preventing them from being thrown off balance.

- Allow extra time for participants
  - to hear verbal cues and see visual cues;
  - to interpret movements that are hard to perceive, such as an arm or leg crossing the body midline or opposition movements; and
  - to make smooth transitions when changing movement direction and when changing to a new position or movement.

- Cue participants to focus on the pool wall or deck when turning in place to prevent dizziness. If the movement requires turning the head side to side, keep the movement slow, and to prevent dizziness, cue participants to pause an instant and focus their eyes straight ahead—not down—as they cross the centerline. Participants may complain of feelings of seasickness (nausea) after looking down at the water. Cue them to look at a stationary land point of reference, such as a deck, wall, or tree.

- Unless coordination is the lesson, avoid focusing on too many activities or movements in one exercise. Use simple movements, avoiding complex choreography that can be confusing.

- Exercising in the water impairs visual feedback because most of the body is submerged. Holding a special meeting to watch a water exercise video designed especially for older adults (such as the *Golden Waves Functional Water Fitness Exercise Video*) can help participants see correct movement patterns for the exercises. Watching the video can facilitate visualization of correct movement patterns and improve performance (besides just being fun).

For exercise suggestions and modifications related to neurological problems, refer to the "Neurological Conditions" section of chapter 15.

Modifications Related to Changes in Body Composition

Older adults acquire a different body shape due to changes in lean body mass, percent total fat, and percentage of body water. These changes affect the ability to exercise and to function normally.

Remind participants to bring their water bottles and leave them poolside to use during class. Drinking water or juice before, during, and after class helps replace fluids lost during exercise. Dehydration is a common problem among older adults, because their thirst sensation is delayed or impaired and the percentage of total body water drops. Also, older adults (particularly women) frequently withhold fluids in response to their fears of incontinence. Severe dehydration and mental confusion are possible consequences of inadequate hydration.

Water depth, overall intensity, and impact may need to be modified to accommodate differences in body size and shape:

- Those with excess body fat should exercise in shallow water, because they are more buoyant. Inability to control movements, even in shallow water, may make it necessary for them to strap on a weight belt to assist in maintaining contact with the bottom of the pool with the feet. Balance, stability, and control of movements can be improved with the use of weights.

- Intensity of exercise should begin at a low level by reducing the size or speed of movements or the surface area involved. Gradually increase the workload by first increasing duration, then increasing the size of the movement, the speed or force with which it is performed, or the surface area involved, as tolerated.

- Participants may need to perform water activities in the neutral working position instead of the rebound or suspended position to reduce impact and intensity. Older adults who are small in size, thin, or frail (for example, those with osteoporosis) may also need to reduce impact. Advanced osteoporosis can make individuals very susceptible to fracture, even during daily activities. These frail individuals may need to wear a flotation belt during water exercise to reduce impact and prevent fractures.

Modifications Related to Cardiorespiratory Changes

On a functional level, cardiorespiratory changes affect our stamina and energy. Here are some suggested exercise modifications for those who have health conditions related to blood pressure or blood flow and exercise stress.

Adjusting for Blood Pressure and Blood Flow Changes

Provide longer warm-up and cool-down periods to accommodate older adults' slower adjustments of blood pressure, circulation, and heart rate response to changes in exercise intensity.

Encourage normal breathing patterns, and encourage exhaling on effort to counter an increased tendency toward holding the breath. Breath holding is often combined with contraction of the abdominal muscles (the Valsalva maneuver). Initially these actions increase blood pressure and heart rate. But if the breath-holding pattern is continued, blood pressure and heart rate decrease, which may cause dizziness or fainting. Maintaining normal breathing patterns also corrects overbreathing (hyperventilation) problems.

Teach older adults how to modify isometric activities, such as prolonged gripping of water exercise equipment. Isometric activity raises blood pressure, but many normal ADL, such as carrying groceries, painting the house, changing high lightbulbs, moving furniture, or shoveling snow, require isometric contractions. Modifications include reducing the duration of isometric contraction to approximately 10-20 seconds (dependent on health and fitness levels, the choice of daily tasks being practiced, and the physician's guidelines) and reducing the resistance or load to decrease the intensity of muscle contraction. Frequent cues to breathe normally during isometric exercise also help prevent the increase in blood pressure that comes with breath holding. For specific modifications and guidelines for cardiovascular-respiratory diseases, refer to the medical considerations described in chapter 15.

Reducing Exercise Stress

Extremely hot or cold weather and overexertion can increase the stress of exercise to a potentially harmful level (Astrand and Rodahl, 1986). To reduce this stress, take precautions and monitor participants. To compensate for participants' poorer adjustment to warm environments, use caution when leading exercise in hot and humid weather, as participants' heart rates will rise rapidly. In cooler environments, provide vigorous enough activities to keep students warm.

Monitor participants and teach them to be aware of the symptoms of overexertion and illness (ACSM, 1995, p. 293):

- Dizziness
- Paleness
- Labored breathing or unusual shortness of breath
- Nausea
- Fever
- Confusion, disorientation, or difficulty in speaking
- Loss of coordination, unusual stumbling, or clumsiness
- Unusual fatigue
- Excessive perspiration or lack of perspiration
- Pain in the chest, shoulder blades, or radiating down into the arms
- Personality changes

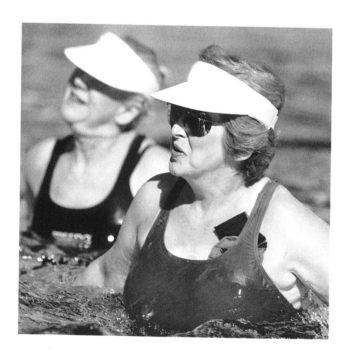

Modifications Related to Musculoskeletal Changes

Educate older adults to sense (to be aware of) a muscle when it contracts and when it stretches. During an exercise, point to a specific muscle and ask if they feel the stretch or contraction at that point. This helps eliminate common performance errors, poor body alignment, and the overstressing of joints.

Due to the increased risk of muscle, tendon, and ligament tearing, modify exercises to eliminate sudden movements, quick hopping or twisting movements, and uncontrolled ballistic or bouncing movements at the outer limit of the range of motion. Progression of muscle strength training also needs to be more gradual.

Changes in joints and bones have the largest impact on the ability to move. Many of these changes appear to be normal and age related. Others are clearly disease related. The popular maxim "Use it or lose it" refers most aptly to all these skeletal changes. Follow these guidelines when you work joints:

- Teach older adults to feel (to be aware of) movement around a joint and to feel a comfortable, full range of motion.
- To avoid overstressing a joint, use only slow movements or static stretching near the outer limits of their range of motion.
- Review and practice finding neutral position for all joints, especially the spine. Neutral position of any joint is the most comfortable position of the joint, and usually it lies within the middle of the available range of motion. (For more on the neutral position of the spine, see chapter 15.)
- So participants can maintain neutral hand position, put foam grips around hand buoys.

Specific information, exercise suggestions, and modifications for musculoskeletal problems can be found in the "Orthopedic Conditions" section in chapter 15.

Modifications Related to Conditions Associated With Sedentary Lifestyles

Conditions such as depression, emotional disorders, constipation, incontinence, low-back pain, hearing or vision impairment, or disease often result in sedentary lifestyles. Sedentary participants benefit greatly from even modest increases in activity level. The biggest risk for these participants is failure; therefore, their immediate success is absolutely essential. Water exercise, which often seems easier than land exercise, is particularly effective.

Modifications Related to Psychological and Social Changes

A most important change that must be recognized in older adult fitness classes is the increased value older adults place on human relationships. Increased opportunity for socialization is essential in all their activities.

Older adults are also very aware of the state of their health and often have fears associated with their health. They have a stronger psychological need for an exercise environment that is supportive and understanding and for instructors whom they trust.

Principles of Exercise

Exercise should be enjoyable, comfortable, and pain free and should produce changes over time, some of which are measurable and others, such as increased self-esteem, that are not. If you understand and apply the scientific principles of exercise, measurable changes will occur. The challenge for you, the instructor, is to set an appropriate and flexible pace for making those changes and to help participants set realistic goals.

Two important principles for designing exercises for older adults are specificity of training and overload.

Specificity of Training

To train a muscle, learn a skill, or alter the condition of a system or its components requires exercise performance that is specific to the task. Older adults enjoy learning the purpose, correct performance, and goal of each particular exercise. This education helps correct common myths about exercise. For example, teach older adults that "spot exercises" will often improve muscle strength but have little effect on local fat deposits.

Overload and Effective and Safe Exercise

As with all adults, the efficiency or strength of a particular muscle or a physiologic system must be overloaded, or worked beyond accustomed levels, to be improved. But the amount of work (that is, the exercise workload) needs to be increased more slowly with older adults.

The concept of effective and safe exercise is useful in setting workload levels. If the overload is insufficient, no change will take place; the exercise is safe, but ineffective. In the past, older adults were considered to be delicate, frail, and breakable. Programs for them were often safe but unchallenging and ineffective. If the overload is too high ("Too much, too soon, too fast"), injury, both immediate and delayed, often results. The exercise is both ineffective and unsafe. If the overload is appropriate, the exercise is both safe and effective. The maxims "Listen to your body," "Train, don't strain," "LSD" (long, slow, distance), and "Take the talk test" provide the appropriate motivation.

To increase the overload safely and effectively, carefully monitor the results of increased intensity, frequency, and duration of exercise. The muscles and joints of older adults tire more easily, and older adults need more time to react to cues and to complete a movement. For these reasons, it is easy to under- or overestimate the appropriate overloads created by the equipment, longer lever arms, water resistance, high exercise repetitions, changes in direction, or stopping and starting movements.

Components of Older Adult Fitness Programs

To an older adult, what does fitness mean? To be considered fit, an individual must be able to function independently, to participate in favorite activities, and to complete the tasks of daily life. This section centers on the following components of physical fitness and how they relate to older adults (Serfass, 1980):

- Cardiorespiratory fitness
- Flexibility
- Muscular strength and endurance
- Performance of ADL

Developing Cardiorespiratory Fitness

Cardiorespiratory fitness improves the efficiency of the heart and lungs and of oxygen delivery to and use in the working cells. It is developed through aerobic and anaerobic exercise. Though even modest increases in energy demands by older adults will shift the muscles momentarily to anaerobic processes, the exercises in this phase of a fitness program should be primarily aerobic. Aerobic training in the water can be achieved by continuous rhythmic large-muscle activity, by performing intervals of aerobic activities and active rest, or by performing continuous muscular endurance activities that frequently change muscle groups. Obviously the age, health, and fitness levels of participants will determine the difficulty of the training activities chosen.

For older adults in water fitness programs, the most effective exercise frequency is two short periods a week of muscle strength training and three to five periods a week of combined muscular endurance and aerobic training, flexibility, and ADL training. Duration of exercise usually varies from 10 to 60 minutes, depending on the fitness level and health of the participants.

Deconditioned, frail, or new participants in an aquatic exercise program should begin with approximately 10 minutes of exercise composed of intervals of low-intensity aerobic water exercise lasting 15 to 45 seconds followed by 30 seconds of active rest. The participants should be instructed to stop the aerobic exercise and begin the active rest at 15, 30, or 45 seconds, depending on their individual tolerance. The duration of exercise should gradually be increased in response to improvements in fitness.

The American College of Sports Medicine recommends that healthy older adults exercise at an intensity of approximately 60 percent to 75 percent of the age-predicted maximum heart rate (ACSM, 1995). However, measuring exercise intensity using heart rate is extremely difficult and inaccurate in the pool. Heart rate responses can vary depending on water depth (the deeper the water, the lower the heart rate response) and water temperature (cooler water lowers the heart rate). In addition, many older adults may be taking medications that decrease heart rate, making age-predicted heart rate goals inaccurate. For those participants who need or want to measure heart rate and who wear heart monitors to measure heart rate for intensity, a heart rate chart appears in appendix A.

In older adult water fitness classes, perceived exertion and the "talk test" (being able to talk comfortably while exercising) are more practical measures of exercise intensity. They also increase the individual's awareness of exertion based on how they feel, which can be applied to daily life. A safe intensity level for slightly deconditioned to moderately fit, healthy older adults ranges from "light" (11) to "hard" (15). Extremely fit individuals may choose to work up to the "very hard" (17) level. Participants who are frail, deconditioned, or have medical conditions such as cardiovascular disease, high blood pressure, obesity, or diabetes may require lower intensities as recommended by their physicians. Refer to chapter 15 for general recommendations and guidelines.

Older adults can set safe and realistic workload goals such as increasing the number of laps walked or the amount of time they can work or the number of repetitions they can sustain during exercise. Initially increasing the duration of exercise before increasing the intensity reduces the likelihood of injury in older adults.

Note that aerobic water exercise is difficult to sustain without a baseline level of muscular endurance. Therefore, muscular endurance training should be a primary focus early in an aerobic training program.

Developing Flexibility

Flexibility is an attribute of joints and muscles. It is the ability of the muscles surrounding the joint to allow the joint to move through its full range of motion. Flexibility exercises involve two components: joint range of motion, moving each joint through its full range of motion, and muscle flexibility, or stretching the muscle. Flexibility exercises should be part of the warm-up for exercise and part of the cool-down following muscular, cardiorespiratory, and ADL training.

Joint range of motion is very important for older adults. It involves moving the joint slowly, in a fluid and continuous movement, through its entire range. Circling the ankles, making fists and opening them, and reaching the arms overhead are common joint range-of-motion exercises. They are usually incorporated into the warm-up or cool-down portions of the exercise program.

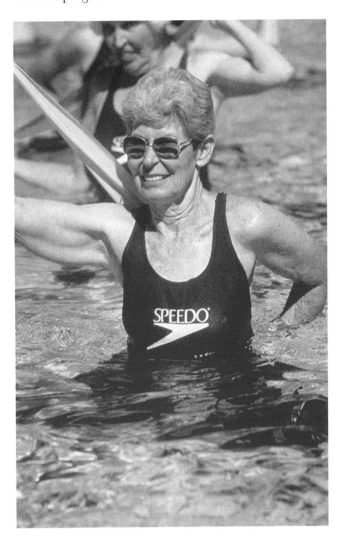

Muscle flexibility exercises in water exercise programs are static stretches, dynamic flexibility exercises, or passive stretches that use water currents to assist. Static stretching involves stretching a muscle slowly to its longest position (or the point of tension). Static stretching can be held from 6 to 15 seconds once or twice per muscle (longer if in warm water pool). The cooler temperatures of most pools used for fitness classes require a decrease in the length of time the stretch is held (around 6 seconds) and movement of other muscles during the stretch to maintain body warmth. For example, when participants stretch the upper body, they should jog lightly, or when they stretch the lower extremities, they should scull. Participants can use buoyancy or buoyancy equipment to help stretch limbs, as in a hamstrings stretch.

Most daily activities are performed within a relatively narrow range of motion, particularly among sedentary older adults. Dynamic flexibility exercise increases this range of active flexibility. It is achieved by performing active, controlled movements within the inner 90 percent of the joint range of motion (avoiding the outer limits or end of range of motion). Walking with progressively larger steps or leaping sideways from the neutral position (light toe contact on the bottom of the pool floor) are examples of dynamic flexibility exercises.

A passive stretch can be accomplished by stretching a muscle slowly to its longest position by the application of external force. The currents of the water can provide a gentle passive stretch to muscles that can be varied by the speed and direction of movements. Turning the body in a clockwise or counterclockwise direction while letting the arm drag behind is an example of gentle passive stretching of the pectorals. The force of the stretch should be monitored carefully. Partners can also work together to do passive stretches. For example, holding a resistance band while facing away from each other, partners can gently lean away from each other and perform a passive pectoral stretch. To prevent injury during partner passive stretching, the partners must communicate.

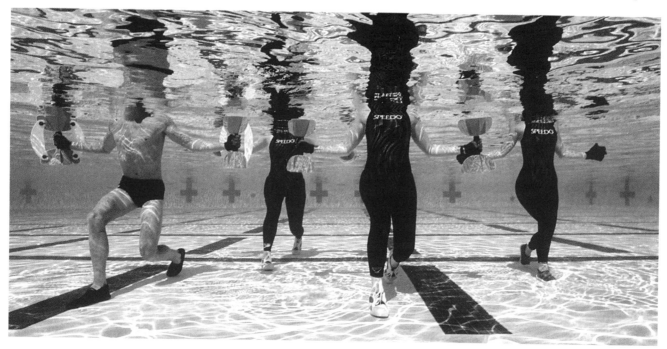

Important points to consider with stretching exercises include the following:

- The participants feel the stretch in the appropriate muscle.
- The surrounding joints are in a comfortable position.
- The end of range is approached slowly during static stretching.
- Dynamic stretching is performed within the inner 90 percent of the available joint range of motion, avoiding the extremes of the end of joint range of motion to prevent injury.

Developing Muscular Strength and Muscular Endurance

The two components of muscle conditioning are muscular strength and muscular endurance. Muscular strength is the ability to apply force through the recruitment of the maximum possible number of muscle fibers to overcome a resistance. All the fibers must recover before another contraction is possible. To build muscular strength, the amount of resistance is increased and the number of sets is gradually decreased. Training for increased muscular strength in the water requires the use of equipment to provide sufficient overload to the muscle. For example, using fitness paddles and following the cue "power back" is an effective way to strengthen the latissimus dorsi.

Note that with fast or forceful exercise in the water, the momentum created by inertia can easily push a joint beyond the normal end of range of motion. This can cause overstretching to the joint or muscles involved. Cue participants to stop or reverse the movement when they reach 60 percent to 70 percent of the range of movement. This slows the momentum and stops the extremity before it reaches the end of the range of motion, avoiding injury.

Muscular endurance is the ability to perform several repetitions of a submaximal contraction without undue fatigue. Muscle endurance also modestly improves muscular strength. Variables used in providing resistance for muscular endurance exercises include using the resistance of the water, adding equipment to increase surface area or buoyancy, and adding size or speed to a movement or length to a lever arm. For new or deconditioned participants, the resistance of the water is frequently the only appropriate resistance that can be tolerated initially.

The primary muscle-conditioning objective in older adult fitness is to build endurance. The changes that occur with muscle endurance training are increases in neuromuscular efficiency, in capillary density, and in the efficiency of enzyme systems related to energy production, as well as a modest increase in fiber size, though not number. To increase muscular endurance, the number of repetitions per set or the resistance is increased. Give the participants options that allow them to vary the number of repetitions and increase resistance to meet their individual needs.

Developing Ability to Perform Activities of Daily Living (ADL)

The ultimate goals of the older adult water fitness program are to increase the amount and variety of activities that participants can do on land and the ease with which they can do them. These programs should be designed to maintain or improve the quality of people's lives, minimizing age-related disability and maximizing physical activity, independence, and general well-being.

Activities selected to be performed in the pool should incorporate the components of ADL that are commonly performed by the individuals in the class. Identify specific activities that require practice by administering the Functional ADL Field Assessments to members before they start the exercise program (see chapter 16) or by asking them about functional challenges in daily tasks. The various components of

ADL can be practiced individually—lunging, balancing, coordination, push-pull, squat, isometric holds and lifting, starting and stopping, directional changes, jumping on and off a step (curb), stepping over the rope (into the tub)—or combined together into the specific tasks.

Practicing land-based functional activities in the water not only improves physical performance of the tasks on land, but also instills confidence. It also can help prepare participants for "surprise" situations. Land exercise programs are limited in performing activities that can cause participants to lose their balance and fall. The water is the perfect environment to allow participants to feel the challenges to balance or coordination and learn how to self-correct. Teach and practice recovery of balance skills in the water with all participants prior to starting the exercise program.

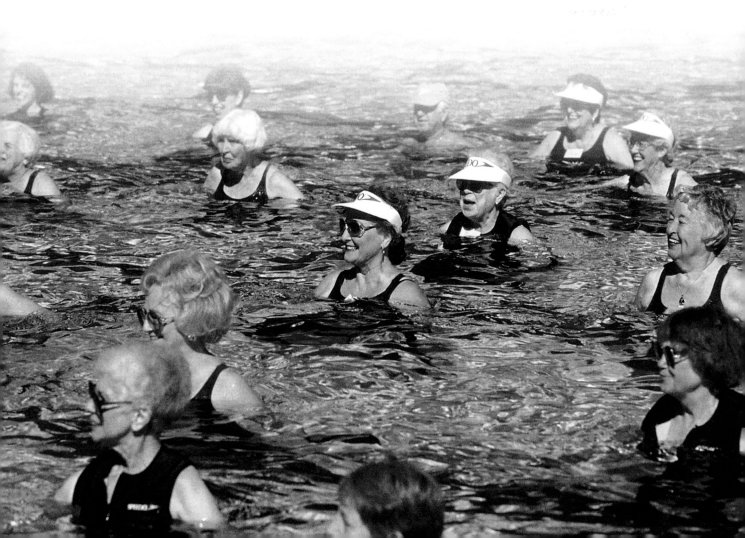

Health Screening

YMCAs offer a variety of types and levels of exercise programs for a diverse population of participants. In order to ensure exercise that is as safe as possible for its participants, the YMCA of the USA recommends a basic health screening for all older adult members (PAR-Q, see appendix A). This provides essential information for exercise instructors and also alerts participants to the potential risks of exercise. Participants with identifiable risk should also complete medical clearance and informed consent forms. Because the health status of older adults generally changes more frequently than does that of younger adults, have them complete health assessments regularly, at least once a year or following a change in health status.

It is prudent to maintain up-to-date information files for individual participants in fitness programs. You should have a class summary sheet listing each participant's name, emergency contact person and phone number, and information from the screening health form. This summary sheet should be kept on a clipboard and taken to every class.

Exercise Safety and Injury Prevention

By selecting safe movement patterns, activities, and exercises, you can prevent most injuries in older adult fitness classes. Here are some general guidelines:

SAFETY

- Check that the area between the parking lot and the pool deck is uncluttered and safe for walking.
- Tell participants who wear hearing aids to consult with their hearing aid adviser about wearing them in the pool. Some hearing aids can be worn in the water.
- If the class is held outdoors, try to avoid scheduling it between the hours of 11 A.M. and 3 P.M. daylight savings time (10 A.M. and 2 P.M. standard time), when exposure to ultraviolet rays is most intense. Encourage participants to wear sunscreen, sunglasses, and hats, and give them frequent water breaks.
- Have participants wear aquatic exercise shoes to prevent slips and falls in the locker room, on the pool deck, and in the pool.
- If the pool does not have a ramp, lift, or stair entry, you will need a volunteer or aide to assist with participant entry and exits. If webbed

gloves are to be worn, be sure participants put them on *after* the entry to avoid slipping.
- Get into the pool to guard and assist all those who need help entering the pool by the ladder or ramp.
- If participants are afraid of water, be sure to teach them basic water skills such as a safe entry, recovery to a stand, and sculling for balance. Wearing flotation belts in shallow water may help them feel secure and maintain an upright stance. (Reference *The Golden Waves*™ videos for basic safety skills). Check that group movements do not create strong currents that float them off their feet.
- Instruct participants to drink water before, during, and after class; to eat at least a light breakfast before a morning exercise session; and not to drink alcohol or eat a heavy meal less than one hour before exercise.
- Teach participants to be aware of (and to tell you of) the signs of exercise intolerance, which may occur between exercise sessions: inability to sleep at night; increased swelling; symptoms such as weakness, numbness, or tingling; inability to recover throughout the day from a workout; persistent aches or pains; unusual weight loss; or a decline in physical or functional abilities. Encourage participants to be conservative, particularly if they are new to the class, do not feel "up to par," or are recovering from an illness or injury. Encourage them to listen to their bodies on a daily basis and to make appropriate adjustments.
- Be aware of environmental conditions. Have participants wear thermal vests or tights to help them stay warm in cooler water temperatures. Instruct participants to start warming up as soon as they enter the water to stay warm. If exercising in an outdoor pool, instruct participants to wear sunscreen, visors or sunglasses, and extra layers of clothing if necessary.
- Enforce all safety rules.
- Encourage participants to bring their water bottles poolside, and provide frequent water breaks.

EXERCISE DESIGN

- Limit splashing and exercises that require getting the entire head wet. Most people prefer to perform "head out of the water" activities. Leave swimming skills for swimming sessions.

- Approach the end of the range of motion for static stretching exercises. Use dynamic exercise in the inner 90 percent of the available range of motion.

- Use gradual progression and overload in both strength and endurance training. Be aware of these signs of overuse, strain, and fatigue: dizziness; paleness; labored breathing or unusual shortness of breath; nausea; fever; confusion, disorientation, or difficulty in speaking; loss of coordination, unusual stumbling, or clumsiness; unusual fatigue; excessive perspiration or lack of perspiration; pain in the chest, shoulder blades, or radiating down into the arms; or personality changes.

- Be aware of and teach participants to be aware of modifications and guidelines for any pertinent medical or special conditions. Keep chapter 15 handy poolside for quick reference for modifications and guidelines.

- If you work with older adults or people with medical conditions, you should have an understanding of and be able to practically apply principles of anatomy, physiology, and kinesiology. You should be willing to spend the extra time to become more knowledgeable in these areas and use available resources to develop a working knowledge about exercise for people with special needs.

LEADING CLASS

- Teach proper movement patterns for activities (even as basic as walking) and how these movements are different when performed in the water.

- Regularly monitor movement mechanics and the body alignment (including neutral joint position) of all participants. Be aware of errors of movement and teach the participants to become aware of errors and how to self-correct.

- Use clear, precise demonstration movements to encourage correct movement patterns, and consciously eliminate distracting extraneous movements. Limit verbal cues to the few words essential to directing the movement.

- Perform exercises away from the pool wall if possible to simulate normal balance responses used for daily tasks on land. This will also prevent neck and shoulder injuries that result from sustained muscular contraction required by hanging onto the wall. Finger touch for balance can be used when balance is so compromised that a light touch is necessary for safety.

- Teach participants who have balance problems to avoid looking down at the water. Instead, tell them to focus their gaze on the poolside or the deck.

- Cue frequently for neutral gaze and proper breathing.

- Monitor exercise intensity frequently using observation, perceived exertion levels (Borg scale), and the "talk test." Heart rate guidelines may be used when appropriate and the participant wears a heart rate monitor.

- Older adults often hesitate to admit that an exercise causes pain or discomfort or is not enjoyable or effective. To overcome this gap in communication, you need to be observant; to be open to comments, questions, and suggestions; and to ask participants about the appropriateness and effectiveness of specific exercises. Of course, when participants have specific recommendations from their physicians for exercise modifications, they should follow those recommendations.

- Instruct participants in how to find proper water depth and how to know when water depth should change.

- Provide appropriate equipment for modification of activities (padded grip handles for those who have arthritis, ski poles with tennis balls on the bottom, or buoyancy dumbbells to assist with balance).

Bibliography

Aldana, S., and W.J. Stone. 1991. Changing physical activity preferences of American adults. *Journal of Health, Physical Education, Recreation and Dance* 62(4): 67–76.

American College of Sports Medicine. 1995. *ACSM's guidelines for exercise testing and prescription* (5th ed). Baltimore: Williams and Wilkins.

Astrand, P.-O., and K. Rodahl. 1986. *Textbook of work physiology: Physiological bases of exercises.* New York: McGraw-Hill.

Birrer, R. 1989. Prescribing physical activity for the elderly. In *Physical activity, aging and sports: Scientific and medical research*, eds. R. Harris and S. Harris, pp. 75–93. Albany, NY: Center for the Study of Aging.

Borg, G. 1973. Perceived exertion: A note on history and methods. *Medicine and Science in Sports and Exercise* 5(2): 90–93.

Caplow-Lindner, E., L. Harpaz, and S. Samberg. 1979. *Therapeutic dance/movement: Expressive activities for older adults.* New York: Human Sciences Press.

Garnet, E.D. 1982. *Movement is life: A holistic approach to exercises for older adults.* Princeton, NJ: Princeton Book.

Ryan, P. (ed.). 1998. Solutions, survey results: What's the secret of facilities with good retention? *IDEA Fitness Manager*, 10 (1): 7–12.

Knopf, K.G., and S.B. Downs. 1989. *Fitness over fifty.* Dubuque, IA: Kendall/Hunt.

Kurabayashi, H., K. Kubota, I. Machida, K. Tamura, H. Take, and T. Shirakura. 1997. Effective physical therapy for chronic obstructive pulmonary disease. *American Journal of Physical Medicine and Rehabilitation* 76(3): 204–207.

National Center for Health Statistics. 1975. *Vital and health statistics: Exercise and participation in sports among persons 20 years of age and over* (DDHS Publication No. HRA 77-1543). Washington, DC: U.S. Government Printing Office.

National adult physical fitness survey. 1973. *President's Council on Physical Fitness and Sports Newsletter* (May): 1–27.

Ornstein, R., and D. Sobel. 1989. *Healthy pleasures.* Reading, MA: Addison-Wesley.

Ostrow, A.C. 1984. *Physical activity and the older adult.* Princeton, NJ: Princeton Book.

Piscopo, J. 1985. *Fitness and aging.* New York: Wiley.

Sanders, M., and C. Kennedy. 1998. Water fitness research findings. *IDEA, The Health and Fitness Source* 16(6): 33–39.

Sanders, M., and C. Maloney-Hills. 1998. *The Golden Waves Functional Water Training for Health Program and The Golden Waves Functional Water Training for Health, Leadership Program* videos. 30 min. and 45 min. Produced by the Sanford Center for Aging, University of Nevada, Reno. Available from the YMCA of the USA Program Store.

Sanders, M., and N. Rippee. 1994. *Speedo aquatic fitness system, instructor training manual.* IDEA, London: Speedo International.

Schoenborn, C.A. 1986. Health habits of U.S. adults, 1985: The "Alameda 7" revisited. *Public Health Reports* 101: 571–580.

Serfass, R. 1980. Physical exercise and the elderly. In *Encyclopedia of physical education, fitness and sports: Training environment, nutrition, and fitness*, eds. G.A. Stull and T.K. Cureton. Salt Lake City: Brighton.

Shephard, R.J. 1978. *Physical activity and aging.* London: Croom Helm.

Smith, E.L., and R.C. Serfass. 1981. *Exercise and aging: The scientific basis.* Hillside, NJ: Enslow.

Stephens, T. 1987. Secular trends in adult physical activity: Exercise boom or bust? *Research Quarterly for Exercise and Sport* 58(2): 94–105.

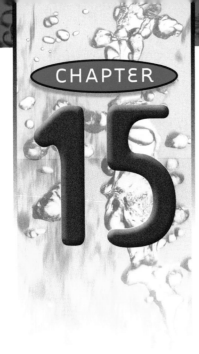

Guidelines for Working With Special Populations

CATHY MALONEY-HILLS AND MARY E. SANDERS

Objectives:

To give water fitness instructors information for working with participants who have the following types of medical conditions:

- Orthopedic conditions
- Neurological conditions
- Cardiovascular-respiratory diseases
- General medical conditions (pregnancy, obesity, diabetes, post-mastectomy)

This chapter is meant to help you design safe and effective water programs for post-rehabilitation participants and participants with special medical considerations. For each of 27 medical conditions, it provides guidelines to ensure proper screening and exercise modifications for helping participants to personalize their programs. It also includes information to help you understand how exercise affects each condition and to explain how to teach participants to monitor and modify exercise intensity and tolerance. Abnormal responses to exercise and recommendations for altering exercise after the abnormal responses are listed, as well as instructions on when to refer participants back to the health care practitioner.

The conditions, which are divided into four areas, are as follows:

ORTHOPEDIC CONDITIONS

1. Arthritis
2. Muscle Strain/Tendinitis
3. General Postsurgical
4. Total Hip Replacement
5. Knee: ACL Post-Rehabilitation
6. Knee: PCL Post-Rehabilitation
7. Knee: Total Knee Replacement
8. Knee: Meniscal Tear/Surgery
9. Knee: Chronic Anterior Knee Pain
10. Shoulder: Rotator Cuff Tear/Impingement/Post-Surgical

11. Shoulder: Adhesive Capsulitis (Stiff Shoulder/Frozen Shoulder)
12. Shoulder: Chronic Dislocation
13. Lateral Epicondylitis (Tennis Elbow)/Carpal Tunnel Syndrome
14. Neck Pain
15. Low-Back Pain
16. Fibromyalgia
17. Osteoporosis

NEUROLOGICAL CONDITIONS

18. Multiple Sclerosis
19. Cerebrovascular Accident (Stroke)
20. Parkinson's Disease

CARDIOVASCULAR-RESPIRATORY DISEASES

21. Cardiovascular Disease
22. Pulmonary Diseases
23. Hypertension

GENERAL MEDICAL CONDITIONS

24. Prenatal
25. Obesity
26. Diabetes Mellitus
27. Post-Mastectomy

Participants may have more than one condition or may have a condition not described in this chapter. Consult with participants' health care practitioners, your Y's medical advisory committee, or local physical therapists for extra advice or assistance if questions arise. Always inform the participant of this information as guidelines and modifications are outlined. Remember that your role as an instructor is to help participants help themselves.

We advise that you follow the recommendations of participants' health care providers (physician, physical therapist, chiropractor). Especially in cases involving the hip, knee, and shoulder, recommendations for postoperative treatment will vary according to each case and individual surgeon's guidelines. *Keep this chapter handy at poolside and use it, along with health care provider recommendations, to help participants who have special needs.*

All YMCA class participants should complete a PAR-Q Form. Results will indicate if a medical condition or special situation exists that requires specific guidelines or program modifications. It is the participant's responsibility to contact her or his health care provider for consent to participate and for specific guidelines if they apply (see sample Medical Clearance Form in appendix A).

The PAR-Q Form is located in appendix A. Feel free to make copies and use it as a tool for assessing your participants' readiness for exercise.

- Increase socialization
- Increase the perceived quality of life
- Increase program adherence
- Increase quality of sleep
- Increase level of fitness or wellness

You might hold classes for any of the following types of participants:

- Older adults
- Those who have low-back pain
- Deconditioned athletes
- Those with chronic illness
- Those recovering from surgery or injury
- Pre- and postpartum women
- Children
- Others who are referred to you by medical professionals

The methods you should use are verbal, written, or hand cues; encouragement, praise, and support; and demonstration. You should design and teach programs that do the following:

- Promote wellness or fitness
- Preserve or improve independence and function

Your Role as Water Fitness Instructor

Helen M. Tilden, RN, Director of Education, Building Bridges Aquatic Consulting in Atlanta, Georgia, has made a statement defining the role of water fitness instructors as part of the health care of participants who have medical conditions. As a water fitness instructor, your objective is to enhance and support the physiological and psychological aspects of rehabilitation following participants' discharge from therapy as a result of illness, injury, surgery, or disease. Your function is to teach water fitness classes to increase participants' efficiency of movement and ability to perform activities of daily living and to keep their minds and bodies healthy. Your goals should be the following:

- Reduce the risk of heart disease and other diseases that may result from a sedentary lifestyle
- Reduce the risk of complications of chronic illness or disability
- Reduce stress, isolation, and depression
- Increase self-esteem and feelings of well-being

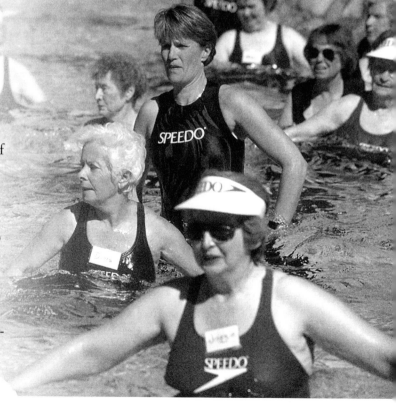

Table 15.1 *Comparison of Water Fitness Instructor to Physical Therapist*

Water fitness instructor	Physical therapist
Participant performs exercises	Therapist may manipulate limbs, provide resistance, change exercises, add weights, and so on.
Water temperatures are 80—88 degrees F.	Water temperatures may exceed 88 degrees F.
Focus on fitness, independence, and mobility	Focus on quantifiable functional restoration
Broad fitness assessments	Evaluation, testing, application of modalities, documentation, referral, and discharge information
Broad, general goals	Specific to need and ability
Does not draw conclusions from data	Uses data for functional, financial, and other outcomes for independence and restoration
Usually works in a group setting	Provides one-on-one care in acute, habilitative, rehabilitative, and preventive stages

From Tilden, H.M. 2000. Aquatic Exercise Instructor, In Norton, C., L. Jamison (eds.), *A Team Approach to the Aquatic Continuum of Care*, Woburn, MA: Butterworth-Heinemann.

- Reduce the incidence or severity of complications of long-term disease, illness, or injury
- Promote muscle strength and overall body conditioning
- Educate and inform participants
- Strategically partner you with medical professionals

See table 15.1 for a comparison of the roles of water fitness instructors and physical therapists.

Common Terms

Before we move to the specific guidelines for each medical condition, you need to know the meanings of some frequently used terms.

The neutral or functional posture/position of the spine is the least painful, most stable position of the spine for each particular activity or exercise. The position is dynamic and can be variable (Morgan, 1988).

To find the neutral or functional posture/position of the spine, have participants stand with feet shoulder-width apart, back to the wall, and heels about 18 inches away from the wall. They should slide down the wall into a slight squat, then flatten or push the low back against the wall by tightening the abdominal and gluteal muscles. Once they've done that, tell them to relax and rock the low back away from the wall, creating an arch in the low back. The movement of the low back through the entire range avail-

able from rocking to arching is called the *functional range of motion of the low back*. Ask them to practice arching and flattening the back, being aware of areas of pain or discomfort, and find the most comfortable position(s) within this range. Then have them vary the amount of knee flexion and extension and shoulder flexion and extension and note how each changes the resting spinal position.

The easiest way to find neutral spinal position is to learn it while lying on the deck with knees bent, feet flat on the deck. Have participants follow the same sequence outlined before, arching, then flattening the low back until they find the most comfortable position(s). Have them try the progression in a squat position against the wall after mastering the task lying down, then try other postures such as sitting, standing, and lunging.

Finally, review the task with them standing in the pool against the wall, then have them move away into the center of the pool and cue them to tighten their abdominals and gluteals to stabilize their trunks. Tell them to use sculling and coordinated hand moves to stabilize the positions while water pushes and pulls against the body.

The *neutral position* of any joint is the most comfortable position of that joint and usually lies within the middle of the available range of motion. The most important point to remember is to avoid positioning the joint at the extreme end of range of motion during active exercise or stretching. This can stress the joint and surrounding soft tissues. The joints that are most commonly cued for neutral or mid-range position include the spine, wrists, hands, knees, and elbows. Some equipment may need modification (putting foam grips around hand buoys) to accommodate neutral hand (grip) position for a participant with arthritis.

The end of range of motion can be approached with static stretching; however, ask the participants where the stretch is felt. For example, if the exercise is stretching the quadriceps, participants should point to the quadriceps muscle. However, if they are pointing to the back of the knee, chances are the knee joint is being stressed.

The acute phase of injury includes the time period from the initial injury to 72 hours after the injury. It is characterized by the four cardinal signs of inflammation:

1. Pain
2. Swelling
3. Redness
4. Heat or increased local temperature

PRICE is used to care for the injury:

> **P** = **Protection** (use of crutches, braces, supports, or similar devices)
>
> **R** = **Rest** (exercising should be postponed or exercises involving the injured area should be modified)
>
> **I** = **Ice**
>
> **C** = **Compression** (elastic bandage or other compressive supports)
>
> **E** = **Elevation** (above the level of the heart to reduce swelling)

The subacute or repair phase of injury can last from 48 hours up to six weeks after the initial injury. The previously noted signs of inflammation should be decreasing during this phase as the injury heals (Kellett, 1986). Exercise can resume if modifications are provided to prevent re-injury and promote healing.

The remodeling phase lasts from 3 weeks to 12 months or more after the initial injury. During this phase, the signs of acute inflammation may be resolved while strength and flexibility are being restored to the injured area (Kellett, 1986). The participant may be able to participate fully in the exercise program, without modification. However, you, as instructor, should be certain to monitor the participant's response to exercise of the involved area so he or she can avoid re-injury.

A *chronic condition* is one in which the pain and dysfunction associated with injury continue beyond the normal time of healing. The participant's ability to perform certain exercises or activities may be limited. He or she may require exercise modifications, and her or his tolerance to exercise should continue to be monitored. Instruct the participant to use modifications as needed for exercises involving the injured area.

Proper body mechanics can be described as the safest, most efficient position of the body for performing any given activity. Here are some descriptions of proper body mechanics for some activities of daily living (ADL):

- Rising from a chair is performed most efficiently if the individual moves the body to the front of the chair. This can be accomplished by scooting or alternately elevating each hip to "walk" the body forward. The person should not push the back against the chair to slide the body forward. Once the body is forward, the individual should position the feet with one forward and one slightly back (staggered stance) to assist with balance. Hands may be free or may push down against the armrests, the seat of the chair, or his or her thighs. Finally, the person should lean the head and shoulders forward, bending at the hips while keeping the back straight before standing up.

- Rolling over from a supine position (lying on the back) requires that the person bend one or both knees. If rolling to the right, the individual should reach across with the left arm, rotating the shoulders, hips, and knees to the right. If in bed, the individual should drop the feet off the side of the bed and simultaneously push down with the right elbow and left hand. This will lift the trunk while the legs are lowered as the person sits up. If the person is on the floor, he or she can follow the previous directions to assume a side-sitting position.

- To stand from the floor, the individual should start by placing both hands on the floor, shoulder-width apart. He or she should pivot the hips up to get on hands and knees (quadruped position), then walk the hands backward so that they rest on the thighs. From there, the individual should lift up the stronger leg to get into a half-kneeling position. The toes of the "kneeling leg" should be tucked under to help with balance and pushing up. If the person is holding onto a chair or resting on the thigh, he or she should push down against the chair or thigh with one hand while standing up.

- To lift an object from the floor, a person should stand close to the object, with feet shoulder-width apart or in a staggered-stance position. Keeping the back straight and the shoulders over the hips, he or she should squat down and extend the arms down while maintaining a neutral spine. The person then should pull the object close to the body, squeeze the gluteal and abdominal muscles, and stand up. He or she should keep the abdominals tight and the object close to the body while walking.

- Pushing an object should be performed in a staggered-stance position. The individual should bend the knees and push the object by leaning forward from the hips, pushing with the legs, and keeping the back and elbows straight, but not locked. He or she should keep the neck and back in alignment.

- Pulling also starts from a staggered-stance position. The individual should bend the knees and pull the object back by leaning back, shifting weight from the front to the rear leg.

- Picking up an object from a shelf may require a staggered stance to pull the object closer (to the edge of the shelf). The person should squat down as far as necessary to grasp the object, hold it close against the body, and stand. If turning, he or she should not twist the torso. Instead, the person should turn the shoulders, hips, and feet together while holding the object close to the body.

In general, an individual should keep abdominals and gluteals tight during lifting, pushing, pulling, or reaching up or forward to prevent the low back from extending (arching). He or she should keep a slight curve in the low back or maintain neutral position during all activities, especially lifting. When moving forward or backward, the person should use a staggered-stance position and shift the body weight forward and backward from the legs, keeping the back straight. If leaning over is absolutely necessary, the individual should use one arm or the chest to support the body weight.

Gait is simply the way a person walks. For example, an antalgic gait is a walk with a limp or lean due to pain with walking.

Range of motion (ROM) is the amount of motion (measured in degrees) that occurs at any particular joint during movement (Hooke, 1986). With fast or forceful exercise in the water, the momentum created by inertia can easily push a joint beyond the normal end range of motion. This can cause overstretching to the joint or muscles involved. Participants should be cued to stop or reverse the movement when they reach 60 percent to 70 percent of the range for that movement. This slows the momentum and stops the extremity before it reaches the end of the range of motion.

Orthopedic Conditions

1. Arthritis

Arthritis can be defined as inflammation of a joint and may be caused by a number of disease processes. The most common forms of arthritis include osteoarthritis, rheumatoid arthritis, and juvenile rheumatoid arthritis.

Osteoarthritis (OA), also called degenerative joint disease (DJD), is the most common form of all joint disorders (see figures 15.1 and 15.2). Almost all people by age 40 have some degree of degeneration in weight-bearing joints, but few have pain (Berkow, 1987). DJD is the degeneration or breakdown of the cartilage covering the ends of the bones making up a joint. It can be caused by a number of factors, such as injury to a joint or the wear and tear of daily life. Athletes such as

Figure 15.1   *Structure of a joint*

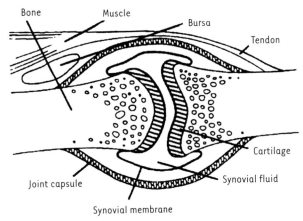

From The Arthritis Foundation and the YMCA of the USA *Arthritis Foundation YMCA Aquatic Program (AFYAF and AFYAP PLUS): Instructors Manual.* 1996. Atlanta: Arthritis Foundation.

Figure 15.2 *Arthritic joint*

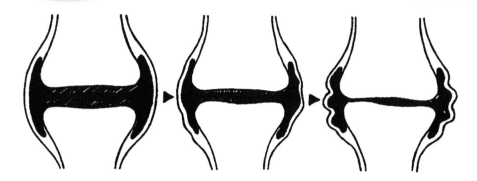

The shaded area (cartilage) gradually thins and is lost until bone contacts bone. These diagrams show progressive damage.

From The Arthritis Foundation and the YMCA of the USA *Arthritis Foundation YMCA Aquatic Program (AFYAF and AFYAP PLUS): Instructors Manual.* 1996. Atlanta: Arthritis Foundation.

long-distance runners surprisingly show no greater incidence of OA than nonathletes their age (Berkow, 1987). Pain and stiffness, which are the primary symptoms, usually improve with exercise or activity.

Rheumatoid arthritis (RA) is different from osteoarthritis in that it is a disease process that affects the entire body, as opposed to a specific joint. It is more common among women than men. The cause is not known and involves the joint surfaces and surrounding soft tissues and ligaments. RA commonly affects the joints bilaterally (equally affecting both sides), with the hands and feet common sites (Berkow, 1987). Joint deformity is usually the outcome, with the most obvious patterns of deformity being slanting of the fingers away from the thumb and toes away from the big toe. Joint pain and inflammation can increase and decrease in a cyclic pattern. During the periods of increased pain and inflammation, the joint is most vulnerable to damage, and exercise tolerance should be closely monitored. Physician's guidelines for activity levels are recommended during this time.

Juvenile RA is similar to adult RA in that it is a disease process affecting the entire body. It starts in children under the age of 16 and usually affects the large joints of the body, interfering with normal growth and development. Guidelines and precautions are similar to RA. As with all forms of arthritis, exercise has been shown to improve functional abilities and strength (Berkow, 1987).

SCREENING

- Check the range of motion of the affected area.
- Observe the participant's willingness to move and points of restriction.
- Watch for signs of pain (grimacing).

SAFETY TIPS AND SUGGESTED EXERCISE MODIFICATIONS

- Decrease range of motion, surface area, and speed if movements are painful or restricted.
- Approach the end of the range of motion only to assist the stretch if it's pain free.
- Check water depth and increase depth to decrease weight bearing.
- Avoid ballistic moves and limit rebounding if necessary.
- Have the participant perform exercises in neutral joint position (have them use smaller sculling motions to maintain the neutral joint position of the wrists).
- Minimize having the participant grip equipment or the pool edge if the hands or wrists are affected.
- Encourage the participant to wear water shoes to prevent jarring and avoid falls.
- Include frequent rest periods in your program.
- Provide gradual progressions.

ABNORMAL RESPONSE TO EXERCISE

- Red, hot, or swollen joints
- Moderate or greater pain during or after exercise
- An inability to move an extremity without pain

RECOMMENDATIONS AFTER ABNORMAL RESPONSE

- Advise the participant to ice and rest the involved joint.
- Recheck exercise performance to see whether the participant is holding the joint in a neutral position.
- Allow the participant to return to exercise when he or she can move without pain.

 Refer the participant back to his or her health care provider if symptoms persist or intensify.

2. Muscle Strain/Tendinitis

A muscle strain is an injury to the muscle involving any portion of the muscle from the belly to the junction of the muscle and tendon. Severity can range from microscopic tears to a complete rupture. Tendinitis is the inflammation of a tendon due to injury or overuse (Berkow, 1987). Severity can vary depending on the degree of damage or inflammation. Rupture of a muscle or tendon would result in the inability of that muscle to contract and perform its designated movement. Individuals who experience pain with movement of a strained muscle or tendinitis should not perform resisted exercises or stretching (if painful) involving that muscle or tendon. Performing resisted exercises when muscles or tendons are painful only perpetuates the problem or causes re-injury. The participant can resume resisted exercises of the affected muscle or tendon when there is no longer pain with movement.

 SCREENING

- Observe the movement of the affected area on the deck and in the pool and note the participant's pain response.
- Ask the participant about symptoms when he or she exits the pool at the end of class.
- Ask the participant how he or she feels just before the beginning of the next class.

 SAFETY TIPS AND SUGGESTED EXERCISE MODIFICATIONS

- Avoid having the participant perform resisted exercise (especially eccentric) in the involved area if it's painful for the muscle or tendon. Reduce the intensity of the exercise by asking him or her to move more slowly, and avoid or minimize the use of overload equipment.

- Instruct the participant to not stretch the affected muscle to the point of pain. If necessary, the participant may have to stop stretching that muscle until it is free of pain.
- For patellar tendinitis, ask the participant about pain during squats, step work, or rebound moves (knee extension). If there is pain, reduce the exercise intensity or eliminate the moves.
- Help the participant strengthen the opposing muscle groups by resisting against buoyancy. Then use buoyancy for assisted or passive recovery of the involved group.

 ABNORMAL RESPONSE TO EXERCISE

- Increase in pain or symptoms during exercise

 RECOMMENDATIONS AFTER ABNORMAL RESPONSE

- Tell the participant to rest and ice the injured area.
- Modify exercises to avoid causing symptoms (change direction of power phase, decrease speed or surface area, remove webbed gloves, check the direction of buoyancy resistance on the area).
- Exercise the rest of the participant's body without affecting the injured area.

 Refer the participant back to her or his health care provider if symptoms persist or intensify.

3. General Post-Surgical

Any surgery is an invasive procedure in which the skin and underlying tissues are entered from the outside environment. Obviously, the larger and deeper incisions, especially those through muscle and bone, are the most invasive procedures and require longer healing time. Recovery can also be prolonged by other factors such as infection, general health of the individual, and other medical complications.

Arthroscopic surgery is much less invasive in that it requires only small slits in the skin. Rigid tubes are inserted through the slits that enable the physician to insert and see through a tiny video camera and microscopically perform the necessary repairs through the tubes. Recovery time is considerably shorter, scars are much smaller, and rehabilitation usually progresses faster with arthroscopic repairs. Arthroscopic surgery is most commonly performed on the shoulder and knee.

SCREENING

- The participant should wait 2 to 4 weeks after arthroscopy and 8 to 12 weeks after open surgery (until the wound is completely healed) before participating in a community-based aquatic exercise program (if no complications exist).
- The participant should have a full range of motion and be free of pain before exercising.
- The participant should have medical clearance specifically for aquatic exercise.

SAFETY TIPS AND SUGGESTED EXERCISE MODIFICATIONS

- Have the participant perform ranges of motion in straight planes (no rotation).
- Avoid having the participant perform rotary (breaststroke kick) or ballistic (rebound) moves of the involved joints.
- Decrease the size and speed of moves.
- Avoid end-range (movements at the extreme end of range of motion) movements of the involved area, unless they are static stretches in warm water.
- Follow the physician's guidelines.

 ABNORMAL RESPONSE TO EXERCISE

- Moderate or greater pain during or after exercise
- Increase in swelling

 RECOMMENDATIONS AFTER ABNORMAL RESPONSE

- Decrease the size, speed, and/or surface area of the movements.
- Decrease the length of time the participant exercises in the pool.
- Tell the participant to rest and ice the area on which surgery was performed.

 Refer the participant back to his or her health care provider if he or she experiences an increase in pain, swelling, redness, or heat in the area of surgery or develops a fever.

4. Total Hip Replacement

A total hip replacement (THR) is the surgical removal of the head and neck of the femur and the acetabulum. These structures are replaced with man-made metal or plastic implants. A THR is usually performed because of a fracture to the femoral neck, loss of blood supply to the femoral head, or arthritis. Severe pain and loss of function are the primary criteria for performing a THR on someone with arthritis.

Medical clearance and guidelines are required for any exercise participant who has had a THR. Participants follow the guidelines for all water exercises and functional activities such as dressing and getting in or out of the pool. Cardiovascular conditioning exercises, lower extremity strengthening (especially gluteals), and training for functional activities are essential program elements for individuals participating in a community-based fitness program who have had a THR.

SCREENING

- Observe the participant's level of difficulty and independence in entering or exiting the pool.
- Have the participant wait until the wound is healed and there is minimal swelling of the involved lower extremity before exercising.
- The participant should wait 12 weeks after surgery before participating in a community-based aquatic exercise program (if no complications exist). (See the postsurgical section.)
- Ask the participant about any previous or current low-back injury or pain (see the low-back pain section).
- The participant should have medical clearance specifically for aquatic exercise.

SAFETY TIPS AND SUGGESTED EXERCISE MODIFICATIONS

- Instruct the participant to not perform hip flexion greater than or equal to 90 degrees.
- Avoid the combination of hip flexion, adduction, and internal rotation (check the surgeon's guidelines).
- Avoid having the participant cross midline in front or behind.
- Decrease the lower-body range of motion and the speed of moves.
- Include exercises that strengthen hip extensors and abductors.

- Monitor the participant when he or she enters and exits the pool. Watch the individual's hip range of motion when he or she uses a ladder.
- Encourage participants to wear water shoes to prevent jarring and avoid falls.

 ABNORMAL RESPONSE TO EXERCISE

- Moderate or greater pain during or after exercise
- Low back pain
- Excessive fatigue

 RECOMMENDATIONS AFTER ABNORMAL RESPONSE

- Decrease the range of motion and speed for exercises of the lower extremities.
- Cue the participant to find and maintain the low back in neutral position (review on land, then check in water) (see low-back guidelines). If necessary, eliminate kicking to the rear to prevent hyperextension of the low back.
- Decrease overall exercise intensity.

 Refer the participant back to his or her health care provider if any one of the following occurs:

- Sudden leg swelling and/or pain
- Fever
- Severe pain in the hip
- Signs of hip dislocation, which can include severe pain, a sudden inability to move the leg, or sudden shortening of the leg

5. Knee: ACL Tear (Sprain) and Reconstructive Surgery

The anterior cruciate ligament (ACL) (see figure 15.3) plays an important role in stabilizing the knee by preventing the tibia from sliding forward on the femur (giving way). Injury to the ACL most frequently occurs during sporting activities involving cutting (changing direction) or coming down from a jump with the knee straight. Tear of a meniscus (knee cartilage) frequently occurs with a complete tear of the ACL. The primary goal of care is to prevent the knee from giving way. Recurrent episodes lead to increased wear and tear on the knee and ultimately arthritis. Activities that put the knee at high risk for giving way are those in which the knee is nearly straight. High-risk activities include cutting, jumping, or walking on uneven ground, down a slope, hill, or stairs (Torrey, 1996).

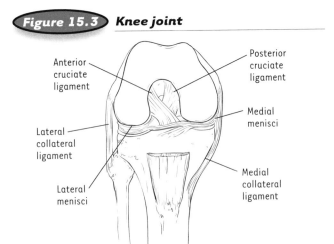

Figure 15.3 *Knee joint*

Reproduced with permission from Snider R.K. (ed): *Essentials of Musculoskeletal Care.* Rosemont, IL, American Academy of Orthopaedic Surgeons, 1997.

Complete rupture of the ACL can sometimes be managed without surgery by avoiding high-risk activities that might cause the knee to give way, strengthening the lower extremity, and wearing a custom knee brace during all activities. The brace prevents the knee from straightening completely and stabilizes the knee joint. Reconstructive surgery is the suggested option for those individuals who cannot or do not want to give up high-risk activities associated with giving way. During reconstructive surgery, an ACL graft is inserted into the tibia and femur. Today, successful knee stabilization occurs in 90 percent of ACL reconstructive surgeries. Stress or load on the graft (especially in straight-knee positions) can lead to irreversible stretching of the graft and knee instability. Medical clearance and guidelines are required for any participant still receiving medical care following ACL injury or reconstructive surgery (Torrey, 1996).

 SCREENING

- The participant should have full, pain-free range of motion in the injured knee as compared to the other knee.
- The participant should wait at least 12 weeks after surgery before participating in a community-based aquatic exercise program (depending on wound healing).
- The participant should have minimal swelling in the injured knee.
- The participant should have medical clearance specifically for aquatic exercise.

SAFETY TIPS AND SUGGESTED EXERCISE MODIFICATIONS

- Avoid using breast stroke or rotary-type kicks.
- Avoid ballistic moves (rebounding off the bottom or pushing off the pool wall).
- Avoid quick changes of direction or turning for six to eight months (check post-surgical guidelines).
- Follow the bracing guidelines of the health care provider. The participant may need to wear a brace in the pool.

 ABNORMAL RESPONSE TO EXERCISE

- Moderate increase in pain and symptoms
- Swelling
- Loss of ROM
- Loss of function
- Increase in local temperature at the knee

RECOMMENDATIONS AFTER ABNORMAL RESPONSE

- Tell the participant to ice and rest the injured knee.
- Move the participant to a deeper water depth to decrease weight bearing.
- Reduce the size and/or speed of movement.
- Have the participant perform lower extremity exercises in straight planes.
- Avoid the end of the range. Watch that water currents do not push the limb past the end of the knee range of motion.

Refer the participant back to his or her health care provider if any one of the following occurs:

- Persistent increase in pain and swelling
- Loss of movement due to pain
- Development of a limp

6. Knee: PCL Reconstructive surgery

The posterior cruciate ligament (PCL) (see figure 15.3) is injured much less frequently than the anterior cruciate ligament. A direct blow to the front of the knee is frequently the cause of PCL injury. Damage to other ligaments surrounding the knee can occur in conjunction with a PCL tear. Most PCL tears that occur without injury to other ligaments can be rehabilitated without surgery. Complete rupture of the PCL alters the normal joint mechanics and increases stress on the knee joint, which can lead to premature arthritis. Reconstructive surgery is recommended if arthritic changes are present or if PCL injury is combined with other ligament or meniscal injuries. Rigid adherence to surgical guidelines is essential to avoid stretching the PCL graft (Torrey, 1996).

Following a complete PCL tear, the injured individual must wear a custom-fit brace for activities that include cutting, pivoting, and jumping. Medical clearance and guidelines are required for a participant still receiving medical care for a PCL injury.

 SCREENING

- The participant should have full, pain-free range of motion in the injured knee as compared to the other knee.
- The participant should wait until 12 to 16 weeks after surgery before participating in a community-based aquatic exercise program (depending on wound healing).
- The participant should have minimal swelling in the injured knee.
- The participant should have medical clearance specifically for aquatic exercise.

 SAFETY TIPS AND SUGGESTED EXERCISE MODIFICATIONS

- Do not allow the participant to engage in pool exercise until 12 to 16 weeks after surgery due to guidelines restricting active hamstring contraction (knee flexion) for three months.
- Emphasize lower-extremity strengthening and flexibility, cardiovascular endurance, and coordination activities for the lower extremities.

ABNORMAL RESPONSE TO EXERCISE

- Moderate increase in pain and symptoms
- Swelling
- Loss of ROM
- Loss of function
- Increase in local temperature at the knee

RECOMMENDATIONS AFTER ABNORMAL RESPONSE

- Tell the participant to ice and rest the injured knee.
- Move the participant to a deeper water depth to decrease weight bearing.
- Reduce the size and/or speed of movement.
- Have the participant perform lower-extremity exercises in straight planes.
- Avoid the end of the range of motion. Watch that water currents do not push the limb past the end of the knee range of motion.

Refer the participant back to his or her health care provider if any one of the following occurs:

- Persistent increase in pain and swelling
- Loss of movement due to pain
- Development of a limp

7. Knee: Total Knee Replacement

A total knee replacement (TKR) is performed when all conservative measures to treat arthritis of the knee have failed. Pain and loss of function are the main criteria for performing a total knee replacement. A TKR involves resurfacing the ends of the bones of the knee joint with a metal or metal-backed plastic insert. The distal end of the femur, the proximal end of the tibia, and the patella are replaced in a TKR. Some patients receive a hemiarthroplasty (one-half of a knee replacement) if only one end of the joint is arthritic (Torrey, 1996).

Benefits of a TKR include relief of pain, increased ability to perform daily tasks, increased knee range of motion, and improved alignment of the leg. Infection, blood clots, and mechanical loosening of the prosthesis (implants) are some of the potential risks associated with a TKR. The most important precautions following knee replacement surgery are to avoid activities that increase rotational force or impact loading to the knee.

Vigorous activities that involve running or jumping are not advised following a knee replacement. Swimming, biking, and golfing (if done carefully) are safe activities to perform. Knee replacements typically last 10 years or more (Torrey, 1996).

SCREENING

- Observe the available range of motion of the involved knee as compared to the other knee.
- The participant should not exercise if there are significant signs of inflammation, including moderate or greater swelling or pain.
- The participant should have medical clearance specifically for aquatic exercise.
- Observe whether the participant can enter and exit the pool independently or needs assistance.
- Follow postsurgical guidelines and remind the participant to do so as well.

SAFETY TIPS AND SUGGESTED EXERCISES MODIFICATIONS

- Check that the participant performs movement and work within the *available* knee range of motion only.
- Decrease the size and/or speed of movement.
- Use strengthening exercises for the lower extremities (especially quadriceps and hamstrings) and trunk, which are essential for improving functional activities.
- Avoid rotational stress on the knee and minimize impact loading of the knee.
- Practice functional activities such as standing from a sitting position, going up and down steps, balancing, and dressing.

ABNORMAL RESPONSE TO EXERCISE

- Moderate or greater pain during or after exercise
- Moderate knee joint swelling
- Loss of ROM
- Loss of function
- Increase in local temperature of the knee

RECOMMENDATIONS AFTER ABNORMAL RESPONSE

- Tell the participant to ice and rest the injured knee.
- Avoid end-of-range knee movements.
- Increase water depth and/or use the neutral position (with feet sliding along the pool floor).

Refer the participant back to his or her health care provider if any one of the following occurs:

- Persistent increase in pain and swelling
- Loss of movement due to pain
- Development of a limp

8. Knee: Meniscal Tear/Surgery

Each knee contains two meniscii, one on the medial and one on the lateral side of the joint. The meniscii are made of a type of cartilage and have a number of functions. They provide shock absorption and lend stability to the knee. A tear or removal of a meniscus can lead to the development of arthritis. The meniscii are most susceptible to injury when a rotary force occurs during flexion or extension of the knee (Torrey, 1996). A torn meniscus usually requires arthroscopic surgery. Meniscal injuries can sometimes be repaired; however, removal of the damaged area is frequently necessary. Medical clearance and guidelines are required for individuals who are still seeing their health care provider following meniscal tear or surgery.

SCREENING

- The participant should have full, pain-free range of motion in the injured knee as compared to the other knee.
- The participant should wait two to four weeks after surgery before participating in a community-based aquatic exercise program (depending on wound healing). (See surgical guidelines.)
- The participant should have medical clearance specifically for aquatic exercise.

SAFETY TIPS AND SUGGESTED EXERCISES MODIFICATIONS

- Avoid using rotary, quick-snapping knee moves.
- Avoid complicated choreography.
- Decrease the size and/or speed of movement.
- Work to the end of range of motion during static stretches only (in warm water).
- Use gradual progressions for squats and step work.

ABNORMAL RESPONSE TO EXERCISE

- Moderate increase or greater pain during or after exercise
- Increased swelling
- Loss of ROM
- Loss of function
- Increase in local temperature at the knee

RECOMMENDATIONS AFTER ABNORMAL RESPONSE

- Tell the participant to ice and rest the injured knee.
- Have the participant perform lower-extremity exercises in straight planes.
- Simplify the exercises.
- Move the participant to a deeper water depth to decrease impact.
- Decrease the size, speed, and surface area for the involved leg movements.
- Eliminate squats, rebounding, and step work if necessary.

 Refer the participant back to his or her health care provider if any one of the following occur:

- ➤ Persistent increase in pain and swelling
- ➤ Loss of movement due to pain
- ➤ Development of a limp

9. Knee: Chronic Anterior Knee Pain

Chronic **anterior** knee pain is a general term used to describe a number of conditions that can affect the anterior (front of) the knee. These dysfunctions are usually a result of overuse or poor training, but can also be influenced by imbalances in muscle strength, muscle tightness, or problems related to anatomic alignment of the femur, tibia, or patella (Koury, 1996).

The group of terms describing pain and dysfunction in the anterior knee is also called patellofemoral syndrome. Some of the conditions that may be involved include these:

Patellar tendinitis. A strain with resulting inflammation of the patellar tendon that usually results from ballistic or repetitive activities such as running or jumping, or resisted open-kinetic chain knee extension exercises. (Open-kinetic chain knee extension exercises are exercises or activities in which the foot is not in contact with a surface such as the ground. An example of an aquatic open-kinetic chain knee extension exercise would be extending the knee from a bent-knee to a straight-knee position [kicking].)

Patellar malalignment. Poor position of the patella that can result from imbalances in muscle strength, muscle tightness (such as in the tensor fascia latae), variances in the anatomy of the femur, and the size or resting position of the patella. All of these factors can lead to problems with smooth gliding of the patella and potential abnormal tracking or dislocation.

Chondromalacia. The softening of the undersurface of the kneecap that results from the increased wear and tear on the patella occurring with patellofemoral syndrome.

Osgood-Schlatter Disease. Inflammation where the patellar tendon attaches at the tibial tubercle. It is seen in adolescents and occurs when strength demands from the quadriceps and patellar tendon pull too hard on the growth plate of the tibia. Resisted knee extension and running and jumping activities are stopped until the growth plate can heal.

Activities to avoid when exercising participants who have anterior knee pain include deep squats and ballistic resisted knee extension. Step work can also increase anterior knee pain. Static squats (progressed from mini-squats to half-squats) of gradually increasing duration and straight-leg kicks should be tolerated. Stretching exercises should focus on tensor fascia latae, quadriceps, hamstrings, and gastrocnemius. Strengthening should emphasize the quadriceps (especially the vastus medialis during the last 30 degrees of knee extension), gluteals, and hamstrings.

 SCREENING

- The participant should have full, pain-free range of motion in the injured knee as compared to the other knee.
- The participant should have minimal swelling in the injured knee.
- The participant should have medical clearance specifically for aquatic exercise and guidelines.
- Check whether the participant has pain during squats, standing from a sitting position, or stair climbing.

 SAFETY TIPS AND SUGGESTED EXERCISES MODIFICATIONS

- Avoid moves that increase knee pain.
- Watch facial responses during leg activities.
- Check whether the participant has pain during and after exercise.
- Gradually progress kicks, squats, and step work. Start with kicking activities that keep the knee extended, then gradually use activities that incorporate knee flexion, as tolerated.
- Avoid rebound movements if painful.
- Avoid using ankle buoyancy cuffs.

- Avoid deep squats and ballistic resisted knee extension.
- Keep in mind that step work can increase anterior knee pain.

STOP **ABNORMAL RESPONSE TO EXERCISE**

- Moderate or greater pain during or after exercise
- Increase in difficulty with land activities such as stair climbing, moving from sitting to standing, and squats

 RECOMMENDATIONS AFTER ABNORMAL RESPONSE

- Eliminate resisted and eccentric knee extension activities (squats, rebounding, step work).
- Work in deep water.

Refer the participant back to his or her health care provider if he or she experiences a persistent moderate to severe increase in pain or swelling.

10. Shoulder: Rotator Cuff Tear, Impingement, Post-Surgical

The four rotator cuff muscles (supraspinatus, infraspinatus, subscapularis, and teres minor) are important for stability and movement at the shoulder. The supraspinatus and infraspinatus muscles are especially prone to injury from activities requiring prolonged or repetitive use of the arms above shoulder level. Pain is typically felt during shoulder flexion and/or abduction in cases of acute or chronic tendinitis. Treatment by a health care provider can relieve pain and restore strength and function.

Progression of symptoms of rotator cuff tendinitis leads to a chronic condition involving inflammation, swelling, pain, muscle atrophy, weakness, and altered shoulder joint mechanics. *Impingement* is a general term used to describe chronic shoulder pain that occurs when the above factors result in pinching of the suprahumeral structures (bursa, supraspinatus, and/or biceps tendon) under the acromion (see figure 15.4). Rotator cuff dysfunction and impingement frequently result in a painful arc occurring during active shoulder abduction (see figure 15.5). Weakness of the rotator cuff muscles, decreased flexibility of posterior shoulder structures, and increased pressure in the subacromial space due to swelling are all potential causes of impingement (Koury, 1996, pp. 159-160). During abduction of the arm, a participant with a

Figure 15.4 *Shoulder impingement*

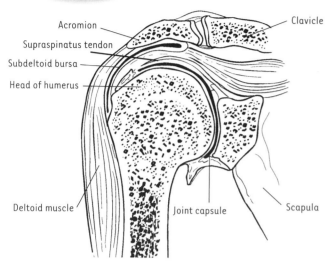

Reproduced with permission from Snider R.K. (ed): *Essentials of Musculoskeletal Care.* Rosemont, IL, American Academy of Orthopaedic Surgeons, 1997.

shoulder impingement may lean away from the injured side in an attempt to help raise the arm and possibly wincing with pain some time during the arm movement. Participants with this type of response to lifting their arm should be referred to their health care provider.

Surgery may be required if conservative care has been unsuccessful in relief of symptoms and/or restoration of function. Arthroscopic or open surgery can be performed to repair a torn rotator cuff muscle or decompress the area below the acromion to allow more space for freedom of movement (Koury, 1996, p. 162). Patients require physical therapy to restore normal motion, strength, and function after surgery.

SCREENING

- Exercise should not be performed if the participant experiences moderate or greater shoulder pain at rest or with activity.
- The participant should feel no radiating arm pain from the shoulder blade to the arm or hand.
- The participant should have medical clearance specifically for aquatic exercise, if postsurgical. (See surgical guidelines if applicable.)
- Observe the participant's shoulder ROM (note any limitations of movement or pain with movement).

Figure 15.5 *Painful arc of motion*

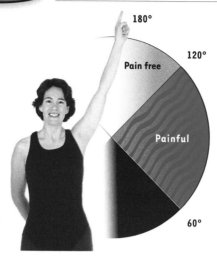

SAFETY TIPS AND SUGGESTED EXERCISE MODIFICATIONS

- If swinging the arms causes the participant pain (as in the cross-country ski move), decrease the length of the arms (levers) by bending the elbows and bringing the arms closer to the body. Speed of movement and surface area can also be decreased if necessary.
- Emphasize resistance to downward and backward arm moves if the person has pain with arm movements (power down and back), and use a passive recovery (assisted by buoyancy or water currents).
- Use minimal or no overhead activities, arm elevation, or reaching up or forward.
- Modify sculling and move deeper in the water for neutral shoulder position. Work with hands near the hips or hold hands in the "tabletop" position for balance.
- Focus initially on strengthening the trunk/shoulder girdle (scapular muscles, abdominals, low-back muscles). Strengthening exercises involving arm elevation can be initiated later, as tolerated by the participant.
- Assess tolerance to upper extremity movement in transitional and deep water depths; may need to stay in shallow water.
- Have the participant begin exercising without gloves and assess over time whether she or he can tolerate wearing gloves during exercise.

 ABNORMAL RESPONSE TO EXERCISE

- Moderate or greater increase in pain during or after exercise
- Leaning sideways while raising the arm (indicating weakness)
- Complaints of neck pain during or after exercise
- Inability to move the involved arm without moderate or severe pain

 RECOMMENDATIONS AFTER ABNORMAL RESPONSE

- Tell the participant to ice and rest the injured arm and shoulder.
- Decrease exercise intensity.
- Eliminate or minimize use of the injured extremity.
- Immobilize (sling) the injured extremity during exercise.

 Refer the participant back to his or her health care provider if any one of the following occurs:

- Moderate to greater increase in shoulder pain
- Inability to move arm
- Radiating arm pain

11. Shoulder: Adhesive Capsulitis (stiff shoulder/frozen shoulder)

Adhesive capsulitis is a common disorder occurring most often in women and middle-aged or older people. In adhesive capsulitis, the shoulder loses passive movement in a "capsular" pattern. Abduction may be limited up to 90 degrees, external rotation can be completely limited, and internal rotation may be limited up to 30 degrees. Sometimes the stiffness occurs following trauma, surgery, or immobilization of the arm. Some cases of frozen shoulder occur unrelated to trauma or surgery. It is speculated that changes in the alignment of the shoulder blade and head of the humerus that occur with hunching over (thoracic kyphosis) can lead to the shoulder stiffness. Most people don't notice the loss of motion until it affects daily tasks such as washing their hair, fastening a bra, or reaching into a back pocket (Hertling and Kessler, 1990). Physical therapy is often necessary to stretch the joint capsule, increase the joint ROM, and then strengthen the shoulder, scapulae, and trunk muscles.

 SCREENING

- Observe the available shoulder range of motion.
- The participant should have no radiating arm pain.
- The participant should have medical clearance specifically for aquatic exercise.

 SAFETY TIPS AND SUGGESTED EXERCISE MODIFICATIONS

- Cue and teach the limits of shoulder movements, encouraging the participant to stay within the available range of motion.
- Work in warm water.
- Avoid repetitive movements at the end of the range of motion (perform movements slowly early in the motion to minimize the water current's carrying effect on the limb).
- Approach the end of range of movements only during static stretches in warm water.

 ABNORMAL RESPONSE TO EXERCISE

- Moderate or greater increase in pain during or after exercise

 RECOMMENDATIONS AFTER ABNORMAL RESPONSE

- Tell the participant to ice and rest the injured shoulder.
- Avoid all end-range movements.
- Refer the participant to a health care provider if group exercise is not appropriate.

Refer the participant back to his or her health care provider if he or she experiences a sudden, severe increase in pain or an inability to move the extremity.

12. Shoulder: Chronic Dislocation

A majority of shoulder dislocations occur in an **anterior-inferior** direction due to forced external rotation when the arm is abducted. The problem, especially among athletes, is that it can recur. Eventually recurrent shoulder dislocation can result from minimal force. The position of instability for a person with anterior-inferior shoulder dislocation is the "I surrender" position. (The "I surrender" position is with arms at shoulder level, elbows bent, and palms forward.) Immediate treatment and rehabilitation of a dislocation can help prevent recurrence (Koury,

1996). In the case of chronic dislocations, surgery is frequently the treatment of choice. Surgical treatment can result in a loss of some ROM in external rotation. This is necessary for maintaining stability and should not be stressed during activities.

 SCREENING

- The participant should have full, pain-free range of motion except for decreased external rotation if after surgery.
- Ask about the direction of the dislocation (95 percent are anterior-inferior).
- Participants who have had surgery or recurrent dislocations should obtain medical clearance and guidelines. Follow postsurgical guidelines.

 SAFETY TIPS AND SUGGESTED EXERCISE MODIFICATIONS

- For those who have anterior dislocations, avoid pectoral stretching (dragging the arms, "I surrender" position, or throwing positions, especially when traveling forward).
- For those who have posterior dislocations, avoid push-up movements such as wall push-ups.
- Avoid extreme end-of-range external rotation (use slow speed, mid-range movements to reduce the effect of water currents on the limb).
- Focus on first strengthening the internal rotators and adductors. Then progress to general strengthening and conditioning exercises.
- Incorporate sports and functional activities into the exercise program.
- Those who have not had surgery and have had an anterior shoulder dislocation should avoid shoulder abduction with external rotation ("I surrender") position of the involved shoulder.

🛑 **ABNORMAL RESPONSE TO EXERCISE**

- Moderate or greater increase in pain during or after exercise

 RECOMMENDATIONS AFTER ABNORMAL RESPONSE

- Decrease the intensity of armwork and avoid using overload equipment on the affected arm.
- Stabilize the arms in front of the body, especially during travel moves, or minimize travel.

Refer the participant back to his or her health care provider if he or she experiences recurrent dislocations.

13. Lateral Epicondylitis (Tennis Elbow), Carpal Tunnel Syndrome

Tennis elbow is a strain and inflammation of the lateral muscles of the forearm (extensors of the fingers and wrist) or their tendinous attachment into the humerus (see figure 15.6). It is typically caused by repetitive movements (turning a screwdriver, playing tennis, entering data into a computer) and is most commonly seen in middle-aged people (Berkow, 1987). Intense pain may be disabling and if not treated successfully can become chronic. There is usually pain with active or resisted supination or extension of the wrist and/or fingers or passive wrist flexion. Physical therapy is usually effective in decreasing pain and inflammation. Resting the muscles and tendons is difficult, because they are used so often in daily tasks. A strap worn just below the elbow is helpful in taking the load off the injured area. Until the muscles and tendons have healed and pain is no longer present with active or resistive wrist and finger extension or supination, resistive exercise will only make the condition worse.

Carpal Tunnel Syndrome (CTS) results from compression of the median nerve as it passes through a small bony and ligamentous tunnel in the wrist. It is more common in women and occurs frequently in jobs or home tasks that require repeated or forceful wrist flexion (Berkow, 1987). Pregnant women can be more likely to have CTS due to increased fluids or swelling. Once the baby is born, caring for the infant can place increased stress on an already painful con-

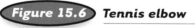 **Figure 15.6** *Tennis elbow*

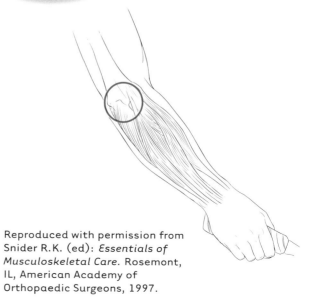

Reproduced with permission from Snider R.K. (ed): *Essentials of Musculoskeletal Care.* Rosemont, IL, American Academy of Orthopaedic Surgeons, 1997.

dition. Pain (occurs commonly at night) and changes in sensation (numbness and/or tingling) in the thumb and first two fingers, palm of the hand, or wrist can be very debilitating. There may also be weakness of thumb opposition (touching thumb to little finger). Like tennis elbow, CTS is an overuse injury, and activities producing pain or symptoms only aggravate the condition. Prolonged gripping activities should be avoided.

 SCREENING

- Observe the range of motion at the elbow, wrist, or hand. Check for an increase in pain or decrease in range of motion while moving the joint through its range of motion.
- Assess the participant's tolerance to sculling and repetitive upper-body moves.

 SAFETY TIPS AND SUGGESTED EXERCISE MODIFICATIONS

- Tell the participant to keep the wrist in neutral joint position while sculling.
- Use caution with repetitive upper-body work and give the participant rests.
- Cue a loose grip or hook equipment through the web space of the thumb to avoid repetitive gripping. Cue to release the grip frequently.
- Pad the grip area of handheld equipment.
- If necessary, modify arm activities to a slicing motion if any resistance causes pain in webbed or cupped hand positions.

 ABNORMAL RESPONSE TO EXERCISE

- Moderate or greater increase in pain during or after exercise

RECOMMENDATIONS AFTER ABNORMAL RESPONSE

- Tell the participant to ice and rest the injured arm, hand, or wrist.
- Decrease the size and speed of movements.
- Modify the scull (have the participant move it lower, down near the hips) and reduce upper-body intensity.
- Eliminate sculling and have the participant use webbed hands passively like rudders for balance.
- Eliminate wearing a webbed glove on the affected limb.

 Refer the participant back to his or her health care provider if he or she experiences a severe increase in pain and symptoms.

14. Neck Pain

Neck pain has a number of potential causes. Some of these can include pinched nerves (due to disc herniations or bone spurs), joint or ligament injury (after a car accident), and muscular pain. Pinched nerves in the cervical spine usually cause pain or numbness or tingling to travel down the arm. The small size of the bones in the neck make it very susceptible to physical stress and strain (see figure 15.7). The neck is unique because it works so closely with the shoulder and arm, with this relationship being a very important consideration in exercise. Increased load on the neck can result from direct exercise or movement of the neck, as well as indirect stress or movement of the long levers of the arms.

When exercisers currently have neck pain or have a past history of neck pain, it can be important to control the intensity of armwork to the level the person can tolerate. Avoid excessive, repetitive overhead movements and resisted arm exercises. Keeping the head and neck in a neutral alignment is also essential during all activities.

Figure 15.7 *Anatomy of the spine*

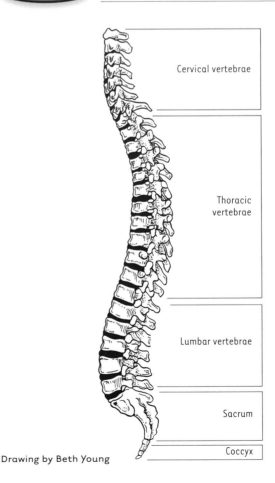

Cervical vertebrae

Thoracic vertebrae

Lumbar vertebrae

Sacrum

Coccyx

Drawing by Beth Young

SCREENING

- The participant should feel no radiating pain in the upper extremity (shoulder blade to arm or hand).

- The participant should feel no numbness or tingling.

- The participant should have a full upper-extremity range of motion.

- The participant should have medical clearance specifically for aquatic exercise if he or she has a current or recent history of significant neck pain.

- Observe the posture of the participant's head, neck, and back.

SAFETY TIPS AND SUGGESTED EXERCISE MODIFICATIONS

- Decrease the speed, surface area, size, and general intensity of all arm movements.

- Have the participant exercise with the arms close to the body, decreasing stress on the neck (by shortening the lever arms).

- Cue for proper posture. When you are on deck, place the participant at the back of the class, crouch low to the water to cue, and cue the participant to use a neutral gaze to avoid cervical hypertension while trying to see you.

- Stress power phase down and back (latissimus, trapezeii, and rhomboids).

- Start the participant exercising without gloves, and gradually add overload equipment, such as gloves, monitoring the effects.

- Avoid repetitive overhead activities.

- Have the participant perform gentle active neck range of motion within his or her pain-free range.

- Deep breathing and gentle upper trapezius stretching exercises can be helpful in reducing stress and increasing neck motion.

- Decrease impact to help prevent headaches.

- Have the participant perform shoulder circles (backwards) or pain-free neck range of motion to relieve muscle spasms.

- Move exercises to transitional or deep water to decrease the work of the muscles supporting the head, neck, and trunk.

ABNORMAL RESPONSE TO EXERCISE

- Moderate or greater increase in pain during or after exercise

- Numbness, tingling, or radiating pain symptoms during or after exercise

RECOMMENDATIONS AFTER ABNORMAL RESPONSE

- Tell the participant to ice and rest the neck.

- Minimize or modify upper-extremity movements.

- Gradually progress overload.

- Watch the participant's neck alignment.

Refer the participant back to his or her health care provider if he or she experiences a moderate or severe increase in pain, or any numbness, tingling, or radiating symptoms into the arms.

15. Low-Back Pain

The causes of low-back pain can vary from disc herniations and bulges to arthritis and spurs, to narrowing of the canal of the spinal cord (stenosis). Muscle strain and spasm can also be a factor in causing low back pain. Weakness of the low-back muscles is common with low-back pain.

While the causes can vary, commonalities exist in approaches to exercise for rehabilitation following injury to the low back. Using guidelines based on functional sensitivities (or functional loss) (Vollowitz, 1988) can simplify the approach the exercise instructor takes when guiding exercises for individuals with low-back pain. Basic guidelines for exercising participants who have low-back pain include the following:

- Maintain the low back in neutral spinal position for all activities. Persons with low-back pain may be sensitive to repetitive extremes of position in flexion (flattening) or extension (arching).

- Unload the spine. Persons with low-back pain can also tend to be sensitive to the effects of compression or load on the spine. This makes the water a perfect medium for exercising load-sensitive back pain participants.

- Change activities frequently. Some participants with back pain may experience an increase in symptoms if they remain in one position for too long and may need to change positions/activities frequently.

Following exercise guidelines based on these functional sensitivities can lead to successful exercise programs for those with low-back pain. The exercise instructor should remember that neutral spine position can vary from person to person, day to day, and activity to activity. If participants do report increased symptoms during or after exercise, make sure that they are able to find and then maintain their neutral position of the spine throughout the activity.

 SCREENING

- The participant should have no radiating pain, numbness, or tingling into the legs.

- Observe the participant's hip range of motion, especially extension, to identify restrictions of motion.

SAFETY TIPS AND SUGGESTED EXERCISE MODIFICATIONS

- Understand and be able to teach neutral spinal position.

- On the deck, train the participant to find one's neutral spinal positions and review those positions in the pool (have the participant work with the back against the pool wall if he or she is having problems).

- Limit the size of lower-extremity moves, especially hip extension.

- Use coordinated hand moves for balance.

- Cue the participant to keep the spine in a neutral position, and check frequently to see if he or she is in that position.

- Progress depths. Begin in shallow, move to transitional, and finally move to deep, as the participant demonstrates adequate control of neutral spinal position with activities at each depth.

- Assess the participant's comfort. If he or she is load sensitive, have the participant wear a flotation belt in shallow water to decrease impact, relieve symptoms, and assist with balance. The participant can start in deeper water and progress gradually to shallow water as tolerated.

- Use straight-plane moves, then progress to diagonal and multiplane moves if tolerated.

- Train the participant in using correct body mechanics for daily tasks.

- Be a good example by moving properly and reinforcing the use of correct body mechanics at all times.

 ABNORMAL RESPONSE TO EXERCISE

- Moderate or greater increase in back pain during or after exercise

- Any pain, numbness, or tingling radiating to the buttocks or legs

 RECOMMENDATIONS AFTER ABNORMAL RESPONSE

- Tell the participant to ice and rest the low back.

- Start all hip extension movements in flexion and stop them at neutral (0 degrees hip extension).

- Review the neutral spinal position on deck and in the pool.

- Decrease the size and speed of movements and minimize or eliminate travel.

- Eliminate rotation and twisting of the spine.

 Refer the participant back to his or her health care provider if any one of the following occurs:

- Severe increase in pain

- Decrease in functional activity level

- Pain, numbness, or tingling in the legs

16. Fibromyalgia

Fibromyalgia is a chronic disorder of unknown origin characterized by widespread musculoskeletal pain and fatigue. Other common symptoms include sleep disturbances, irritable bowel syndrome, chronic headaches, morning stiffness, and cognitive and memory impairments (Thorson, 1992). Fibromyalgia is diagnosed based on the following criteria:

- The person has widespread pain on both sides and above and below the belt.

- The person reports pain felt in 11 of the 18 specified tender point sites where the tester is touching (see figure 15.8)(Bennett, Smythe, and Wolfe, 1992).

Fibromyalgia may be brought on or made worse by physical or mental stress, poor sleep, trauma, exposure to dampness or cold, or an infection. It is most commonly seen in women, although it can occur in people of any age or gender (Berkow, 1987). Persons with fibromyalgia have been shown to have decreased coordination and muscle strength and significantly lower cardiovascular endurance (Goldenberg, 1992, p. 249). However, McCain found improvements in pain symptoms and cardiovascular fitness in a group of fibromyalgia patients who performed cardiovas-

Figure 15.8 *Tender point sites in fibromyalgia*

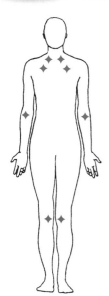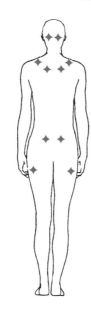

cular fitness training three times per week for 20 weeks (McCain, 1986, p. 76). The water is an ideal environment for persons with fibromyalgia to exercise in, due to the wide variability of intensities that can be achieved and the reduction of impact for persons with pain. It is prudent to begin a person with fibromyalgia at a low intensity and duration, then gradually increase the duration depending on the participant's tolerance. Exercise instructors should be aware that people suffering from fibromyalgia experience frequent ups and downs in symptoms and are subject to depression. Tolerance of activities should be monitored before and after every class. Careful guidance in intensity, regular monitoring, and regular encouragement are vital to successfully exercising a person with fibromyalgia.

SCREENING

- Assess the participant's tolerance to activities on a class-by-class basis.
- Check screening guidelines for the areas that are most painful (refer to the appropriate sections in this chapter, such as neck pain or low-back pain)
- Ask the participant about current level of activity and fitness.

SAFETY TIPS AND SUGGESTED EXERCISE MODIFICATIONS

- Encourage the participant to wear water exercise shoes to prevent slips and falls.
- Start with low intensity and duration and increase duration first. Gradually increase duration and intensity as tolerated.
- Teach the participant how to adjust intensity and do not push him or her to keep up with the group.
- Allow the participant to respond to current conditions and encourage feedback with modifications.
- Vary activities (stretch, use interval, etc.).
- Incorporate functional activities.
- Avoid overexertion. Instruct the participant to pace herself or himself.
- Work in warm water.
- Ask the participant to keep an exercise journal to track progress (review it and provide feedback).

ABNORMAL RESPONSE TO EXERCISE

- Increase in pain or symptoms
- Decrease in function
- Exhaustion, inability to perform daily tasks

RECOMMENDATIONS AFTER ABNORMAL RESPONSE

- Change the water depth to increase exercise tolerance.
- Decrease duration or use intervals with adjusted work/rest cycles.
- Add range-of-motion work such as Tai Chi moves.

Refer the participant back to his or her health care provider if he or she experiences a severe increase in pain or decline in function.

17. Osteoporosis

Osteoporosis is a disease characterized by a loss of bone tissue, making bones more fragile. This fragility or weakness of the bone makes one more susceptible to breaks or fractures. Some fractures occur during a fall, while others can happen spontaneously without any trauma, during normal daily tasks. The most common areas of fracture due to osteoporosis, in order of frequency of occurrence, are the hip, the spine, and the wrist. Postmenopausal women are most susceptible to developing osteoporosis and related fractures, although this disease can also affect men. The most common features of those at risk for osteoporosis include a small build, fair hair and skin, blue eyes, being of Northern European or Asian descent, having a family history of osteoporosis, and being postmenopausal. All individuals should complete an individual risk assessment for osteoporosis (See Appendix A.).

The best treatment for osteoporosis is prevention via exercise, adequate calcium intake, and postmenopausal use of estrogen replacement therapy. Exercise is essential from early in life in order to build strong bones through increased mechanical loading. Exercises should include general strengthening, cardiovascular conditioning, and balance training (Swezey, 1996). Other helpful tips to reduce risks for osteoporosis are to avoid smoking and limit intake of animal protein, alcohol, and caffeine.

SCREENING

- Observe the participant's shoulder and neck range of motion.
- Observe the participant's posture (check for a forward head, a rounded mid-back, forward shoulders, or a dowager's hump).
- Give the participant a complete osteoporosis risk assessment by checking for the risk factors mentioned previously.
- Screen for ADL safety during use of locker room and entry and exit from the pool.

SAFETY TIPS AND SUGGESTED EXERCISE MODIFICATIONS

- Teach the participant to "know the environment," increasing her or his awareness of the pool, locker room, and home environments. Keep the pool and locker room environments clutter free and safe to prevent collisions and falls.

- Encourage the participant to wear water shoes to prevent slipping and falling in the locker room area and pool.
- Work in shallow water and encourage the participant to use rebound exercises to provide sufficient load.
- Use postural exercises such as keeping a neutral spine; chin tucks; exercises involving the latissimus dorsi, rhomboids, lower traps, and triceps; and pectoral stretches.
- Incorporate lower-extremity strengthening, endurance, and coordination exercises, especially for ankle movements.
- Train to increase the participant's muscle strength and power, using a high load and low reps to increase mechanical loading and stimulate bone growth.
- Include activities that challenge balance, stepping activities, and activities that train both slow- and fast-twitch (reaction) muscles in order to prepare the participant for the unexpected.

SAFETY TIPS AND SUGGESTED MODIFICATIONS FOR THOSE WITH FRAIL OSTEOPOROSIS

Participants with "frail osteoporosis" are those who could fracture without trauma during normal activities. These individuals require the following special modifications:

- To decrease weight bearing and help with comfort, increase the water depth to a level where the participant can still maintain balance and control. Use an inflatable flotation belt to adjust weight bearing as needed. An inflatable belt is less rigid than a foam belt and can be adjusted to the individual, so it is more comfortable and it can afford better protection from excessive force that could cause a fracture.
- To help the participant enter/exit the pool, use a lift or use two assistants. One assistant should stand at the top of the ladder to help with entry, and the other should be positioned in the pool at the bottom of the ladder to help the participant lower into the water.

- Limit using equipment overhead or using overhead armwork, which may compromise the participant's balance and place more weight on the lower body. Avoid having the participant grip for extended periods of time. Also, limit exercise intensity at first, but gradually increase duration, then intensity as tolerated.

- Make sure all locker room and pool deck surfaces are not slick. Check that the water shoes the participant has chosen provide a good grip, even when wet.

 ABNORMAL RESPONSE

- Moderate or greater pain during or after exercise

 RECOMMENDATIONS AFTER ABNORMAL RESPONSE

- Tell the participant to ice and rest any painful areas.

- Avoid forceful movements or holds at the end of range in painful areas.

- Decrease exercise intensity.

 Refer the participant back to his or her health care provider if he or she experiences a moderate or severe increase in pain or a decrease in his or her functional activity level.

Neurological Conditions

18. Multiple Sclerosis

Multiple sclerosis (MS) is a chronic, frequently progressive disease of the central nervous system involving the brain and spinal cord. The term multiple sclerosis refers to the multiple areas of scarring (sclerosis) that result in patches of breakdown in the myelin sheath that covers the nerves. It is usually detected betweeen the ages of 20 and 40, and women are affected more often than men. In a majority of cases, people with MS go through periods when symptoms become more severe (exacerbation) and then less severe (remission). Exacerbation may occur spontaneously or be triggered by an infection, and it can be followed by months or years without further symptoms (Berkow et al., 1997). The cause and cure of MS are unknown, although a genetic predisposition is possible and is being studied.

Common symptoms of MS are abnormal fatigue; weakness; heat intolerance; tremors with movement; difficulty with balance and coordination; gait distur-

bances; slurred speech; bladder, bowel, and sexual dysfunction; numbness, tingling, or pain; visual disturbances; and spasticity of the extremeties or trunk. Symptoms may be intensified by very warm weather, a hot bath or shower, or a fever (Berkow et al., 1997). About 50 percent of people with MS experience cognitive deficit, although the majority of these cases are mild. The most common forms of cognitive dysfunction involve abstract reasoning, short-term memory loss, and impaired concentration. Symptomatic management is possible, and certain immunoregulatory agents reduce the relapse rate and may prove to slow disease progression (NMSS, 2000).

Many people with MS benefit from rehabilitation and participation in a regular exercise program. Some can return to prior function after an exacerbation and others have varying levels of disability, but most people with MS have a normal life span (Berkow et al., 1997). The course of the disease is unpredictable, which can be very difficult emotionally. Group interaction offers support for some individuals.

 SCREENING

- Observe how the participant enters and exits the pool.

- Check the participant's coordination, control of movements, and ability to perform transfers and get in and out of the pool. Is assistance necessary?

- Ask if he or she has visual problems, such as double vision.

- Note the participant's walking pattern (if wobbly or wide-based) and if he or she uses any assistive devices, such as a cane.

 SAFETY TIPS AND SUGGESTED EXERCISE MODIFICATIONS

- Use shallow water to increase weight bearing, sensory input, and stability.

- Use the 4S's to set and pace the level of intensity and prevent overexertion. Base intensity and pacing on participants' ability and current energy levels.

- Start with larger, slower movements. Increase intensity by gradually progressing to movements in combinations or patterns. Sculling can be modified by performing large, slow figure-eights or by holding the arms out as rudders. Monitor intensity for excessive arm movements, as that can lead to overexertion.

- Provide buoyancy equipment or ski poles to assist with balance and stability. Use one-pound ankle weights to maintain foot contact on the pool floor.

- Avoid fast directional changes, cue neutral gaze stabilization, and minimize turbulence to reduce the incidence of dizziness, nausea, or rapid eye movement (REM).

- Focus on using trunk stabilization muscles and maintaining neutral posture, which can reduce energy expenditure, improve trunk control, and promote good breathing patterns.

- Avoid extreme water temperatures, which may cause overheating or chilling and lead to fatigue or cramping. The National Multiple Sclerosis Society recommends an ideal temperature range of 80–84 degrees Fahrenheit (NMSS, 2000). Suggest that participants bring items such as vests and tights that can be adjusted for comfort, and encourage them to drink water frequently to help regulate body temperature.

- Remind participants to check regularly for areas of skin breakdown and tolerance to pool chemicals. Prednisone, a common medication prescribed intermittently for MS, can cause the skin to become thin, making it more susceptible to bruising and tearing.

- Use Tai Chi movements, gentle stretching, or slower movements performed while standing or walking in place for active rest.

- Offer deep-water activities using a buoyancy support, such as bicycling, that enable participants to perform self-paced cardiovascular training. Wearing inflatable buoyancy belts (with individual pockets) will allow participants to add buoyancy as needed around the body for a custom fit. Such belts can provide participants with adequate support and positioning, prevent tipping, and allow participants intermittent periods of active rest.

- The water is an ideal medium for working on balance, walking, and daily living activities. Incorporate changing directions, pivoting, and varying the size and speed of steps, as tolerated. Increased muscle strength and stability can lead to safer performance of land activities.

 ABNORMAL RESPONSE TO EXERCISE

- Abnormal fatigue or exhaustion
- Inability to perform normal daily tasks
- Abnormal changes in muscle tone or control
- Excessive dizziness or visual disturbance

 RECOMMENDATIONS AFTER ABNORMAL RESPONSE

- Decrease duration and intensity.
- Provide more rest breaks.

Refer the participant back to his or her health care provider if he or she experiences a prolonged decrease in strength or control of movement, or an increase in difficulty performing functional activities.

19. Cerebrovascular Accident/Stroke

A cerebrovascular accident (CVA), or a stroke, occurs due to disease of the blood or blood vessels in the brain or trauma. Stroke typically occurs between the ages of 50 to 70, but it can occur at any age. The following are the three major types of CVA (Chusid, 1982):

- Cerebral thrombosis, a blood clot that stops the blood flow

- Cerebral hemorrhage, a rupture of one of the blood vessels of the brain (usually from arteriosclerosis; see Cardiovascular Disease)

- Cerebral embolism, the blockage of a blood vessel in the brain by a small piece of blood clot, tumor, fat, air, bacteria, or other substance.

A stroke usually occurs suddenly, although some people may have had headaches, dizziness, drowsiness, or confusion prior to the event. Victims of a stroke may lose consciousness or have difficulty with speaking, comprehension, movement, vision, or loss of sensation. Symptoms can last from a few seconds to an indefinite period (Chusid, 1982). As many as 35 percent of stroke victims die while in the hospital, with the chance of death increasing with age (Berkow, 1987, p. 1385). Some stroke survivors may remain in a coma indefinitely, while others progress to rehabilitation and ultimately return home, requiring various degrees of assistance. Return of function varies, depending on the location and severity of the stroke. The areas of the brain affected by the stroke can affect voluntary movement, sensation, ability to speak or understand the spoken word, sensation, comprehension, memory, balance, coordination, and vision on the side of the body opposite the CVA.

Some individuals with minor involvement return to normal function or have some spasticity (increased muscle tone) with movement. Other individuals may be unable to speak (aphasia) after a stroke, but can understand what someone says and write a response. Visual problems can include blindness in a portion of the visual field. An individual can even completely ignore one side of the body, unaware of its existence unless cued or encouraged to look at it (called neglect). Exercise instructors should ask anyone who has had a stroke if he or she has any difficulty with vision, speaking, understanding, control of movement, or balance.

SCREENING

- The participant should have medical clearance specifically for aquatic exercise.
- Observe how the participant walks and enters and exits the pool.
- Check the participant's ability to perform transfers (e.g. moving from sitting to standing).
- Note which side of the body appears weaker. If it is not apparent, ask the participant if an extremity feels weaker with activities or exertion.
- Check the participant's control of movement.
- Check whether the participant can successfully recover from loss of balance forward, backward, and to the side in water.

SAFETY TIPS AND SUGGESTED EXERCISE MODIFICATIONS

- Have the participant exercise in shallow water for increased stability and control.
- Focus on the quality of movement, using slower speeds and appropriate-sized movements.
- Cue for posture and hand coordination for balance.
- Check the participant for dizziness, cue neutral gaze stabilization, avoid quick direction changes, work in quiet and calm water, and minimize travel.
- Use teaching methods that address challenges in communication.
- If necessary, start balance activities at a lower level and progress them gradually.

- If the participant has a flaccid arm (floppy, with no voluntary movement or tone), he or she should wear a sling to support the arm while in the water.
- To stretch tight, spastic (increased muscle tone) muscles in the arm and shoulder blade area, try arm activities crossing to the opposite side of the body and forward. Cue the participant to clasp the hands together to move a spastic arm that cannot move by itself (most practical for slow movements or stretching) and to help with neglect.
- If the participant wears a plastic foot brace in her or his shoe on land, encourage him or her to wear it in water shoes while exercising in the water.
- Use walking activities in all directions to help with general strengthening and balance.

STOP ABNORMAL RESPONSE TO EXERCISE

- Exhaustion or increased pain during or after exercise
- Pain in a joint (shoulder, knee), neck, or back (refer to the appropriate area in this chapter)

RECOMMENDATIONS AFTER ABNORMAL RESPONSE

- Decrease exercise intensity and duration.
- For shoulder pain (flaccid arm), secure the arm using an elastic wrap to the body.

Refer the participant back to his or her health care provider if any one of the following occurs:

- Progressive weakness
- Decrease in functional activity
- Any disorientation or confusion
- Speech or visual disturbances, even if temporary
- Complaints of joint or spinal pain that persist or intensify

20. Parkinson's Disease

Parkinson's disease is a chronic degenerative disease involving one or more areas of the brain associated with voluntary movement. The onset occurs most often in persons in their 50s or 60s and affects more men than women. Parkinson's disease may also occur in individuals who have had encephalitis, head trauma, stroke, or carbon monoxide or manganese poisoning. This disease starts gradually and progresses slowly. Common characteristics of this disease include the following (Chusid, 1982, pp. 362-365):

- "Pill-rolling tremor" in the hands and tremors that usually occur when an extremity is at rest
- Difficulty starting any movement
- A masklike, expressionless face
- Muscular rigidity, which can best be felt as a resistance to passive movement in any direction (this rigidity can cause fatigue and pain)
- A shuffling gait that can easily break into a run, with difficulty stopping
- Speech that can be slurred, slowed, low in volume, and monotonous
- Changes in mental abilities (during the later stages of the disease)

SCREENING

- Check the participant's posture (it can be stooped, head forward, arms fixed at side).
- Check the participant's ability to walk and perform transfers safely. Balance can be a problem. The participant may require assistance in the locker room and in entering and exiting the pool.
- Check the participant's general range of motion (ROM), noting her or his ability to control starting and stopping movements.
- Check whether the person's participation in a group exercise class is appropriate. Someone who needs frequent assistance would not be safe in a group setting.

SAFETY TIPS AND SUGGESTED EXERCISE MODIFICATIONS

- Warm water is preferable to help relax rigid muscles.
- Encourage the participant to wear water shoes to prevent slips and falls.
- Emphasize rotational movements to help decrease rigidity and help initiation and control of movement.
- With water walking, cue for longer strides, increased arm swing, and upright posture. Have participants practice stopping on the lane line (this will be difficult for some).
- Incorporate functional activities into the program.
- Start with smaller movements and gradually increase their size if the participant can maintain control.
- Use balance activities, which are safer in the water (see screening to assess whether participation in a group exercise setting is appropriate).
- Use warm water stretching, which is important for increasing the quadriceps, hamstrings, calves, pectorals, and hip flexors in those with Parkinson's disease.
- Include postural exercises (chin tucks; strengthening the latissimus, rhomboids, and lower traps).
- Monitor intensity. Fatigue can increase tremors.
- Use deep breathing exercises to help increase chest expansion and posture.
- Request notification if the participant is taken off medication ("drug holiday"). It may diminish control or significantly affect her or his abilities. The participant may need to be reassessed for class appropriateness or assistance while temporarily off medication.
- Because medications for Parkinson's disease may lower the participant's blood pressure, stand by and be ready to assist her or him with pool entry or exit.

STOP ABNORMAL RESPONSE TO EXERCISE

- Excessive fatigue
- Increased tremors
- Moderate or greater pain during or after exercise

RECOMMENDATIONS AFTER ABNORMAL RESPONSE

- Decrease exercise intensity.
- If pain involves the spine or extremities, refer to the appropriate section in this chapter for guidelines.
- Monitor the participant for control of movements and stretching.

Refer the participant back to his or her health care provider if he or she experiences a decline in functional abilities, control, or balance, or if pain persists or intensifies.

Cardiovascular-Respiratory Diseases

21. Cardiovascular Disease

General cardiovascular disease (CVD), also known as atherosclerosis or arteriosclerosis, is a general term used to describe diseases in which the walls of the arteries become thick and lose elasticity. It is the leading cause of death in the United States and other Western countries, as it is associated with stroke, kidney failure, loss of blood flow and subsequent amputation of extremities, and diminished function of many vital organs of the body. The primary risk factors for developing cardiovascular diseases include the following:

- Hypertension
- High cholesterol/blood lipids
- Cigarette smoking
- Diabetes mellitus
- Obesity
- Male gender (although with the increase in women smokers, there has been an increase in CVD, strokes, and heart attacks in women).

Other factors that can increase the likelihood of developing CVD are family history, physical inactivity, aging, and certain behavioral patterns (such as having a type A personality) (Berkow, 1987).

SCREENING

- The participant should have medical clearance specifically for aquatic exercise.
- Follow post-surgical guidelines (if applicable).

SAFETY TIPS AND SUGGESTED EXERCISE MODIFICATIONS

- Teach the participant to monitor intensity by assessing heart rate and/or rate of perceived exertion (RPE) response.
- Increase the warm-up/cool-down time.
- Frequently monitor intensity.
- Follow the intensity guidelines from the physician. Increase duration before increasing intensity.
- Cue the participant to keep her or his own pace. The participant may need to work from a stationary position while the group travels.
- Reduce armwork intensity, which may elevate blood pressure and increase ventilation demands.
- Have the participant practice breathing against hydrostatic pressure when the lungs are submerged.
- Encourage the participant to perform relaxation exercises by incorporating Tai Chi and deep breathing into the class.

STOP ABNORMAL RESPONSE TO EXERCISE

- Pain, pressure, aches, numbness, or tingling in the neck, chest, shoulders, arms, or legs
- Shortness of breath
- Exhaustion during or after exercise
- Nausea

RECOMMENDATIONS AFTER ABNORMAL RESPONSE

- Decrease intensity (decrease the speed, size, or surface area of the movement).
- Use interval work with longer rests.
- Allow the participant to leave the pool to rest and stay warm.
- Allow the participant to use her or his own medication according to the physician's advice.

If the participant finds that symptoms do not subside with rest and self-administration of the prescribed medication, activate your Emergency Medical Response System.

22. Pulmonary Diseases: Asthma, Emphysema, Chronic Bronchitis, and Chronic Obstructive Pulmonary Disease

Asthma is a hypersensitivity of the bronchial airways produced by swelling and muscular spasm of the bronchial passages and excessive mucus secretion, causing mucus plugs. Symptoms of asthma include difficulty breathing, coughing, wheezing, and expectoration of thick mucus. Symptoms may be mild or life threatening and can become progressively more severe with age. In half of asthmatics, attacks are triggered by infection, irritating inhalants, cold air, exercise, and emotional upset. Medications (bronchodilators) that relax bronchial spasm and open up air passages, facilitating normal breathing, are very effective (Berkow, 1987).

Exercise-induced asthma (EIA) is a form of asthma that is provoked by exercise and occurs frequently in those who have no history of regular asthma. Coughing is the most common symptom of EIA; however, frequent complaints also include chest tightness, wheezing, and shortness of breath. Many individuals with EIA don't know they have it and think they are just out of shape. Symptoms usually begin with strenuous exercise and can persist for as long as one hour after exercise has stopped. Pollen, ragweed, exhaust, smoke, chemical odors, air pollution, dust mites, dander, and cold air are all potential irritants. Aquatic exercise can be helpful for all those suffering from asthma. The increased air humidity of the pool helps to keep airways open. The use of bronchodilators 15-20 minutes before exercising and avoiding environmental irritants are the most effective ways to treat EIA (McLaughlin, 1997).

Chronic bronchitis is a long-term inflammation of the bronchial tubes (small airways in the lungs). It is characterized by a chronic productive cough not caused by an acute upper respiratory infection. Cigarette smoking is the most common cause; however, air pollution, certain occupations, and bronchial infections can also be factors. Persons with chronic bronchitis are called "blue bloaters" because they usually have a stocky build and are "blue" because of lack of oxygen. Bronchitis causes production of thick, tenacious sputum that is difficult to expectorate. Respiratory rate is usually increased, along with use of accessory breathing muscles (scalenes, pectorals, sternocleidomastoid, and intercostals). These patients should avoid bronchial irritants and drink large amounts of water to keep secretions thinner, easing expectoration (Berkow, 1987).

Emphysema is a disease of the smallest airways and alveolar sacs of the lungs, where the exchange of oxygen from air to the blood occurs. Swelling, inflammation, and thickening of the walls of the bronchioles can occur, along with enlargement of the alveolar sacs. The disease is progressive and the survival rate at five years is around 50 percent. Difficulty breathing is the most common complaint of persons with emphysema. Other common symptoms include coughing, bouts of wheezing, weakness, lethargy, severe weight loss, and increased use of accessory breathing muscles (resulting in "barrel chest"). The normal elastic recoil of the lungs is lost, making exhalation also difficult. Purse-lipped breathing is a technique used to facilitate and increase the time of exhalation. Persons with emphysema are referred to as "pink puffers" because of the increased respiratory work that must be done to maintain adequate oxygen. The most common cause of emphysema is exposure to cigarette smoke while heredity is also a factor (Berkow, 1987).

Emphysema can commonly occur with chronic bronchitis, especially in older people. The term chronic obstructive pulmonary disease (COPD) is the term used to designate those individuals who have some combination of chronic bronchitis, emphysema, and asthma.

SCREENING

- The participant should have medical clearance specifically for aquatic exercise.
- Ask about specifically prescribed breathing techniques (diaphragmatic, nose and/or purse-lipped breathing with exhalation).
- Follow surgical guidelines (if appropriate).
- Check the participant for a history of asthma, allergies, and environmental triggers to asthma.

SAFETY TIPS AND SUGGESTED EXERCISE MODIFICATIONS

- Have the participant practice breathing against hydrostatic pressure.
- Suggest that the participant keep medications labeled with her or his name and dose available poolside.

- Increase the duration of the warm-up and cool-down (in gradual progressions).
- Give frequent water breaks during class.
- Reduce arm intensity to decrease ventilation demands.
- Follow the physician's intensity guidelines.
- Monitor exercise intensity frequently (use the "talk test" or RPE).
- Keep pool air warm for asthmatics.
- Limit or prevent exposure to known environmental triggers.
- Suggest that the participant take her or his medications for asthma either 15 to 20 minutes prior to exercise or as recommended by her or his health care provider.
- Emphasize diaphragmatic breathing, which can be used with relaxation activities and trunk or shoulder range-of-motion exercises.
- Include postural exercises (chin tucks and strengthening for the latissimus, rhomboids, and lower traps).
- Place participants who can tolerate low-intensity exercise only in a warm water class.

 ABNORMAL RESPONSE TO EXERCISE

- Inability to speak, gasping for air
- Moderate to severe shortness of breath, wheezing, excessive coughing, or chest tightness
- Blue nailbeds or lips
- Excessive use of accessory breathing muscles

 RECOMMENDATIONS AFTER ABNORMAL RESPONSE

- Decrease exercise intensity and duration (use rest intervals).
- Screen for potential environmental irritants. Postpone exercise if air quality is poor.
- Have the participant use her or his own medications and leave the pool to rest.

 If the participant finds that symptoms do not subside with rest and self-administration of the prescribed medication, activate your Emergency Medical Response System.

23. Hypertension

Hypertension (HTN), or high blood pressure, is an increase (above normal) of systolic and/or diastolic blood pressure. The upper limit of normal blood pressure in adults is 140/90. The cause of HTN is not known, although heredity can be a predisposing factor. The first line of treatment is weight reduction, eating less salt in the diet, and exercise. Cigarette smoking should be avoided and drinking of alcoholic beverages minimized. Medications are prescribed by the doctor if the above measures do not restore normal blood pressure. At least 35 percent of persons in the United States have HTN that is properly controlled, with up to 25 percent of U.S. citizens not even aware that they have it. Untreated HTN increases the risk of heart failure, heart attack, stroke, or kidney failure (Berkow, 1987).

The American College of Sports Medicine (ACSM) recommends that those with HTN exercise at moderate intensity (10 to 12 on the Borg Scale [RPE]) 4 to 5 times per week for 30 to 60 minutes.

 SCREENING

- The participant must obtain medical clearance from a physician prior to starting an exercise program.
- Encourage the prescribed use of medication.

SAFETY TIPS AND SUGGESTED EXERCISE MODIFICATIONS

- Limit overhead armwork to 15 to 20 seconds for each exercise (single armwork is preferable).
- Cue for a light grip on equipment and limit gripping to 15 to 20 seconds, then rest, relax, and release.
- Cue breathing to avoid the Valsalva maneuver (breath holding and bearing down that can occur with exercise or exertion).
- Allow the participant to adjust slowly to the hydrostatic pressure of the water. Begin in shallow water and then, if tolerated, gradually move into deep water as adjustment to hydrostatic pressure progresses.
- Focus on endurance training and dynamic exercise.
- Teach the participant how to self-monitor and modify exercise intensity.

- Increase the warm-up and cool-down time.
- Gradually increase exercise duration. Increase duration before increasing intensity.
- Use Tai Chi and relaxation exercises to help reduce stress. Cue the participant to "feel" the muscles tighten and relax when inhaling and exhaling.
- Avoid isometric activities lasting more than 15 seconds, especially with arms.
- If a participant takes medications, the RPE (8-14 on 20-point Borg Scale), not pulse rate, should be used to monitor intensity.

 ABNORMAL RESPONSE TO EXERCISE

- Exhaustion
- Dizziness (may relate to medications or be a postural response)

 RECOMMENDATIONS AFTER ABNORMAL RESPONSE

- Move to more shallow water.
- Decrease exercise intensity.
- Ask the participant to have his or her physician check his or her medications.
- Remove the participant from the pool.
- Allow the participant to rest.
- Refer the participant to a physician if necessary.

 Refer the participant back to his or her health care provider if the symptoms listed under "Abnormal Response to Exercise" persist or he or she shows the same signs as those for stroke (see "Cerebrovascular Accident/Stroke" in this chapter).

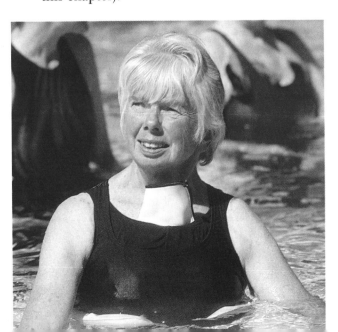

General Medical Conditions

24. Prenatal

Prenatal literally means before birth. During the estimated 40 weeks of pregnancy, a woman's body undergoes many changes. Within weeks of conception hormones are released that relax the ligaments throughout the body, resulting in decreased joint stability. Blood volume increases by as much as 50 percent, which increases the amount of blood the heart has to pump with each beat. Respiratory rate increases due to greater oxygen demand and consumption. Additional pressure of the uterus on the diaphragm increases respiratory rate and general work of breathing. Additional weight adds load and increases joint stress. The increase in surface area of the body creates more drag in the water. Changes in posture and a more forward center of gravity present new challenges to balance. The increase in basal metabolic rate requires extra caloric (300 calories/day) and fluid intake, especially before exercising (Manos, 1995).

The American College of Obstetricians and Gynecologists (ACOG) states that pregnant women who are without obstetric or medical complications can perform a moderate level of physical activity to maintain cardiorespiratory and muscular fitness during and after pregnancy (ACOG Technical Bulletin, 1994). Women who currently participate in an exercise program can continue training throughout pregnancy (intensity and duration naturally decrease as pregnancy advances). Women who begin exercising after becoming pregnant are advised to start with a low intensity and low- or nonimpact activities. Duration or intensity of the exercise should not be increased before the 15th week or after the 25th week of pregnancy. Exercising three or more days per week is safer than an intermittent schedule. For women who don't have specific guidelines from their physician, intensity should be based on maternal symptoms. RPE guidelines would be 12-14 (somewhat hard) on a 20-point scale. Heart rate guidelines vary from a maximum of 140 (ACOG) to 144 (AFAA) beats per minute (bpm) to a maximum based on maternal age (Quinn, 1994). ACOG guidelines also suggest exercises be stopped at fatigue and that women not exercise to exhaustion. Duration varies from 15 minutes for previously sedentary women to 45 minutes for fit women. Vigorous exercise should be limited to 15 to 20 minutes (Manos, 1995).

Studies have shown that women who perform non-weight-bearing exercise (swimming or biking) were able to maintain a moderate or greater intensity of exercise throughout the third trimester. Pregnant women engaging in weight-bearing modes of training (running, aerobics) typically stopped all exercise by the third trimester. This supports the aquatic environment as an ideal medium for exercise during pregnancy (McLaughlin, 1997).

SCREENING

- Acquire medical consent for each participant, with specific guidelines if necessary.

- Screen for other current or previous injuries to the spine or other areas of the body.

- Observe the participant's posture for the presence of increased neck or low-back extension (lordosis), forward head and shoulders, or knee hyperextension.

- Observe the participant's gait for signs of pain (limping) and general ability to move (getting in and out of the pool, in and out of chairs).

- Postpone exercise if the participant has a fever.

- Ask the participant about previous and current fitness levels (how many times she exercises each week, how long, and how often).

SAFETY TIPS AND SUGGESTED EXERCISE MODIFICATIONS

- Keep the pool temperature at 83–86 degrees F (28–30 C), which is ideal (Brecker, 1993, p. 13). Avoid exercising in pool temperatures that exceed 90 degrees F (32 degrees C) (Addington, 1996). Maintaining comfortable body warmth is important to prevent nipple stimulation, which could induce labor. If the participant feels chilly, have her work the legs more vigorously to generate more heat or wear a thermal vest and supplex tights to reduce heat loss. Even if the class is conducted in the recommended water temperature, individual response will vary and should be monitored.

- Encourage the participant to wear water shoes in the locker room and pool to avoid slips and falls and to use the ladder or ramp for pool entry and exit. Have her check her balance as she exits the pool slowly, pausing as needed to regain her "gravity legs" as she adjusts to a different center of balance. Stand nearby to assist if necessary.

- Teach neutral spine and neutral position for all joints, reviewing the spinal position frequently during exercise. Cue and help the participant adjust sculling (hand movements) to acquire effective balance skills. As pregnancy advances, sculling positions for basic moves may need to change in response to a new body shape and center of buoyancy. Limit hip extension past neutral, because buoyancy assists the leg upward as it moves back into extension and this may strain the broad ligament of the uterus. It is easy to hyperextend the hip and cause hyperextension at the low back (which can also occur during scissors moves). In general, limit the size of hip movements and cue the participant to scull at "table top" position (low in the water and in front), using soft webbed gloves for extra support. Remind the participant to tighten the gluteals and abdominals, to keep the neck in neutral, and to avoid twisting at the waist, which increases strain on the round ligament of the uterus.

- Teach proper body mechanics and incorporate them into the class. Encourage proper body mechanics with ADL at home and work. Have the participant practice and train in the pool for lifting the baby, pushing the buggy or stroller, and transferring the baby or buggy/stroller from place to place.

- Emphasize strengthening for gluteals, abdominals, quadriceps, hamstrings, pelvic floor muscles, and upper extremities. Don't forget those Kegel exercises!

- Incorporate postural exercises (chin tucks, strengthening for latissimus dorsi, rhomboids, and lower traps).

- Stretching exercises should include hamstrings, iliopsoas (hip flexors), hip adductors (avoid maximal stretch), quadriceps, erector spinae (low back), gastrocnemius (calves), and pectoralis muscles.

- Cue breathing frequently to avoid breath-holding, and have the participant practice breathing for relaxation during warm-up or cool-down (Tai Chi, diaphragmatic breathing).

- Suggest wearing a jog bra or other support to decrease bouncing and potential nipple stimulation (can induce labor).

- Work at a proper water depth, where the participant can control position, movements, balance, and impact. Modify movements as needed. As pregnancy progresses, traveling sideways may be modified by moving diagonally. Suspended or rebound moves may need to be modified by being worked in neutral position. Transitioning from horizontal to vertical positions may become more difficult. Eliminate these types of moves or teach coordinated arm movements that make the transitions safe and effective, allowing the participant extra time to complete the work.

- Include balance activities (the step can be used). Anterior knee pain occurring during step or squat activities may indicate knee tendinitis or other anterior knee problems (refer to chronic anterior knee pain guidelines in this chapter). If the participant has anterior knee pain, remove the step and replace that activity with small static squats (adjusting water depth for weight bearing) according to tolerance.

- Allow the participant to set exercise intensity according to her previous fitness level and comfort. The "talk test" and RPE Scale can be used to monitor intensity. If heart rates are included as part of the intensity check, have the participant wear a monitor.

- Keep drinking water and snacks available to maintain hydration and proper blood sugar levels.

- Limit or avoid exercises using long levers, and avoid the use of buoyancy devices on the extremities. The properties of water increase resistance to movements, and both of these situations can increase force and stress on ligaments and joints. In general, keep movements small and controlled and avoid sudden changes of movement. Work basic moves slowly through the progressions, checking for neutral joint position.

- Make the transition to gravity as gradual as possible by having the participant walk in the shallowest water possible, feeling gravity, before exiting the pool.

 ABNORMAL RESPONSE TO EXERCISE

- Shortness of breath
- Leg pain
- Joint pain
- Low-back ache/pain
- Menstrual-like cramps or uterine contractions
- Dizziness/nausea

RECOMMENDATIONS AFTER ABNORMAL RESPONSE

- For contractions or cramps, if the participant is in the first or second trimester, stop exercise; if the participant is in her third trimester, decrease intensity and reassess.

- For spinal pain, check that the participant is holding the spine in a neutral position (refer to low-back pain guidelines in this chapter) and check the methods used by the participant to maintain balance during exercise performance. Correct or modify the movements and frequently cue the participant to use trunk stabilizers to improve effectiveness.

- For any joint or muscular problems, refer to the participant's health care provider (refer to the appropriate section in this chapter for guidelines).

- Stress that the participant should exercise at her own pace.

- Encourage the participant to drink to hydrate and eat to restore adequate blood sugar levels after class.

 Refer the participant back to her health care provider if any one of the following occurs (Manos, 1995):

- Joint or spinal symptoms persist or intensify
- Persistent menstrual-like cramps or uterine pain
- Progressive abnormal decrease in functional abilities
- The participant's water breaks (rupture of membranes)
- Any bloody or abnormal vaginal discharge
- Sudden swelling of ankles, hands, or face
- Persistent severe headache and/or visual disturbances

- Swelling, pain, and redness in the calf of one leg
- Increased heart rate or blood pressure persisting after exercise
- Excessive fatigue, palpitations, or chest pain
- Unexplained abdominal pain
- Pubic pain
- Absence of fetal movement

25. Obesity

Obesity is functionally defined as the percent body fat at which the risk for disease increases (ACSM, 1995). Some of these diseases include hypertension, diabetes, and cardiovascular disease. Excess body fat can also limit a person's ability to perform simple daily tasks such as walking up a flight of stairs, carrying groceries, or dressing. Body fat can be reduced by consuming fewer calories than are used. The most effective way to lose body fat is by both decreasing the amount of food (calories) eaten and increasing the amount of calories used through exercise. Fasting and extreme reduction of eating (starvation or semi-starvation diets) result in loss of water and tissues other than fat. A decrease in calories due to exercise results in weight loss consisting mainly of fat. Successful weight loss programs also incorporate behavioral modification techniques to modify eating habits and result in gradual progressive weight loss through lifetime changes in physical activity and dietary habits (Berkow, 1987).

Exercises for an obese person should be based on low intensity and a progressive increase in duration of activities (ACSM, 1995). The individual should choose exercise activities that are enjoyable, low impact, and at an easy skill level to perform. Exercising with a group or partner increases support and camaraderie. It is essential that those who are obese clearly understand the purpose of exercise in relation to their weight management program and the implications of stopping exercise (remaining obese, the increased risk of disease, and progressive decrease in the ability to perform daily tasks).

SCREENING

- Check whether the participant has any medical conditions, such as diabetes, hypertension, cardiovascular disease, or any orthopedic problems (refer to the appropriate sections of this chapter for screening guidelines). We strongly recommend a medical release for those who have medical conditions. Follow your YMCA's regulations on this.
- Check whether the participant can successfully recover balance in the water in all directions.

SAFETY TIPS AND SUGGESTED MODIFICATIONS

- Encourage the participant to wear water exercise shoes to prevent slips and falls.
- Exercise in waist-deep water for greater control of movement.
- To reduce impact and intensity, the participant may need to perform exercises in neutral instead of rebound or suspended working position.
- Keep intensity low and gradually increase first the duration, then intensity as tolerated.
- Include functional activities.
- Base intensity on heart rate (HR) when using a monitor and/or a combination of the "talk test" and RPE (use the Borg Scale).
- The participant should understand that the exercise program is individualized and should be self-paced exercise.
- Encourage the participant to drink fluids before, during, and after exercise for proper hydration and to prevent overheating.
- Have the participant wear a weight belt to keep her or his feet in contact with the bottom of the pool and improve balance and stability.
- Recommend to the participant that she or he stave off hunger after exercise by taking a nutritious carbohydrate snack to eat immediately after exercise.

STOP **ABNORMAL RESPONSE TO EXERCISE**

- Complaints of moderate or greater muscle or joint pain
- Excessive fatigue or exhaustion during exercise or later in the day
- Any other problems that are related to other diseases associated with obesity (refer to the appropriate sections in the chapter)

RECOMMENDATIONS AFTER ABNORMAL RESPONSE

- Tell the participant to ice and rest the involved painful joint or muscle.
- Decrease exercise intensity and/or duration and have the participant monitor intensity more frequently.
- Decrease impact by eliminating any rebound moves (if applicable).
- Monitor the participant's caloric intake to check that caloric intake is sufficient (to discourage exercising while fasting).

Refer the participant back to his or her health care provider if he or she experiences moderate or greater muscle or joint pain that persists or intensifies or presents symptoms of extreme intolerance related to cardiovascular disease, hypertension, or diabetes (if applicable).

26. Diabetes Mellitus

Diabetes mellitus (DM) is a chronic disorder of carbohydrate, protein, and fat metabolism. Classic symptoms include frequent urination, excessive thirst, and increased appetite. Diabetics have a higher than normal fasting blood glucose (sugar) level and are at greater risk for heart and kidney disease, blockage of the blood vessels of the legs and feet, and loss of nerve function (Berkow, 1987).

A number of subgroups of diabetes exist, including the following (Berkow, 1987):

- *Insulin-dependent diabetes mellitus* (IDDM or type 1). IDDM is also called juvenile onset diabetes and is caused by a lack of insulin. The cause of IDDM is unknown. These individuals need insulin injections.
- *Non-insulin dependent diabetes mellitus* (NIDDM or type 2). This type of diabetes usually starts during adulthood. These individuals can control their diabetes through diet, exercise, and/or medications .

- *Gestational diabetes.* Pregnant women can develop glucose intolerance. It can frequently be controlled by diet and exercise but sometimes requires the use of insulin.

Complications of diabetes can include diabetes-induced blindness, kidney disease, nerve damage, cardiovascular disorders, and foot ulcers. Tobacco should be avoided because it constricts the blood vessels in the extremities, compounding the effects of DM. Reduced blood supply and nerve damage associated with DM contribute to diabetic foot ulcers (Berkow, 1987). Feet should be checked regularly and should be kept clean, warm, and free of anything that may impair circulation.

Exercise is beneficial for all types of diabetics. Regular exercise can decrease the amount of insulin needed, increase cardiovascular health and glucose tolerance, and help with weight loss. Physician's consent and guidelines are essential for appropriate placement into a fitness program.

SCREENING

- The participant should obtain a physician's consent and guidelines. IDDM diabetics must be under adequate control before starting an exercise program (ACSM, 1995, p. 214).
- The participant with DM should always have a source of simple sugar available poolside.
- Inquire about any visual problems and, if the participant has them, put him or her in the front of the class for a better view.
- Inspect the participant's feet and calves. Check for open wounds; if they exist, your facility's rules may prevent the participant from entering the pool. If the skin on the calves seems shiny, has lost hair, or has a bluish color, this may indicate circulatory problems. If any of these conditions appears, suggest to the participant that she or he discuss the problem with her or his health care provider.

SAFETY TIPS AND SUGGESTED EXERCISE MODIFICATIONS

- Recommend that the participant wear well-fitting, nonconstrictive shoes and clothing.
- Avoid putting buoyancy equipment or resistive bands around legs and feet.
- Follow the guidelines for CVD (many who have diabetes also have HTN and CVD).
- Increase the time spent on warm-up and cool-down, and progress intensity gradually.
- Monitor exercise intensity frequently. To increase the training level, increase duration first, then intensity.
- Warn the participant not to exercise if she or he is feeling hypoglycemic (low blood sugar).
- Remind the participant to drink water frequently.
- Encourage the participant to wash and carefully dry feet after class also checking for abrasions.
- The participant should ask her or his physician about decreasing insulin or eating extra food prior to and/or after exercise.
- Read instructions on medic alert bracelets that any participant wears.
- Have the participant use the RPE and the "talk test" in addition to heart rate to monitor intensity (ACSM, 1995).

⛔ ABNORMAL RESPONSE TO EXERCISE

- Excessive fatigue
- Nausea/vomiting
- Shortness of breath, feeling lightheaded or dizzy
- Pain, pressure, aches, numbness, or tingling in the neck, chest, shoulders, and arms
- Mental confusion

RECOMMENDATIONS AFTER ABNORMAL RESPONSE

- Decrease intensity or allow rest.
- Refer to the sections on hypertension and cardiovascular disease in this chapter if pertinent.
- Allow the participant to exit the pool to stay warm and to eat simple sugars.

If the abnormal responses to exercise listed previously do not subside with rest or sugar, or the participant loses consciousness, activate your Emergency Medical Response System. Refer the participant back to his or her health care provider if he or she experiences progressive fatigue, severe thirst, frequent urination, nausea, or vomiting.

27. Post-Mastectomy

Breast cancer is the most common form of cancer in women, and it is found in 4 of every 10 women today. Of all cancers affecting women, breast cancer and lung cancer claim the most lives. Years ago, women underwent a radical mastectomy, in which the breast was removed, along with the lymph nodes from under the arm and the pectoralis muscle. Today, the choice is generally between a modified radical mastectomy, in which the breast and lymph nodes are removed, or a partial mastectomy, a lumpectomy in which the lump and the lymph nodes are removed. A lumpectomy is less invasive, with less scar tissue and potentially fewer complications. The success rate is about the same for both surgeries. After surgery, treatment consisting of radiation therapy and/or chemotherapy may continue (Berkow, 1987).

Aquatic exercise can be started after postsurgical and/or postradiation skin changes have healed. Group exercise is helpful for camaraderie and general emotional support. Possible complications after surgery can include wound infection, frozen shoulder, lymphedema (swelling of the arm due to removal of the lymph nodes), and reflex sympathetic dystrophy (RSD), which is when hypersensitivity, pain, and swelling inhibit voluntary use of an extremity.

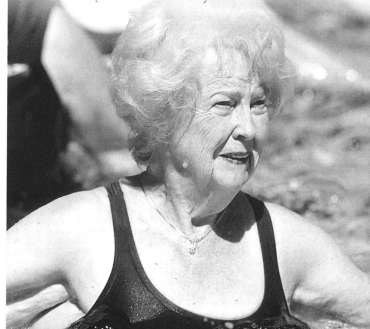

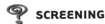

SCREENING

- Observe the participant's range of motion of the neck and arms.
- Observe the participant's sculling technique.
- Follow postsurgical guidelines.
- Inquire about the participant's current activity level and stamina.

SAFETY TIPS AND SUGGESTED EXERCISE MODIFICATIONS

- A post-mastectomy participant may be deconditioned after surgery or following radiation or chemotherapy. Decrease exercise duration and intensity if necessary and progress as tolerated.
- If necessary, initially limit the size, speed, and surface area of upper-body moves. Focus on control and quality of movements.
- Incorporate postural exercises.
- Incorporate gentle arm, neck, pectoral, general body stretching (avoid overstretching). Tai Chi, relaxation and breathing exercises can be used for stress reduction.
- Keep arm and neck movements within pain-free ranges of movement.

STOP **ABNORMAL RESPONSE TO EXERCISE**

- Moderate or greater increase in pain during or after exercise
- Pain in the shoulders, arms, or neck
- Excessive fatigue.

RECOMMENDATIONS AFTER ABNORMAL RESPONSE

- Decrease the size, speed, and surface area of upper-body activities.
- Modify sculling (smaller and lower in the water or stationary on the affected side).
- Decrease the exercise intensity.

Refer the participant back to his or her health care provider if he or she experiences persistent pain or swelling or the inability to move the arms.

Bibliography

Addington, J. 1996. Presentation at the European Aquatic Fitness Conference, Karlsruhe, Germany.

American College of Obstetricians and Gynecologists. 1994. Exercise during pregnancy and postnatal period. Technical Bulletin No. 189. Washington, D.C.

Arthritis Foundation and National Council of YMCA of the USA. 1990. *Arthritis Foundation YMCA Aquatic Program (AFYAP) and AFYAP Plus Instructor's Manual.* Atlanta: The Arthritis Foundation.

Bennett R., H. Smythe, and F. Wolfe. 1992. Recognizing fibromyalgia. *Patient Care*, 15 March.

Berkow, R., ed. 1987. *Merck manual of diagnosis and therapy.* Rahway, NJ: Merck.

Berkow, R., M. Beers, and A. Fletcher, eds. 1997. *The Merck manual of medical information: Home edition.* Whitehouse Station, NJ: Merck Research Laboratories.

Brecker, L. 1993. Easing the load with aquatic exercise for women prenatal/postpartum. *Advance For Physical Therapists*, 21 June.

Chusid, J.G. 1982. *Correlative neuroanatomy and functional neurology*, 18th ed. Los Altos, CA: Lange Medical Publications.

Frownfelter, D. 1978. *Chest physical therapy and pulmonary rehabilitation: An interdisciplinary approach.* Chicago: Year Book Medical Publishers.

Goldenberg, D. 1992. Fibromyalgia, chronic fatigue, and myofascial pain syndromes. *Current Opinion in Rheumatology* 4: 247-257.

Hertling, D., and R. Kessler. 1990. The shoulder and shoulder girdle. In *Management of Common Musculoskeletal Disorders*. Philadelphia: J.B. Lippincott.

Hills, C., and M. Sanders. 1999. Aquatic rehabilitation for low back dysfunction. *Spinal rehabilitation*. Stamford: Appleton & Lange.

Hooke, A. 1986. *Therapeutic group exercise for older adults: An alternative approach.* St. Paul, MN.

Kellett, J. 1986. Acute soft tissue injuries-a review of the literature. *Medicine and Science in Sports and Exercise* 18(5).

Koury, J. 1996. *Aquatic therapy programming guidelines for orthopedic rehabilitation.* Champaign, IL: Human Kinetics.

Krupp, M, and M. Chatton. 1980. *Current medical diagnosis and treatment.* Los Altos, CA: Lange Medical Publications.

Lewis, C. 1995. *Aging, the health care challenge: An interdisciplinary approach to assessment and rehabilitation of the elderly.* Philadelphia: F.A. Davis.

Lewis, C., and K. Knortz. 1993. Orthopedic assessment and treatment of the geriatric patient. St. Louis: Mosby Yearbook.

Manos, T. 1995. Exercise and pregnancy. Presentation at the Aerobics and Fitness Convention, Taiwan, ROC.

McCain, G. 1986. Role of physical fitness training in the fibrositis/fibromyalgia syndrome. *American Journal of Medicine* 81 (suppl. 3A).

McLaughlin, C. 1996. Recognizing symptoms of exercise-induced asthma. *Advance for Physical Therapists,* 16 December.

McLaughlin, C. 1997. Exercising for two: Good for mom and baby. *Advance for Physical Therapists,* 14 April.

Morgan, D. 1988. Concepts in functional training and postural stabilization for the low-back injured. *Topics in Acute Care and Trauma Rehabilitation* 2(4): 8-17.

NMSS Information Resource Center and Library. 2000. *Multiple Sclerosis Information Sourcebook.* **www.nmss.org.**

Pate, R., M. Pratt, S. Blair, W. Haskell, C. Macera, C. Bouchard, D. Buchner, W. Ettinger, G. Heath, A. King, A. Kriska, A. Leon, B. Marcus, J. Morris, R. Paffenbarger, K. Patrick, M. Pollock, J. Rippe, J. Sallis, and J. Wilmore. 1995. Physical activity and public health: A recommendation from the Centers for Disease Control and Prevention and the American College of Sports Medicine. *JAMA* 273(5): 402–407.

Quinn, T. 1994. Exercise during pregnancy: Practical implications for prescription. Presentation at New England Chapter of American College of Sports Medicine, September, Foxboro, Massachusetts.

President's Council on Physical Fitness and Sports. 1995. Osteoporosis and Physical Activity. Series 2, no. 3, September.

Saal, J., and J. Saal. 1989. Nonoperative treatment of herniated lumbar intervertebral disc with radiculopathy: An outcome study. *Spine* 14(4): 431-437.

Sanders, M., and C. Maloney-Hills. 1998. Aquatic exercise for better living on land. *ACSM's Health & Fitness Journal* 2(3): 16–23.

Sanders, M., and N. Rippee. 1994. *Speedo aquatic fitness system, instructor training manual.* London: Speedo International.

Swezey, R. 1996. Exercise for osteoporosis—Is walking enough? The case for site specificity and resistive exercise. *Spine* 21(23).

Thorson, K. 1992. The fibromyalgia syndrome facts and political case statement. *Fibromyalgia Network* (March).

Tilden, H. M. 2000. Aquatic Exercise Instructor, In C. Norton, L. Jamison (eds.), *A Team Approach to the Aquatic Continuum of Care,* Woburn, MA, Butterworth-Heinemann.

Torrey, D. 1996. Current Concepts in Knee Rehabilitation Seminar. Folsom Physical Therapy, Folsom, California.

Vollowitz, E. 1988. Future prescription for the conservative management of low-back pain. *Topics in Acute Care and Trauma Rehabilitation* 2(4): 18-37.

YMCA of the USA. 1987. *Aquatics for special populations.* Champaign, IL: Human Kinetics.

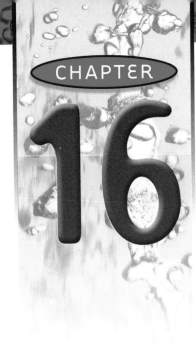

Functional ADL Field Assessments

MARY E. SANDERS AND CATHY MALONEY-HILLS

Objectives:

To provide the protocols for testing participant's abilities on nine activity of daily living (ADL) tasks:

- Static balance
- Dynamic balance
- Agility
- Aerobic endurance

- Standing from a sitting position
- Arm curling
- Chair sit and reach

- Back scratch
- Stair climb

Functional field assessments can help you appropriately place participants into the variety of programs offered at the YMCA (see chapter 13). Administer a health screening to all older adults and to potential participants in the Arthritis Foundation YMCA Aquatic Program (AFYAP), AFYAP Plus, or Functional Fitness classes, then perform functional assessments on all those who pass the screening. The test results will help you identify specific goals each participant can work toward. Doing a baseline assessment and periodic reassessments every three to four months will give participants feedback about their individual progress. It also will alert you to any participants who have regressed, so you can refer them to their health care providers. Tracking progress through functional testing can also motivate participants to attend classes and work toward achieving their goals.

The testing procedure does take some time and space and will have some cost if equipment must be purchased. You also should test participants consistently, with the same person always performing the assessments, if the results are to be valid.

Ask participants to wear comfortable tennis shoes and clothing for the assessment. You can test four participants together during a 45-minute period. Schedule the assessments before class, during class, or as a separate appointment at the YMCA. Testing participants after participation in an exercise class is not a good idea, as the results could be inaccurate due to participants' fatigue. Perform all retesting at the same scheduled time with the same testing instructor to ensure the validity of the results.

To ensure scoring accuracy and interpretation, strict adherence to all instructions is essential.

Throughout all testing, participants should be instructed to *do the best they can on the tests but to never push themselves to a point of overexertion or beyond what they think is safe for them.* Prior to testing, participants must do a 5- to 10-minute warm-up and general stretching routine.

People who *should not* take the tests without physician approval are those who

- have been advised by their doctors not to exercise because of a medical condition;
- are currently experiencing chest pain, dizziness, or have exertional angina (chest tightness, pressure, pain, heaviness) during exercise;
- have had congestive heart failure; or
- have uncontrolled high blood pressure (greater than 160/100).

Nine tests are included in the Functional ADL Field Assessments. They should be performed in the same order for pre and post testing, using the procedures described later in this chapter:

1. Static Balance
2. Dynamic Balance
3. 8-Foot Up-and-Go (agility)
4. 6-Minute Walk
5. 30-Second Chair Stand
6. Arm Curl
7. Chair sit and reach
8. Back scratch
9. Stair climb

Use the scoring sheet shown in figure 16.1 to record test results.

Figure 16.1 *Scoring sheet for functional ADL field assessments*

Functional Field Assessments

Name _____

Date _____

Static Balance

Practice _____

Right leg: Time 1 _____ : _____ – _____   Time 2 _____ : _____ – _____

Left leg: Time 1 _____ : _____ – _____   Time 2 _____ : _____ – _____

Dynamic Balance

Practice _____

For each step, circle "step on circle (no.)," then circle the number of seconds balanced (1–4).

Step on circle 1 (4pts) Using watch count 1 2 3 4

Step on circle 2 (4pts) Using watch count 1 2 3 4

Step on circle 3 (4pts) Using watch count 1 2 3 4

Step on circle 4 (4pts) Using watch count 1 2 3 4

Step on circle 5 (4pts) Using watch count 1 2 3 4

Step on circle 6 (4pts) Using watch count 1 2 3 4

Step on circle 7 (4pts) Using watch count 1 2 3 4

Center _____ Balance _____

8-Foot Up-and-Go

Practice _____

Circuit (2x) Time 1 _____ : _____ – _____   Time 2 _____ : _____ – _____

6-Minute Walk

Practice _____

Total number of yards _____

30-Second Chair Stand

Practice _____

Number of stands _____

Arm Curl

Practice _____

Number of curls _____

Fill in the blank with a + or –.

Chair Sit and Reach

Right leg   Trial 1 _____   Trial 2 _____

Left leg   Trial 1 _____   Trial 2 _____

Back Scratch (circle preferred arm R or L)

Left arm   Trial 1 _____   Trial 2 _____

Right arm Trial 1 _____   Trial 2 _____

Stair Climb

Trial 1 _____   Trial 2 _____

Each task must be done exactly the same way every time to ensure accurate assessment.

Before beginning each of the tasks, remind participants that if they feel lightheaded, dizzy, or have any pain, they should stop immediately and tell the person administering the test.

The remainder of this chapter contains the testing instructions for each of the nine assessments. A chart of forms for the stair stand, arm curl, 6-minute walk, chair sit and reach, back scratch, 8-foot up-and-go test is located in Appendix A.

Static Balance

Purpose. To assess static balance

Equipment. Stop watch, scoring sheet, a level surface

Protocol. The participant is asked to do the following:

- Place hands on hips.
- Stand flat footed on the right foot.
- Place the other foot on the supporting ankle.

The tester performs one demonstration, allows the participant one practice trial, and then presents four trials. The support leg for each trial should be alternated.

Timing begins when the participant's foot is on the supporting ankle and stops after 30 seconds. The tester records time to the nearest 1/100th of a second. If the participant's hands come out to the side, timing should stop. The tester can correct the participant on the first trial if he or she is performing the task incorrectly. If the participant's hands come out to the side on the second or subsequent trials, the tester should note it and stop timing at that point.

The tester can cue the participant to tighten stabilizers or to find a focal point of concentration such as an X marked on a wall. If these cues are used during the initial assessment, they should be given during each reassessment for consistency.

Some of the problems that may occur include the following:

- Hands come off the hips.
- The foot comes into the air.
- The toe taps in front of the supporting foot.

Scoring. 30 seconds is a perfect score for each leg. The best time for the correctly performed task for both the left and right legs is to be recorded on the score sheet.

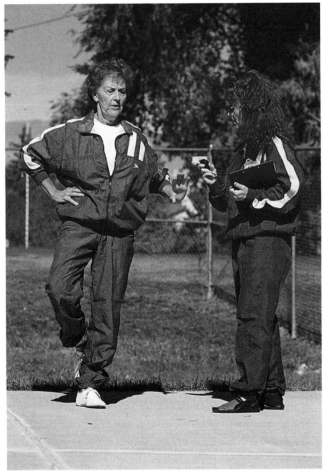

During the static balance test, when the foot comes up in the air, timing stops and is recorded.

Dynamic Balance (based on a modification of the Bass Test of Dynamic balance)

Purpose. To assess dynamic balance

Equipment. Seven 10-inch rubber circles of a non-skid material (for example, made of contact paper), masking tape or chalk, a tape measure

Setup. The rubber circles must be arranged in the following way (figure 16.2):

- There must be 24 inches from the center point of one circle to the next circle.
- Circles number 1, 3, 4, 6, and 7 must be in a straight line.
- Circles number 2 and 5 must be at a 45-degree angle and 24 inches apart.
- There must be 6 inches from the starting line to the first circle.

"Static Balance" and "Dynamic Balance" from Johnson, B. L. and J. K. Nelson. *Practical Measurements for Evaluation in Physical Education,* 4th ed. © 1986 by Allyn & Bacon. Adapted by permission.

Figure 16.2 *Sample stepping pattern (modified by Dr. Art Broten, University of Nevada, Reno)*

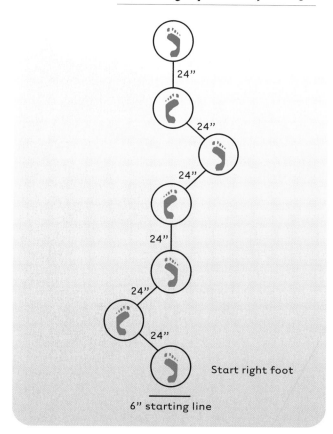

24"

24"

24"

24"

24"

24"

24"

Start right foot

6" starting line

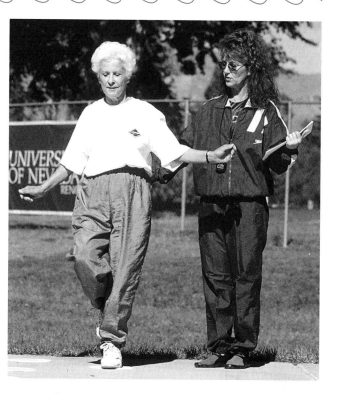

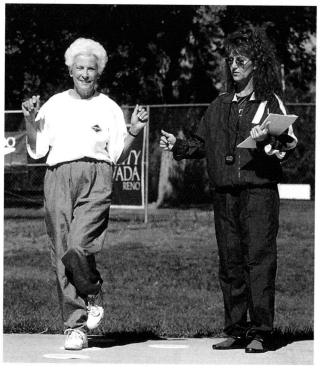

Protocol. The participant is asked to alternate stepping right and left for seven steps, beginning on the right foot. She or he holds for four seconds on each step as the tester counts "one, one thousand, two, one thousand, three one thousand, step (on the fourth count)." On "step" the participant steps forward to the next circle. This procedure continues until he or she has completed all seven steps.

The participant gets one practice run through each of the seven steps, then one trial. The participant should be told to prepare for each run by putting weight on the left foot and putting the right foot in the ready position, with the heel up.

The participant may balance with movement during the holding time, such as moving the arms around. He or she may not prepare before moving into the hold position, that is, may not tap the floor on the way up to the hold position.

Scoring. One point is awarded for stepping in the middle of the circle. One point is awarded for every second the participant balances on the circle with one foot up (it is possible to have a score of 0). The maximum number of points possible is 35.

The non weight bearing foot has to be off the ground in order for the participant to receive points. If the foot does not come directly up to the hold position, the points for the seconds the participant held still are not counted.

8-Foot Up-and-Go (Agility)

Purpose. To assess agility/dynamic balance

Equipment. Stopwatch, tape measure, cone (or similar marker), straight-back or folding chair (seat height approximately 17 inches)

Setup. The chair should be positioned against a wall or in some other way secured so that it does not move during testing. It should also be in a clear, unobstructed area, facing a cone marker exactly 8 feet away (measured from a point on the floor even with the front edge of the chair to the back of the marker). There should be at least 4 feet of clearance beyond the cone to allow ample turning room for the participant.

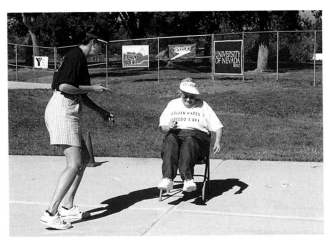

Protocol. The test begins with the participant fully seated in the chair (erect posture), hands on thighs and feet flat on the floor (one foot slightly in front of the other). On the signal "go" the participant gets up from the chair (pushing off thighs or chair is allowed), walks as quickly as possible around the cone (on either side), and returns to the chair. The participant should be told that this is a timed test and that the object is to walk as quickly as possible (without running) around the cone and back to the chair. The tester should serve as a spotter, standing midway between the chair and the cone, ready to assist the participant in case of loss of balance. For reliable scoring, the tester must start the timer on "go," whether or not the participant has started to move, and stop the timer at the exact instant the participant sits in the chair.

After a demonstration, the participant walks through the test one time as a practice and then is given two test trials. Participants should be reminded that the timing does not stop until they are fully seated in the chair.

Scoring. The score is the time elapsed from the signal "go" until the participant returns to a seated position in the chair. Record both test scores to the nearest 1/10th of a second and circle the best score (lowest time). The best score is used to evaluate performance.

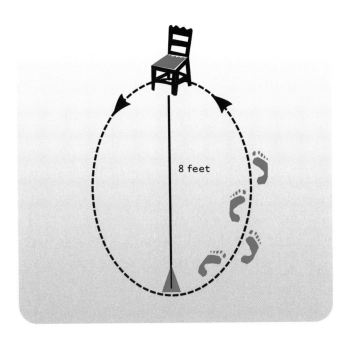

8 feet

6-Minute Walk

Purpose. To assess aerobic endurance

Equipment. Stopwatch, long measuring tape, cones, Popsicle sticks, chalk, masking tape (or some other type of marker). For safety purposes, chairs should be positioned at several points alongside the walkway.

Setup. The test involves assessing the maximum distance that can be walked in 6 minutes along a 50-yard course marked into 5-yard segments (see figure 16.3). The inside perimeter of the measured distance should be marked with cones, and the 5-yard segments with masking tape or chalk. The walking area, which can be indoors or outdoors, should be well lit, with a nonslippery, level surface.

Protocol. To keep track of distance walked, a Popsicle stick (or similar object) can be given to the participant each time he or she rounds a cone, or a partner can mark a scorecard each time a lap is completed. Two or more participants should be tested at a time, with starting times staggered (10 seconds apart) so that participants do not walk in clusters or pairs. When several people are being tested at once, numbers should be placed on the participants to indicate the order of starting and stopping. On the signal "go," participants are instructed to walk as fast as possible (not run) around the course as many times as they can in 6 minutes. If necessary, participants may stop and rest (on provided chairs), then resume walking. The timer should move to the inside of the marked area after everyone has started. To assist with pacing, elapsed time should be called out when participants are approximately half done, when 2 minutes are left, and when 1 minute is left. Encouragement phrases such as "You are doing well" and "Keep up the good work" should be called out at approximately 30-second intervals. At the end of 6 minutes, participants (staggered every 10 seconds) are instructed to stop and move to the right, where an assistant records their

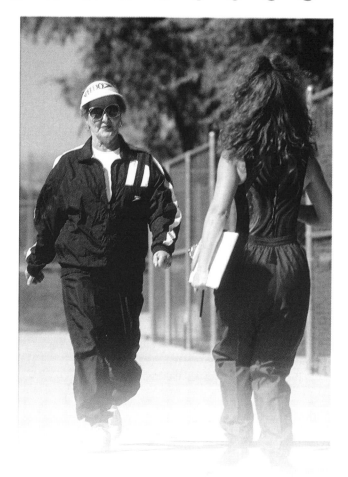

score. To assist with proper pacing and to improve scoring accuracy, a practice test should be given prior to the actual test day.

Safety. The test should be discontinued if at any time a participant shows signs of dizziness, pain, nausea, or undue fatigue. At the end of the test, each participant should slowly walk around for about a minute to cool down.

Scoring. The score is the total number of yards walked in 6 minutes to the nearest 5 yards. The test administrator or aide records the nearest 5-yard mark.

Figure 16.3 *Setup for walking course*

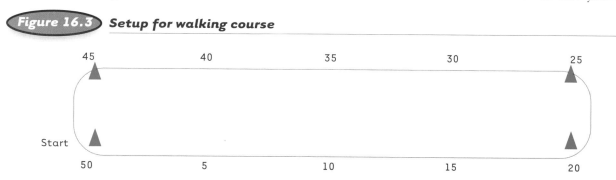

Reprinted by permission, from Rikli, R. and J. Jones. 1999. "Development and validation of a functional fitness test for community-residing older adults." *Journal of Aging and Physical Activity* 7(2): 129–161.

30-Second Chair Stand

Purpose. To assess lower body strength

Equipment. Stopwatch, straight-back or folding chair (without arms), height approximately 17 inches. For safety purposes, the chair should be placed against a wall or in some other way stabilized to prevent it from moving during the test.

Protocol. The test begins with the participant seated in the middle of the chair, back straight and feet flat on the floor. Arms are crossed at the wrists and held against the chest. On the signal "go" the participant rises to a full stand and then returns to a fully seated position. The

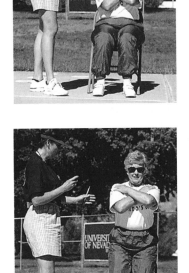

participant is encouraged to complete as many full stands as possible within 30 seconds. After a demonstration by the tester, a practice trial of one to three repetitions should be done to check for proper form, followed by one 30-second test trial.

Scoring. The score is the total number of stands executed correctly within 30 seconds. If the participant is more than halfway up at the end of 30 seconds, it counts as a full stand.

Arm Curl

Purpose. To assess upper-body strength

Equipment. Wristwatch with second hand, straight-back or folding chair (without arms), hand weights (dumbbells—5 pounds for women, 8 pounds for men)

Protocol. The participant is seated on a chair, back straight and feet flat on the floor, with the dominant side of the body close to the side edge of the chair. The weight is held at the side in the dominant hand (handshake grip). The test begins with the arm down beside the chair, perpendicular to the floor. At the signal "go" the participant turns the palm up while curling the arm through a full range of motion and then returns to the fully extended position. At the down position, the weight should have returned to the handshake grip position.

The examiner kneels (or sits in a chair) next to the participant on the dominant-arm side, placing his or her fingers on the person's mid-biceps to prevent the upper arm from moving and to ensure that a full curl is made (participant's forearm should squeeze examiner's fingers). It is important that the participant's upper arm remain stabilized (still) throughout the test.

The examiner may also need to position his or her other hand behind the participant's elbow so that the participant knows when full extension has been reached, as well as to prevent a backswinging motion of the arm.

The participant is encouraged to execute as many curls as possible within the 30-second time limit. After a demonstration by the examiner, a practice trial of one or two repetitions should be given to check for proper form, followed by one 30-second trial.

Scoring. The score is the total number of curls made correctly within 30 seconds. If the arm is more than halfway up at the end of the 30 seconds, it counts as a curl.

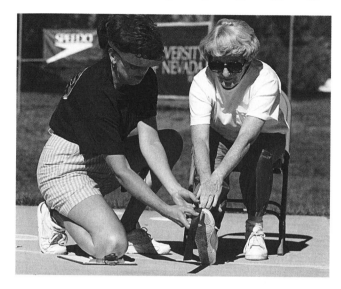

Chair Sit-and-Reach

Purpose. To assess lower body (primarily hamstring) flexibility

Equipment. Straight-back or folding chair (approximately 17-inches seat height), 18-inch ruler. For safety purposes, the chair should be placed against a wall and checked to see that it remains stable (doesn't tip forward) when the participant sits on the front edge.

Protocol. Starting in a sitting position on a chair, the participant moves forward until she or he is sitting on the front edge. The crease between the top of the leg and the buttocks should be even with the edge of the chair seat. Keeping one leg bent and *foot flat on the floor*, the other leg (the preferred leg*) is extended straight in front of the hip, with heel on floor and foot flexed (at approximately 90 degrees).

With the extended leg as straight as possible (but not hyperextended), the participant slowly bends forward *at the hip joint* (spine should remain as straight as possible, with head in line with spine, not tucked) sliding the hands (one on top of the other with the tips of the middle fingers even) down the extended leg in an attempt to touch the toes. The reach must be held for 2 seconds. If the extended knee starts to bend, ask the participant to slowly sit back until the knee is straight before scoring. Participants should be reminded to exhale as they bend forward; to avoid bouncing or rapid, forceful movements; and to never stretch to the point of pain.

---

*The preferred leg or hand is defined as the one that results in the better score. Although it is important to work on flexibility on both sides of the body, for the sake of time only the "better" side has been used in developing norms.

After a demonstration by the tester, the participant is asked to determine the preferred leg. The participant is then given two practice (stretching) trials on that leg, followed by two test trials.

Scoring. Using an 18-inch ruler, the scorer records the number of inches a person is short of reaching the toe (minus score) or reaches beyond the toe (plus score). The middle of the toe at the end of the shoe represents a zero score. Record both test scores to the nearest $\frac{1}{2}$ inch, and circle the best score. The best score is used to evaluate performance. Be sure to indicate "minus" or "plus" on the score card.

Back Scratch

Purpose. To assess upper body (shoulder) flexibility.

Equipment. 18-inch ruler (half of a yardstick).

Protocol. In a standing position, the participant places the preferred hand* behind the same-side shoulder, palm toward back and fingers extended, reaching down the middle of the back as far as possible (elbow pointed up). The participant places the other hand behind the back, palm out, reaching up as far as possible in an attempt to touch or overlap the extended middle fingers of both hands.

Without moving the participant's hands, the tester helps to see that the middle fingers of each hand are directed toward each other. The participant is not allowed to grab his or her fingers together and pull.

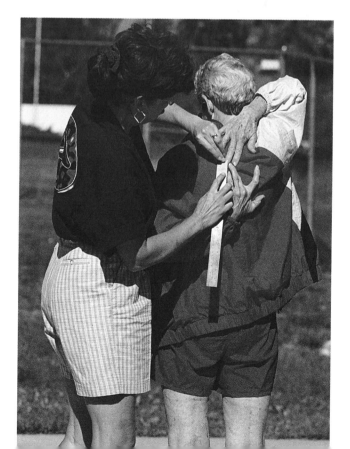

After a demonstration by the tester, the participant is asked to determine the preferred hand, and is then given two practice (stretching) trials, followed by two test trials.

Scoring. The distance of overlap or distance between the tips of the middle fingers is measured to the nearest $\frac{1}{2}$ inch. A minus score (–) is given to represent a distance short of touching: a plus score (+) represents the amount of overlap. Record both test scores and circle the best one. The best score is used to evaluate performance. Be sure to indicate "minus" or "plus" on the score card.

Stair Climb

Purpose. To measure stair climbing and descending speed.

Equipment. A flight of stairs (with handrails if possible) and a stop watch

Protocol. The participant stands at the top of a flight of stairs. The tester tells him or her to walk down the stairs to the bottom, then turn around and walk back to the top. The tester tells the participant to move as quickly as he or she can and still be safe. On the cue "Top to bottom...go," the participant walks down and up the stairs. The participant must step off the bottom step with both feet and turn around.

The participant performs two test trials. Use the same set of stairs for subsequent tests.

Scoring. Record the time to the nearest 1/100th of a second.

Descriptions of the 8-Foot Up-and-Go, 6-Minute Walk, 30-Second Chair Stand, Arm Curl, Chair Sit-and-Reach, and Back Scratch are from Rickli, R., and J. Jones. 1999. Development and validation of a functional fitness test for community-residing older adults. *Journal of Aging and Physical Activity* 7(2): 129-161. This material is ©1999 R. E. Rikli and C.J. Jones.

Bibliography

Corbin, D.E., and J. Metal-Corbin. 1984. *Reach for it! A handbook of health, exercise and dance activities for older adults.* 2nd ed. Reston, VA: AAPHERD.

Rickli, R., and J. Jones. 1999. Development and validation of a functional fitness test for community-residing older adults. *Journal of Aging and Physical Activity* 7(2): 129-161.

Sanders, M., N. Constantino, and N. Rippee. 1997. A comparison of results of functional water training on field and laboratory measures in older women. *Medicine and Science in Sports and Exercise* 29(5): Abstract 630.

APPENDIXES

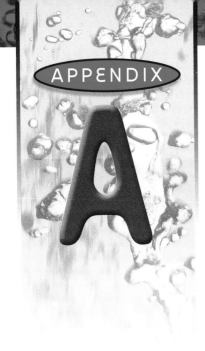

Program Forms

This appendix contains a number of forms that may be useful in your YMCA Water Fitness classes. They include the following:

- PAR-Q & You
- Medical Clearance Form
- Description of Testing for Activities of Daily Living and Exercise Programs
- Informed Consent for Fitness Testing Form
- Informed Consent for Exercise Participation Form

- Waist-to-Hip Ratio and Body Composition Form
- Body Mass Index Table
- Target Heart Rate (THR), Intensity and Rate of Perceived Exertion (RPE) Chart
- Assessing Your Risk for Osteoporosis
- Functional ADL Field Assessments, Normative Scores

The following health screening, medical clearance, and informed consent forms (Forms I through IV) are adapted from forms in *Principles of YMCA Health and Fitness* (1995) and *Y's Way to Physical Fitness* (3rd ed.)(1989). They have been modified to be used with the tests for activities of daily living described in chapter 16 of this book. They can be reproduced and used as needed for your YMCA classes, but, if you choose to use them, please make sure you have them reviewed and approved by your local medical and legal counsel first.

The screening form should be administered when participants enter a program and yearly thereafter. Copies of all completed participant forms should be retained in a records file for at least three years.

Additional forms in Appendix A include the Waist-to-Hip Ratio and Body Composition Form; the Body Mass Index Table; the Heart Rate Chart; and the Functional ADL Field Assessments, Normative Scores.

Form I
Health Screen Form
(Par-Q & You)

Form I is the Physical Activity Readiness Questionnaire developed by the Canadian Society for Exercise Physiology. It asks for general information about the participant's physical condition. Individuals should be instructed to follow the recommendations based on their answers prior to participating in YMCA testing or exercise programs.

Forms II and IIa
Medical Clearance Form and Description of Testing for Activities of Daily Living and Exercise Programs

The Medical Clearance Form is used by the participant's physician to report any restrictions that should be placed on the participant during testing or exercise programs. The physician should see both Form II and Form IIA, which describes generally the YMCA testing and exercise programs and the risks associated with each.

Form III
Informed Consent for Activities of Daily Living Testing Form

The Informed Consent for Activities of Daily Living Testing Form ensures that the participant is aware of the risks involved in the testing procedures. It documents that a description of the testing procedures has been read and that all questions concerning those procedures have been answered satisfactorily.

Form IV
Informed Consent for Exercise Participation Form

The Informed Consent for Exercise Participation Form ensures that the participant is aware of the risks involved in exercise. It documents that the description of the exercise program has been read and all questions concerning the exercise program have been answered to the participant's satisfaction.

When and How to Use the Forms

The Health Screen Form (Form I) should be completed before a participant starts any program, even if it is just an education class. The information obtained in this form is valuable for educating participants on potential health and cardiovascular risk. Note that Form I is not intended to be a medical exam but simply a means to obtain key health information.

If a potential participant requires medical clearance, use Form II. It allows a physician to indicate that he or she thinks the individual is capable of participating in the Y's exercise programs. Form IIA provides a description of the YMCA exercise programs for the doctor.

The informed consent forms (Forms III and IV) are designed to notify participants of the inherent risks of testing and exercise programs. Form III, Informed Consent Form for Testing for Activities of Daily Living Testing, should be given to any person registering for an activities of daily living test. It should be read and signed before testing starts. Form IV, Informed Consent for Exercise Participation, should be given to any participant in a supervised exercise program. It should be read and signed before exercise starts.

PAR-Q & YOU

(A Questionnaire for People Aged 15 to 69)

Regular physical activity is fun and healthy, and increasingly more people are starting to become more active every day. Being more active is very safe for most people. However, some people should check with their doctor before they start becoming much more physically active.

If you are planning to become more physically active thatn you are now, start by answering the seven questions in the box below. If you are between the ages of 15 and 69, the PAR-Q will tell you if you should check with your doctor before you start. If you are over 69 years of age, and you are not used to being very active, check with your doctor.

Common sense is your best guide when you answer these questions. Please read the questions carefully and answer each one honestly: check YES or NO.

YES	NO	
❑	❑	1. Has your doctor ever said that you have a heart condition <u>and</u> that you should only do physical activity recommended by a doctor?
❑	❑	2. Do you feel pain in your chest when you do physical activity?
❑	❑	3. In the past month, have you had chest pain when you were not doing physical activity?
❑	❑	4. Do you lose your balance because of dizziness or do you ever lose consciousness?
❑	❑	5. Do you have a bone or joint problem that could be made worse by a change in your physical activity?
❑	❑	6. Is your doctor currectly prescribing drugs (for example, water pills) for your blood pressure or heart condition?
❑	❑	7. Do you know of <u>any other reason</u> why you should not do physical activity?

If you answered

YES to one or more questions

Talk with your doctor by phone or in person BEFORE you start becoming much more physically active or BEFORE you have a fitness appraisal. Tell your doctor about the PAR-Q and which questions you answered YES.

- You may be able to do any activity you want—as long as you start slowly and build up gradually. Or, you may need to restrict your activities to those which are safe for you. Talk with your doctor about the kinds of activities you wish to participate in and follow his/her advice.

- Find out which community programs are safe and helpful for you.

NO to one or more questions

If you answered NO honestly to <u>all</u> PAR-Q questions, you can be reasonably sure that you can:

- start becoming much more physically active—begin slowly and build up gradually. This is the safest and easiest way to go.

- take part in a fitness appraisal—this is an excellent way to determine your basic fitness so that you can plan the best way for you to live actively.

Delay becoming much more active:

- if you are not feeling well because of a temporary illness such as a cold or a fever—wait until you feel better; or

- if you are or may be pregnant—talk to your doctor before you start becoming more active.

Please note: If your health changes so that you then answer YES to any of the above questions, tell your fitness or health professional. Ask whether you should change your physical activity plan.

Informed Use of the PAR-Q: The Canadian Society for Exercise Physiology, Health Canada, and their agents assume no liability for persons who undertake physical activity, and if in doubt after completing this questionnaire, consult your doctor prior to physical activity.

You are encouraged to copy the PAR-Q but only if you use the entire form.

NOTE: If the PAR-Q is being given to a person before he or she participates in a physical activity program or a fitness appraisal, this section may be used for legal or administrative purposes.

I have read, understood and completed this questionnaire. Any questions I had were answered to my full satisfaction.

NAME _____

SIGNATURE _____   DATE _____

SIGNATURE OF PARENT _____   WITNESS _____
or GUARDIAN (for participants under the age of majority)

Reprinted from the 1994 revised version of the Physical Activity Readiness Questionnaire (PAR-Q and YOU). The PAR-Q and YOU is a copyrighted, pre-exercise screen owned by the Canadian Society for Exercise Physiology.

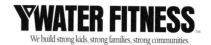

Medical Clearance Form

Dear Doctor:

_____ has applied for enrollment in the testing

(name of applicant)

activities of daily living at the YMCA. The testing program involves the following tests: Static Balance, Dynamic Balance, 8-Foot Up-and-Go (agility), 6-Minute Walk (aerobic endurance), 30-Second Chair Stand (lower body strength), Arm Curl (upper body strength), Chair Sit-and-Reach (lower body flexibility), Back Scratch (upper body flexibility), and Stair Climb. The exercise programs are designed to start easy and become progressively more difficult over a period of time. A more detailed description of the testing and exercise programs is attached in Form IIA. All tests and exercise programs will be administered by qualified personnel trained in conducting exercise tests and exercise programs.

By completing the form below, however, you are not assuming any responsibility for our administration of the testing for activities of daily living and/or exercise programs. If you know of any medical or other reasons why participation in the testing and/or exercise programs by the applicant would be unwise, please indicate so on this form.

If you have any questions about the YMCA testing and/or exercise programs, please call.

Report of Physician

_____ I know of no reason why the applicant may not participate.

_____ I believe the applicant can participate, but I urge caution because

_____

_____

_____ The applicant should not engage in the follow activities:

_____

_____

_____ I recommend that the applicant NOT participate.

Physician signature _____ Date _____

Address _____ Telephone _____

City and state _____ Zip _____

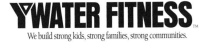

Description of Testing for Activities of Daily Living and Exercise Programs

Dear Doctor:

The YMCA testing for activities of daily living for which the participant has applied are described as follows:

Testing—The purpose of the testing program for activities of daily living is to evaluate balance, cardiorespiratory fitness, flexibility, muscular strength, and stair climbing ability. For balance, both a Static Balance and a Dynamic Balance test are used. The cardiorespiratory fitness test is the 6-Minute Walk. Flexibility is determined by the Chair Sit-and-Reach and Back Scratch tests. Muscular strength is evaluated by the 30-Second Chair Stand and the Arm Curl. The Stair Climb test evaluates stair climbing ability.

Exercise programs—The purpose of the exercise programs is to develop and maintain balance, cardiorespiratory fitness, body composition, flexibility, muscular strength and endurance, and stair climbing ability. A specific exercise plan will be given to the participant based on needs and interests and your recommendations. All exercise programs include warm-up, exercise at target heart rate, and cool-down (except for muscular strength and endurance training, in which target heart rate is not a factor). The programs may involve walking, jogging, swimming, or cycling (outdoor and stationary); participation in exercise fitness, rhythmic aerobic exercise, water fitness, or choreographed fitness classes; or calisthenics or strength training. All programs are designed to place a gradually increasing workload on the body in order to improve overall fitness and muscular strength. The rate of progression is regulated by exercise target heart rate and/or perceived effort of exercise.

In both the testing and exercise programs, the reaction of the cardiorespiratory system cannot be predicted with complete accuracy. There is a risk of certain changes that might occur during or following exercise. These changes might include abnormalities of blood pressure and/or heart rate. YMCA exercise instructors are certified in CPR, and emergency procedures are posted in the exercise facility.

In addition to your medical approval and recommendations, the participant will be asked to sign informed consent forms that explain the risks of testing and exercise participation before the programs are initiated.

Form III

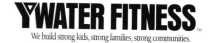

Informed Consent Form for Testing
for Activities of Daily Living

Name _____
(please print)

The purpose of the testing program for activities of daily living is to evaluate balance, cardiorespiratory fitness, flexibility, muscular strength, and stair climbing ability. For balance, both a Static Balance and a Dynamic Balance test are used. The cardiorespiratory fitness test is the 6-Minute Walk. Flexibility is determined by the Chair Sit-and-Reach and Back Scratch tests. Muscular strength is evaluated by the 30-Second Chair Stand and the Arm Curl. The Stair Climb test evaluates stair climbing ability.

I understand that I am responsible for monitoring my own condition throughout the tests, and should any unusual symptoms occur, I will cease my participation and inform the instructor of the symptoms.

In signing this consent form, I affirm that I have read this form in its entirety and that I understand the description of the tests and their components. I also affirm that my questions regarding the testing program have been answered to my satisfaction.

In the event that a medical clearance must be obtained prior to my participation in the testing program, I agree to consult my physician and obtain written permission from my physician prior to the commencement of any tests.

Also, in consideration for being allowed to participate in the testing program, I agree to assume the risk of such testing, and further agree to hold harmless the YMCA and its staff members conducting such testing from any and all claims, suits, losses, or related causes of action for damages, including, but not limited to, such claims that may result from my injury or death, accidental or otherwise, during, or arising in any way from, the testing program.

_____ Date _____
(Signature of participant)

_____ Date _____
(Person administering tests)

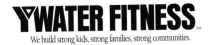

Informed Consent for Exercise Participation Form

I desire to engage voluntarily in the YMCA exercise program to attempt to improve my physical fitness. I understand that the activities are designed to place a gradually increasing workload on the cardiorespiratory system and to thereby attempt to improve its function. The reaction of the cardiorespiratory system to such activities can't be predicted with complete accuracy. There is a risk of certain changes that might occur during or following the exercise. These changes might include abnormalities of blood pressure or heart rate.

I understand that the purpose of the exercise program is to develop and maintain balance, cardiorespiratory fitness, body composition, flexibility, muscular strength and endurance, and the ability to climb stairs. A specific exercise plan will be given to me, based on my needs and interests and my doctor's recommendations. All exercise programs include warm-up, exercise at target heart rate, and cool-down. The programs may involve walking, jogging, swimming, or cycling (outdoor and stationary); participation in exercise fitness, rhythmic aerobic exercise, water fitness, or choreographed fitness classes; or calisthenics or strength training. All programs are designed to place a gradually increasing workload on the body in order to improve overall fitness. The rate of progression is regulated by exercise target heart rate and perceived effort of exercise.

I understand that I am responsible for monitoring my own condition throughout the exercise program and should any unusual symptoms occur, I will cease my participation and inform the instructor of the symptoms.

In signing this consent form, I affirm that I have read this form in its entirety and that I under-stand the nature of the exercise program. I also affirm that my questions regarding the exercise program have been answered to my satisfaction.

In the event that a medical clearance must be obtained prior to my participation in the exercise program, I agree to consult my physician and obtain written permission from my physician prior to the commencement of any exercise program.

Also, in consideration for being allowed to participate in the YMCA exercise program, I agree to assume the risk of such exercise, and further agree to hold harmless the YMCA and its staff members conducting the exercise program from any and all claims, suits, losses, or related causes of action for damages, including, but not limited to, such claims that may result from my injury or death, accidental or otherwise, during, or arising in any way from, the exercise program.

_____ Date _____
(Signature of participant)

Please print:

Name _____ Date of birth _____

Address_____
Street   City   State   Zip

Telephone _____

Name of personal physician _____

Physician's address _____

Physician's phone _____

Limitations and medications _____

Waist-to-Hip Ratio and Body Composition Form

Once you have completed this worksheet, you should have a better understanding of how your body composition is likely to affect your health. While being overweight can raise the risk of disease, especially cardiovascular diseases, your risk is only partially determined by your weight. The distribution of the weight matters as well. The waist-to-hip ratio will allow you to determine your risk for heart disease.

1. Take measurements with a tape measure.

Waist _____ (measure at the narrowest point of the waist)

Hip _____ (measure where the buttocks protrude most)

2. Calculate the waist-to-hip ratio using a calculator.

Waist _____ / Hip _____ = _____ Waist-to-hip ratio

3. Determine your risk classification.

Find the box where your waist-to-hip ratio measurement would be located. Determine your risk classification, then look below for more risk classification information.

High Risk Factors

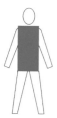

- No visible waistline
- Fat concentration in waist

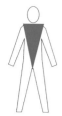

- Broad shoulders
- Narrow hips
- Fat concentration in chest

Family history of disease, sedentary lifestyle, high stress, high-fat diet, smoking, and high blood pressure

Low Risk Factors

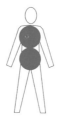

- Broad hips and chest
- Small waist
- Fat concentration in hips and chest

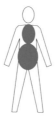

- Narrow shoulders
- Average waist
- Fat concentration in hips and/or thighs
- Small chest

No family history of disease, active lifestyle with regular exercise, low stress, low-fat diet, no smoking, and normal blood pressure

Source: Carol Kennedy. Reprinted with permission.

Body Mass Index Table

Height inches	19	20	21	22	23	24	25	26	27	28	29	30	31	32	33	34	35	36
							Body Weight (pounds)											
58	91	96	100	105	110	115	119	124	129	134	138	143	148	153	158	162	167	172
59	94	99	104	109	114	119	124	128	133	138	143	148	153	158	163	168	173	178
60	97	102	107	112	118	123	128	133	138	143	148	153	158	163	168	174	179	184
61	100	106	111	116	122	127	132	137	143	148	153	158	164	169	174	180	185	190
62	104	109	115	120	126	131	136	142	147	153	158	164	169	175	180	186	191	196
63	107	113	118	124	130	135	141	146	152	158	163	169	175	180	186	191	197	203
64	110	116	122	128	134	140	145	151	157	163	169	174	180	186	192	197	204	209
65	114	120	126	132	138	144	150	156	162	168	174	180	186	192	198	204	210	216
66	118	124	130	136	142	148	155	161	167	173	179	186	192	198	204	210	216	223
67	121	127	134	140	146	153	159	166	172	178	185	191	198	204	211	217	223	230
68	125	131	138	144	151	158	164	171	177	184	190	197	203	210	216	223	230	236
69	128	135	142	149	155	162	169	176	182	189	196	203	209	216	223	230	236	243
70	132	139	146	153	160	167	174	181	188	195	202	209	216	222	229	236	243	250
71	136	143	150	157	165	172	179	186	193	200	208	215	222	229	236	243	250	257
72	140	147	154	162	169	177	184	191	199	206	213	221	228	235	242	250	258	265
73	144	151	159	166	174	1822	189	197	204	212	219	227	235	242	250	257	265	272
74	148	155	163	171	179	186	194	202	210	218	225	233	241	249	256	264	272	280
75	152	160	168	176	184	192	200	208	216	224	232	240	248	256	264	272	279	287
76	156	164	172	180	189	197	205	213	221	230	238	246	254	263	271	279	287	295

Height inches	37	38	39	40	41	42	43	44	45	46	47	48	49	50	51	52	53	54
							Body Weight (pounds)											
58	177	181	186	191	196	201	205	210	215	220	224	229	234	239	244	248	253	258
59	183	188	193	198	203	208	212	217	222	227	232	237	242	247	252	257	262	267
60	189	194	199	204	209	215	220	225	230	235	240	245	250	255	261	266	271	275
61	195	201	206	211	217	222	227	232	238	243	248	254	259	264	269	275	280	285
62	202	207	213	218	224	229	235	240	246	251	256	262	267	273	278	284	289	295
63	208	214	220	225	231	237	242	248	254	259	265	270	278	282	287	293	299	304
64	215	221	227	232	238	244	250	256	262	267	273	279	285	291	296	302	308	314
65	222	228	234	240	246	252	258	264	270	276	282	288	294	300	306	312	318	324
66	229	235	241	247	253	260	266	272	278	284	291	297	303	309	315	322	328	334
67	236	242	249	255	261	268	274	280	287	293	299	306	312	319	325	331	338	344
68	243	249	256	267	269	276	282	289	295	302	308	315	322	328	335	341	348	354
69	250	257	263	270	277	284	291	297	304	311	318	324	331	338	345	351	358	365
70	257	264	271	278	285	292	299	306	313	320	327	334	341	348	355	362	369	376
71	265	272	279	286	293	301	308	315	322	329	338	343	351	358	365	372	379	386
72	272	279	287	294	302	309	316	324	331	338	346	353	361	368	375	383	390	397
73	280	288	295	302	210	318	325	333	340	348	355	363	371	378	386	393	401	408
74	287	295	303	311	319	326	334	342	350	358	365	373	381	389	396	404	412	420
75	295	303	311	319	327	335	343	351	359	367	375	383	391	399	407	415	423	431
76	304	312	320	328	336	344	353	361	369	377	385	394	402	410	418	426	435	443

To use this table, find the appropriate height in the left-hand column. Move across to a given weight. The number at the top of the column is the BMI at that height and weight. Pounds have been rounded off.

Source: National Heart, Lung, and Blood Institute

Target Heart Rate (THR), Intensity and Rate of Perceived Exertion (RPE) Chart

Age	Max Heart Rate (HRmax, 220-age)	Modified Target HR Range for Unfit People/RPE (55% to 65% of maximum) 55% to 65% THR Moderate Intensity 12–13 RPE Scale beats/minute	Target HR Range/RPE (65% to 90% of maximum) 65% to 69% THR Moderate Intensity 12–13 on RPE scale beats/minute	60% to 89% THR Hard Intensity 14–16 RPE Scale beats/minute	90% THR Very Hard 17–19 RPE Scale beats/minute
20	200	110–130	130–138	120–178	180
25	195	107–127	127–134	117–174	175
30	190	104–123	123–131	114–170	171
35	185	102–120	120–127	111–165	166
40	180	99–117	117–124	108–160	162
45	175	96–114	114–120	105–156	157
50	170	93–110	110–117	102–152	153
55	165	91–107	107–114	99–147	148
60	160	88–104	104–110	96–143	144
65	155	85–101	101–107	93–138	139
70	150	82–97	97–103	90–134	135
75	145	80–94	94–100	87–129	130
80	140	77–91	91–96	84–125	126
85	135	74–88	88–93	81–120	121
90	130	71–84	84–90	78–116	117
95	125	69–81	81–86	75–111	112
100	120	66–78	78–82	72–107	108

Note: Target heart rates can vary in water, so be sure to also use rate of perceived exertion and listen to how your body feels to monitor intensity.

Assessing Your Risk for Osteoporosis

For each of the following questions, check either yes or no.   YES   NO

1. Do you have a family history of osteoporosis? (Have any of your relatives broken a wrist or hip or had a dowager's hump?)   ❏   ❏

2. Did you go through menopause or have you had your ovaries removed by surgery before age 50?   ❏   ❏

3. Did your menstrual periods ever stop for more than a year for reasons other than pregnancy or nursing?   ❏   ❏

4. Did your ancestors come from England, Ireland, Scotland, Northern Europe, or Asia, or do you have a small, thin body frame?   ❏   ❏

5. Have you had surgery in which a part of you stomach or intestine was removed?   ❏   ❏

6. Are you taking or have you taken drugs like cortisone, steroids, or anticonvuslants over a prolonged period?   ❏   ❏

7. Do you have a thyroid or parathyroid disorder (hyperthyroidism or hyperparathyroidism)?   ❏   ❏

8. Are you allergic to milk products or are you lactose intolerant?   ❏   ❏

9. Do you smoke cigarettes?   ❏   ❏

10. Do you drink wine, beer, or other alcoholic beverages daily?   ❏   ❏

11. Do you do less than one hour of exercising, such as aerobics, walking, or jogging per week?   ❏   ❏

12. Have you ever exercised so strenuously that you had irregular periods or no periods at all?   ❏   ❏

13. Have you ever had an eating disorder (bulimia or anorexia nervosa)?   ❏   ❏

If you answered "yes" to many of these questions, you may be at an increased risk for osteoporosis.

From *Wellness: Choice for Health and Fitness,* 1st edition, by R. Donatelle, C. S. Harter, and A. Wilcox, . Benjamin/Cummings. © 1995. Reprinted with permission of Wadsworth Publishing, a division of Thomson Learning. Fax 800-730-2215.

Functional ADL Field Assessments, Normative Scores

Women, Age Group

Category	60-64	65-69	70-74	75-79	80-84	85-89	90-94
Chair stand (no. stands)	12–17	11–16	10–15	9–14	8–13	4–11	
Arm Curl (no. reps.)	13–19	12–18	12–17	11–17	10–16	10–15	8–13
6-min walk (yards)	545–660	500–635	480–615	430–585	385–540	340–510	275–440
Chair sit & reach (in.)	(-0.5 to 5)	(-0.5 to 4.5)	(-1.0 to 4)	(-1.5 to 3.5)	(-2.0 to 3)	(-2.5 to 2.5)	(-4.5 to 1)
Back scratch (in.)	(-3 to 1.5)	(-3.5 to 1.5)	(-4 to 1)	(-5 to .5)	(-5.5 to 0)	(-7 to -1)	(-8.0 to -1.0)
8-ft. up & go (seconds)	6–4.4	6.4–4.8	7.1–4.9	7.4–5.2	8.7–5.7	9.6–6.2	11.5–7.3
BMI (kg/m squared)	22.8–29.8	23–30	23.1–29.1	22.5–28.3	22–27.4	21.8–26.8	21.1–27.1

Men, Age Group

Category	60-64	65-69	70-74	75-79	80-84	85-89	90-94
Chair stand (no. stands)	14–19	12–18	12–17	11–17	10–15	8–14	7–12
Arm Curl (no. reps.)	16–22	15–21	14–21	13–19	13–19	11–17	10–14
6-min walk (yards)	610–735	560–700	545–680	470–640	445–605	380–570	305–500
Chair sit & reach (in.)	(-2.5 to 4)	(-3 to 3)	(-3.5 to 2.5)	(-4 to 2)	(-5.5 to 1.5)	(-5.5 to 0.5)	(-6.5 to 0.5)
Back scratch (in.)	(-6.5 to 0)	(-7.5 to -1)	(-8 to -1)	(-9 to -2)	(-9.5 to -2)	(-10 to -3)	(-10.5 to -4)
8-ft. up & go (seconds)	5.6–3.8	5.7–4.3	6–4.2	7.2–4.6	7.6–5.2	8.9–5.3	10–6.2
BMI (kg/m squared)	24.6–30.2	24.7–30.3	24–29.2	23.8–29	23.8–28.4	23.3–26.5	22.4–27.4

Note: Scores reflect average scores across a broad range of ability levels found in general community-residing older adult populations in the United States. Scoring for smaller, specific populations may vary.

Source: Adapted from Functional Fitness Normative Scores for Community-Residing Older Adults. Ages 60–94. *Journal of Aging and Physical Activity*, 1999, 7. 162–181, Human Kinetics: Champaign, IL.

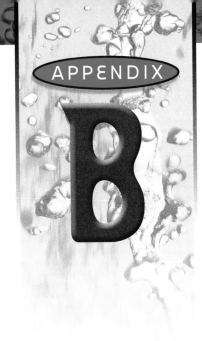
Additional Workouts

The following are notes from workouts presented on video or audio cassette. Watch the videos or listen to the tape to clarify the exercises and see them in action.

Tidal Waves
Tidal Waves *Video*™

1. Buoyancy Warm-Up (5—10 min with 8—12 movement reps)
Apply the **A.** in the **S.W.E.A.T.** formula. All movements are in neutral position.

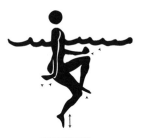

JOGGING
Knees front
Heels side
Heels cross back

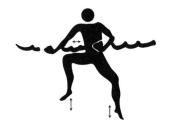

STRADDLE ROCK
Side to side
Windshield wiper arms
Kick back, push forward

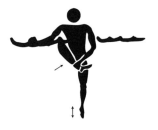

INSTEP KICKS
Push pull arms
Flexuous arms

2. Traveling Cardio Warm-Up (3—5 min) Apply the **T.** in the **S.W.E.A.T.** formula along with **S.**, **E.**, and **A.**

Jog forward, backward, and sideways: scull, fist, cup, web, clap, and row arms. Gradually increase speed and size of movement.

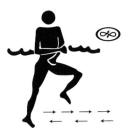

⊗ Sculling

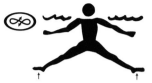

3. Cardio Working Positions (5 min) Work rebound, neutral, and suspended.

Straddle jump

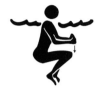

Aerial jax
Reverse aerial jax

Leap frogs

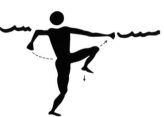

4. Muscular Conditioning (8–12 reps for each exercise) Work the biceps.

Rocking horse with
biceps pull

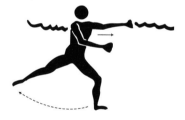

Shovels side
to side
Short to long arms

5. Cardio Travel Set (5 min). Use all working positions (rebound, neutral, suspended) while traveling all moves.

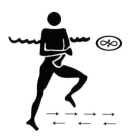

   1. Grapevine sideways
   2. Jog with breaststroke arms, forward and back
   3. Scissors forward, backward, and sideways

6. Muscular Endurance and Cardio Suspended Set (5 min). Use all working positions (rebound, neutral, suspended).
Note: Lengthen the time suspended when using buoyancy gear. Otherwise, change to neutral when participants cannot maintain a suspended position.

   1. Scissors

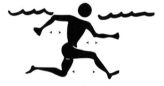

   2. Reverse aerial jax, front clap
   3. Instep kicks, ankle touch (forward, back, side to side)
   4. Cross backs
   5. Tilting
   6. Power pops
   7. Walk the dog

7. Cardio Combo Set: Working positions and traveling (5 min and 8—12 reps)
Work through all **S.W.E.A.T.** elements.

1. Straddle jump, rebound
2. Rocking horse, travel forward
3. Tuck jump, rebound
4. Rocking horse, travel forward
5. Surfboard jumps
6. Hitch kicks, travel backward

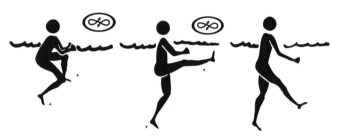

8. Funky Set. Use rebound and neutral positions.

1. Jog, cross arms front, and push back
2. Reverse, jog cross back, pull to front
3. Funky chaplain, toes and hands in . . . then out. Travel backward.
4. Funky Sims, scoot sideways
5. Hammer hands, rock sideways

9. Warm-Down (15 min or 8—12 reps each move) and Stretch

Skipping (light rebound) forward, back, and sideways, reduce size

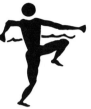

Stretch and range of motion
Straddle stretch
Neutral and suspended

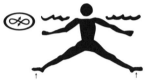

Scissors (for calf and shins)
Neutral and suspended

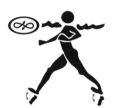

Hamstrings
Neutral

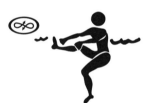

Quadriceps
Standing

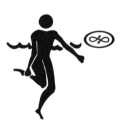

10. Playful Moves to End the Workout Warm!
Use the **A.** in **S.W.E.A.T.**
Easy jax
Soft leaps
Neutral

Tidal Waves, reprinted with permission from Wave Aerobics™

Shallow Wave Workout
The Introduction to the
Speedo Aquatic Fitness System

1. Buoyancy Warm-Up (3—5 min)

Apply **S.E.A.**

Jogging   Kicking   Rocking

2. Cardio Warm-Up (2—3 min)

Apply **S.E.A.T.**

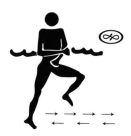 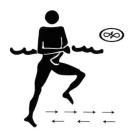

Jogging   Work around the
                  body, straddle jog

3. Muscular Endurance and Light Cardio
(4—6 min)

Apply **S.E.**

Figure eight legs, arms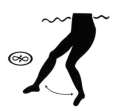

Enlarge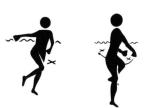

4. Cardio and Muscular Endurance (4-6 min)

Apply **W.A.**

 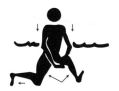

Tuck jumping   Surfboard jumps

5. Cardio, Posture, and Functional Exercise Set
(4—10 min)

Apply **S.E.A.T.**

Walking (heel,
then toes lead)

Walk sideways
and diagonally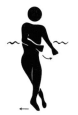

6. Cardio Set (4—6 min)

Apply **S.W.E.A.T.**

Scissors   Scissors to jax
             (work around the hip joint)

7. Cardio Set, Traveling (4—15 min)

Apply **S.W.E.A.T.**

Travel, hold stationary...change working
positions, then travel again...repeat sequence
with the basic moves.

Walking   Rocking   Jumping
Jogging   Kicking

8. Funky Set for Fun! (4 min)

Travel some and do some stationary.

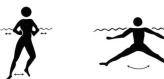

Accordions   Robot jax   Cannon balls

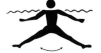

Roger Rabbit   Flexuous Charlie

Piano hands   Hop rope with
                   resistance band

9. Warm-Down (4–6 min)

Apply **S.** (decrease), **E.** (reduce size),
A., and **T.** (easy).

Walking   Leaping   Kicking

10. Range of Motion (4–6 min)

Apply **E.** and **A.**

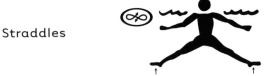

Straddles

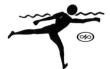

Part horse's mane

Grind corn

Greet the sun

Hip drop

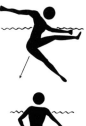

Cross leg

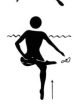

11. Playful Warm-Down

Remove gloves.

Kick   Leap   Skip   Rock

Source: From *Speedo Aquatic Fitness System Instructor Training Manual.*

A.B.Y.S.S.S., Deep Water Workout
Specificity of Training and Deep Water Program *Video*

Orient participants by using **A.B.Y.S.S.S.**:

A. = Adjust the belt for balance by turning them around if necessary for neutral alignment.

B. = Have participants face each other and practice inhalations and exhalations (watch the body rise and fall).

Y. = Yield to buoyancy; practice extensions downward.

S. = Scull for balance and propulsion (travel).

S. = Use synergism. For example, for a scissors move, first work the arm and leg on the same side together, then move arms and legs in opposition, and feel the balance difference.

S. = Practice safety skills such as recovery to vertical from fall supine and prone.

1. Buoyancy Warm-Up and Adjustment to Deep Water (3—5 min)

Jog around the body, kick around the body, with insteps up for active stretch.

2. Cardiovascular Warm-Up (2—3 min)

Bicycle: Vary using **S.W.E.A.T.** Use the lower body.

3. Stabilization and Active Stretching (3—5 min)

Tilt: Vary using **S.E.A.** Scull for balance.

4. Cardiovascular Set 1 (4—6 min)

Jog: Vary using **S.W.E.A.T.** Tilt the body and slowly add the arm overhead for intensity.

Tip If a participant has high blood pressure, have him or her keep the arms in the water.

5. Cardiovascular Set 2 (4—6 min)

Curl unders performed in straddle, power pops, scissors, quad kicks, power pops in scissors

Option: Insert a work or rest set between the cardio work.

- Cardio Interval (1 minute, high intensity) Scissors, legs only. Slice while wearing mitts; let the legs do the work!

- Active Rest (15 sec to 1 min)

Jog easily in a supine or vertical position.

6. Cardiovascular Intervals Set 3 (4—6 min)

Go easy/go hard intervals and apply **S.W.E.A.T.**

Scissors diagonally, go easy, go hard

Bicycle, go easy, go hard, leans

Do crawls and jax, go easy, go hard

Tip Advanced participants can remove their belts and float beside the belts for rest.

7. Cardiovascular Set 4 (4—6 min)

Kicking: Apply **S.W.E.A.T.** Seated, move back (for the quads) and forward (for hamstrings). Go to vertical. Kick wide. Do Cossack kicks. Push back and jog crawl forward.

8. Muscular Endurance Lower-Body Set (8—15 reps for 1-5 sets)

Apply **S.W.E.T.**

Move adductors/abductors, do jax, tilting, sitting, supine.

Travel forward, then back, with toes forward.

9. Cardio Kicking (3—5 min)

Apply **S.W.E.A.T.** With the flotation belt off, do flutters, change belt position, go vertical on the side, go wide, go vertical (scissors) on the other side.

10. Muscular Endurance Upper-Body Set
(8—15 reps for 1—5 sets)

Sculling: Apply **S.E.A.T.** With the flotation belt off, seated, pull forward.

11. Active Range of Motion (2—5 min)

Split the group in half and move one half to shallow water and one half to deep water. Have participants wear flotation belts to assist with range of motion. Perform range-of-motion work or stretches for the following:

Quads/hamstrings/hip flexors
Pectorals/rhomboids
Adductors/abductors
Neck and shoulders
Triceps
Spine (Remove flotation belt, sit on it, and swing to release the spine.)

12. Shallow Warm-Down and Transition
(1—2 min)

Have participants take their gloves off and put their flotation belts away.

Warm down to leave the pool.

Source: From *Speedo Aquatic Fitness System Instructor Training Manual.*

All Depths Workout—Shallow, Transitional and Deep
Specificity of Training and Deep Water Program *Video*

Choose a depth, and practice the moves using all the principles you've mastered! This workout uses basic moves that can be adapted for all depths. Refer to the video to review specific modifications for each depth. Have participants wear gloves until after part 10.

1. Buoyancy Warm-Up (3—5 min)

Apply **S.E.A.**

2. Cardio Warm-Up: Jogging (2—3 min)

Apply **S.W.E.A.T.**

3. Cardio Set 1: The Twist (3—5 min)

Apply **S.W.E.A.T.**

Jump and twist sideways
Grapevine
Twist, one leg bent
Chunky grapevine (knees come up)
Twist, straddle legs
Grapevine, turning the body direction

4. Cardio Set 2: Rock and Kick (3—5 min)

Apply **S.W.E.A.T.**

Rock forward
Hitch kicks
Rock sideways
Hitch kicks sideways

5. Cardio Set 3: Play Baseball (3—5 min)

Apply **S.W.E.A.T.**

Catch a ground ball, scoop.
Move gloves like an umpire signaling "safe."
Catch a fly ball.
Bat the ball and sneak the bases.
Run the bases.

6. Cardio Set 4: The Cancan (3—5 min)

Apply **S.W.E.A.T.**

Kicking through **S.W.E.A.T.**!

7. Cardio Set 5: Scissors and Jax

Apply **S.W.E.A.T.**

Scissors: rebound, neutral, suspended, travel
Jax: rebound, neutral, suspended, travel
Change travel direction.
Go rebound to suspended, but don't sink!

8. Muscular Conditioning: (8—15 reps)

Apply **S.E.T.**

Pull-ups to side (biceps)
Gorilla arm claps under knees, legs jogging (pectorals)
Skateboard (gluteals and trunk)
Lat pull-downs (latissimus dorsi)
Rows (pectorals and latissimus dorsi)

9. Warm-Down: Flexuous Walking (2—5 min)

On toes/on heels
Straddle creep sideways
Toes out/ in
Shoulder rolls
Heel toe/toe heel walks

10. Stretch and Move Combo: Partners

 Gloves can be removed here.

STRETCH MOVES	**WARM MOVES**
Hamstrings/quadriceps	Rock and stir it up
Calf/tibialis anterior	Rock and reach
Shoulders and pectorals	Flexuous kicks
Gluteals and lower back	Leap sideways

11. Post Stretches, Warm-Down, and Exit the Pool

Source: From *Speedo Aquatic Fitness System Instructor Training Manual.*

The Aquatic Step Circuit Workout
The Speedo Aquatic Step Program *Video*

This workout can be performed with or without the aquatic step. Without the step, substitute travel for step work.
Equipment: Aquatic steps and webbed gloves. Have participants place the steps where the water level is at their elbows when they stand on the steps.

1. Buoyancy Warm-Up (off the step) (3—5 min)

   Apply **S.W.E.A.**

Do some easy sculling, jogging, kicks, and rocks.
Practice scissors and jax through easy rebound, neutral, and suspended positions.

2. Step and Cardio Warm-Up (3—5 min)

Rock on

Rock off front

Rock sideways

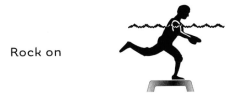

Jog on top

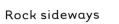

Step out and recover

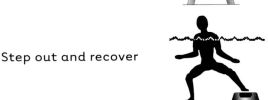

3. Muscular Endurance: Biceps (8—15 reps)
   Apply **S. E.** (**T.** without the step).
   Basic move: Rocking

4. Cardio Set (3-5 min)
   Apply **S. W. E.** (**T.** without the step).

Neutral

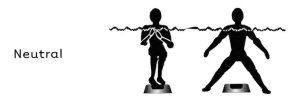

Extended

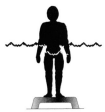

Rebound

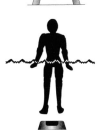

5. Muscular Endurance: Rhomboids and Trapezius (8—15 reps)
   Apply **S. E.** (**T.** without the step).
   Basic move: Rocking

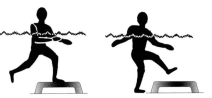

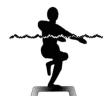

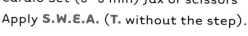

6. Cardio Set (3—5 min) Jax or scissors
Apply **S.W.E.A.** (**T.** without the step).

Neutral

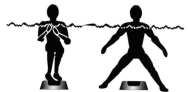

Extended

Rebound

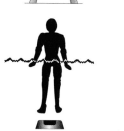

7. Muscular Endurance: Triceps (8—15 reps)
Apply **S. E.** (**T.** without the step).
Basic move: Rocking

8. Cardio Set (3—5 min)

Leap frogs

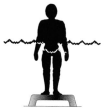

Road runners

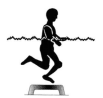

9. Muscular Endurance: Pectorals (8-15 reps)
Apply **S. E.** (**T.** without the step).
Basic move: Rocking

10. Cardio Combo Set (3—5 min)
Apply **S.W.E.A.T.** across the step.

Rock on sideways
3 times

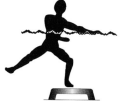

Rock off

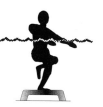

Jog across sideways
4 times

Repeat in the other direction.

11. Muscular Endurance: Sculling Suspended
(2—3 min)

Apply **S.** and **T.** in the suspended position.

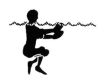

12. Muscular Endurance and Posture:
Skateboard (8–15 reps)

Apply **S.** and **E.**

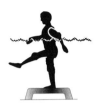

BALANCE
Scull

SQUAT
Power down

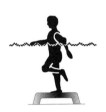

RECOVER
Hands sculling

BALANCE

13. Flexibility and Range-of-Motion
Warm-Down (3–5 min)

Quadriceps

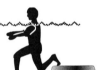

Calf
Heel drops

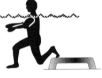

Hip adductors

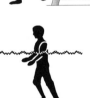

Low back

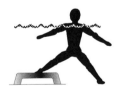

*Optional Cardio Sets to Insert
(from Video Session 6, Group Play)*

A. Interval Sets: "Go Gravity, Go Buoyant"

On step work (75 sec) and suspended work
(30 sec)

Jog on step (75 sec)

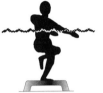

Jog suspended (30 sec)

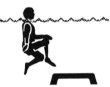

Jax on/off step (75 sec)

Jax suspended (30 sec)

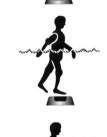

Scissors with step
(75 sec)

Scissors suspended
(30 sec)

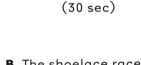

B. The shoelace race! (See the video.)

C. Partners around the world

One partner works on the step, the other wears
a flotation belt in the suspended position to
travel around or travel one length, then "tags"
the stepper, and then they change activities.

The Speedo Aquatic Step Program video, reprinted, with
permission, by Wave Aerobics/Speedo Authentic Fitness.

The Golden Waves Workout #1

The Golden Waves™ Functional Water Program,
Training for Health *Video #1*

Review and practice: Neutral posture, sculling, recovery to a stand, the 4 S's

1. Walking and Visiting Warm-Up (5—15 min)

Undirected free time and walking variations for each day: Backward day then sideways, forward, backward, and diagonal day!

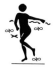

Hips: Walk sideways

2. Basic Moves Review, Practice, and Warm-Up (3—10 min)

Apply **S.E.A.**

Practice coordinated basic moves being used in the workout. Choose from walking, jogging, kicking, jumping, and scissors.

Practice the 4 S's and stabilization. Check, correct, and respond to participants.

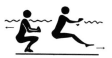

Ankle pops: backward, sideways

Rock through the spine: Walk forward

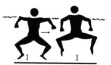

4. Cardio Set: Interval Training, Go Hard, Go Easy! (3—10 min)

Apply **S.W.E.A.T.** to basic moves.

Jog   Suspended

3. Joint Energy: Range-of-Motion Warm-Up (3—10 min)

Apply **S.E.A.T.** Roll each joint through ROM, then travel with hands assisting.

Shoulders: Walk sideways

Rebound

Knees: Walk sideways

Neutral

5. "Freeze Frame" for Balance and Light Cardio (3–10 min)

Apply **S.E.A.T.** Perform walk and hold progression (walk, then stop) variations using two feet:

Freeze positions

Sculling

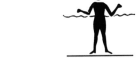

Hands out of water

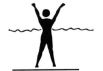

Hands above head

Arms on diagonal

Use lower-body variations to increase intensity. Repeat arm variations:

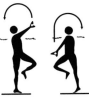

Walk and stop:
1 leg, knee forward; 1 leg, knee to the side

Walk diagonally.

6. Muscular Endurance: Upper-Body Postural Muscles (Trapezius and Rhomboids) (8–15 reps)

Apply **S.E.T.** Have participants wear webbed gloves and progress from slicing the water to clenching the fists to opening the webbing.

Slice
(easier)

Fist
(moderate)

Web
(harder)

Tell participants to find their "Somewhat hard-hard" level and work the reps!

7. Play Ball!: Gripping, reaching, coordination (3–5 min)

Apply **S.** (speed of grip/release) **E. A. T.**
Have participants squeeze and release sponge balls and scoot/jog/walk across the pool. Have them stretch the fingers by pushing the balls across the pool.

Stretch fingers

Jog across pool

Grip and release

Push the ball and jog

Squeeze around
the clock

Jog and push

Squeeze and move it

Chase and push ball

8. Vacuuming! (3–5 min)

Apply **S.E.A.**

Give participants webbed gloves or a paddle and have fun pushing and pulling the "vacuum" in many directions.

Cue participants to keep their shoulders "quiet" and to use their legs to enlarge the movement.

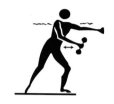

Lunge and vacuum

Sweep, shovel, and hug

9. Fluid Energy for ROM and Relaxation (3–10 min)

Apply **S.E.A.T.**

Fall backward and sideways.

Open the arms to the sides and turn the head to one side or the other for the neck.

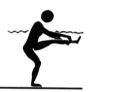
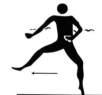

Stretch hamstrings, Tilt hips back

Leap sideways.

Stand and hug a knee to stretch gluteals.

Move the leg to the side, then push the heel down behind the body to stretch the calf.

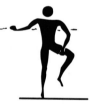

Stretch quadriceps: Stand and scull.

Circle around and drag the arm to stretch the chest.

Relax playfully before exiting.

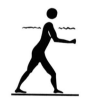

Reach up and massage across the shoulders.

Stretch the calf

The Golden Waves Functional Water Fitness Program, reprinted, with permission, from Wave Aerobics.

Golden Waves Workout #2
Functional Water Fitness Program
The Golden Waves Leadership Program *Video #2*

EQUIPMENT

gloves
aquatic steps
resistance bands
balls (balloons half filled with water or
 medicine balls)
kickboards
sponge balls

1. Warm-Up (3—10 min)

Music: "Return to Innocence"

Balance work using sculling, postural
review, and range-of-motion practice.

Cue gaze stabilization.

Patterns, backward and forward—
walk sideways

Stand on one foot, close the eyes.

2. Finger Work with Sponge Balls (3—5 min)
Music: "Macarena"

Power pops for gripping, grabbing, and
holding

Push, grab, push, grab, cross front,
change hands, push down

3. The Clock Squats (3—5 min)
Music: "Magic Carpet Ride"

Balance, posture, and reaction work

Walking, stop at certain times, hold
Add squats

4. Kickboard Stand, Reach, Fall and Abs
Down Under (3—5 min)

Music: "Typewriter"

Abdominal work in neutral posture. Immerse
a kickboard for the progression, reach, and
stand.

5. Leash and Walk (3—5 min)

Music: "Rum & Coca Cola"

Walk a line with your partner. . . if you can!
Move forward, backward, sideways, and
diagonally.

Transition to pick up aquatic steps at side
of pool

6. Step, Fall, and Recover and Step Clock
Squats Combo (3—10 min)

Music: "Buggy Song"

7. Pothole Shuffles (3—5 min)

Music: "Leroy Brown"

Transition to return steps to side of pool and
pick up resistance bands

8. Stretch and Strengthen Resistance Band
Set (3—5 min)

Music: "Firedance"

Stretch, strengthen (both dynamically
and isometrically), then stretch again.
Stretch first, do range-of-motion work,
and stretch the following:
Upper back
Triceps
Rotator cuff
Biceps
Arms overhead

Transition to return resistance bands to side
of pool and pick up balls

9. Lifting, Reaching, Jumping (3 min)
Music: "The YMCA"

Have participants form a circle. Pass out
balls for lifting, and then have them each
roll their ball around the body to target
range of motion. Reach and jump up for
the YMCA chorus.

Transition to return the balls to side of pool

10. Partner Stretches and Glenohumeral
Stretch (5—10 min)

Music: "Reach"

Warm-down activity combinations

The Golden Waves Leadership Program Video, reprinted,
with permission, from Wave Aerobics.

"One With Nature" Workout

One With Nature Program *Video and Manual by Ghada Muasher*

Venture on a journey of wonder and fitness as you move in harmony with the free-flowing movements of the dwellers of the sea and shore!

One With Nature™ is an impact-free water resistance exercise program that uses easy-to-remember movements that simulate the natural movements of sea creatures and aquatic birds. In *One With Nature*™ you will blend mind and body, imagination and exercise, to experience the natural way to aerobic fitness, muscle toning, physical endurance, and flexibility. This workout can be performed using a flotation belt in shallow water, deep water, or a combination of both. Use the entire workout or select particular exercises to suit your classes.

The complete *One With Nature*™ package includes the following:
* An exercise book
* A 90-minute videotape
* A SandDollar Aqua Belt
* A laminated waterproof cue card
* An 80-minute audiocassette of original music

You can also order the *One With Nature*™ Complete Instructional set (all the above items excluding the SandDollar Aqua Belt). Both can be ordered at the following address:

Greater Success   or Call Toll Free
One With Nature™   1-888-899-1616
P.O. Box 576748
Modesto, CA 95357

Sunrise: The Awakening Warm-Up

The Power of Living: Harmony in Diversity Workout

Upper-Body Workout: Vertical

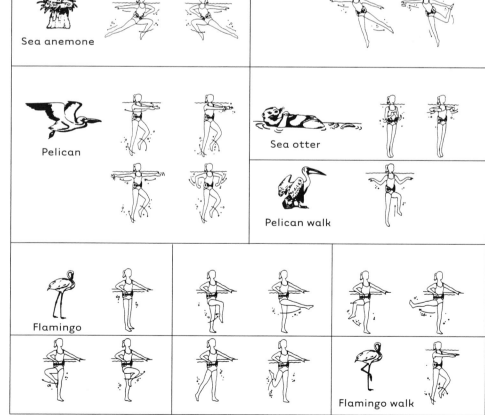

**Full-Body Workout:
Vertical**

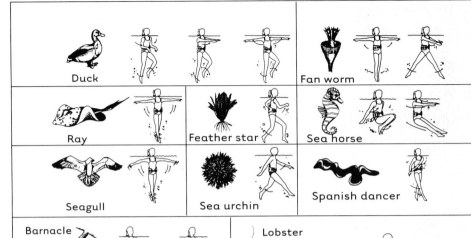

Duck · Fan worm · Ray · Feather star · Sea horse · Seagull · Sea urchin · Spanish dancer

**Full-Body Workout:
Horizontal**

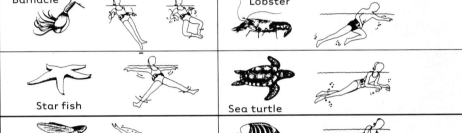

Barnacle · Lobster · Star fish · Sea turtle · Flying fish · Angel fish

**Full-Body Workout:
Sitting and Reclining**

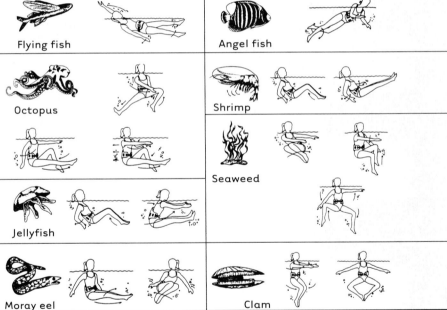

Octopus · Shrimp · Seaweed · Jellyfish · Moray eel · Clam · Squid · Crab

*Sunset:
The Hideaway
Cool-down*

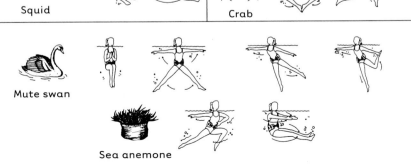

Mute swan · Sea anemone

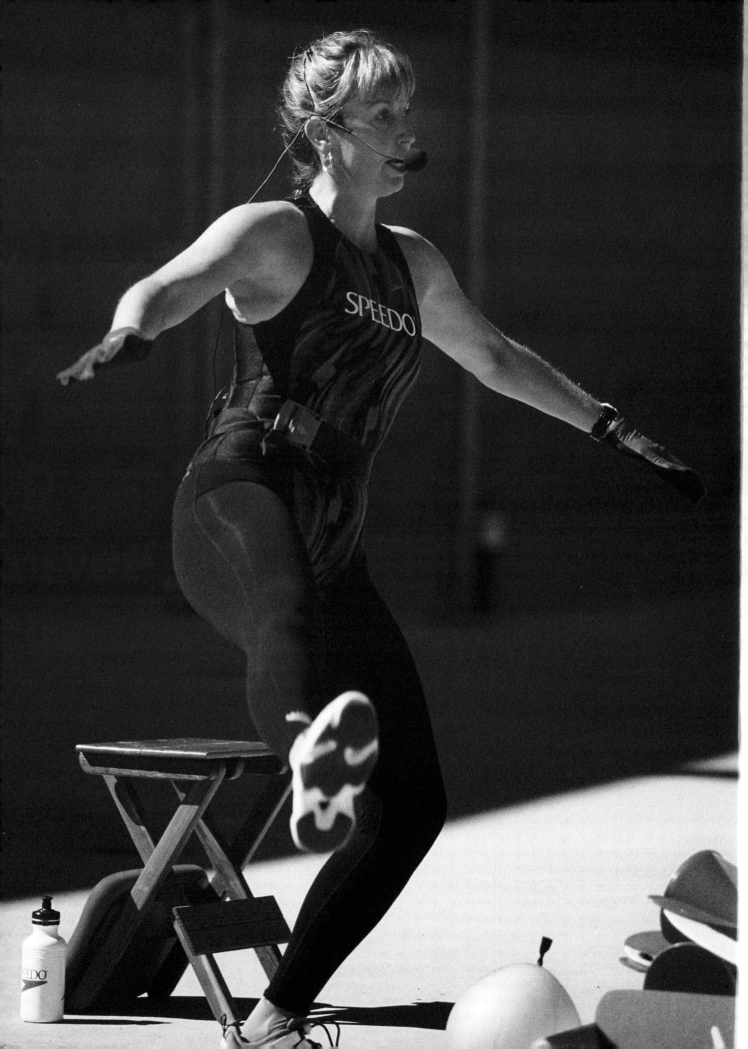

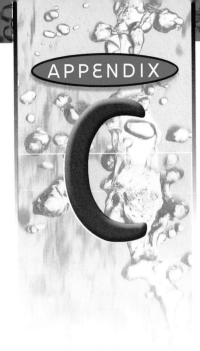

Cue Cards

This appendix contains cue cards to use by the pool during classes. The cards are organized by types of exercise:

◎ Cardiorespiratory endurance and body composition

◎ Muscular strength/endurance flexibility and range of motion

◎ Functional activities of daily living (ADL)

Each category begins with general recommendations for the teaching progression and for regulating exercise intensity, followed by individual cue cards. Each cue card focuses on a specific movement pattern and its variations.

Cardiorespiratory Endurance and Body Composition

Use the following teaching progression:

- Stabilize the basic move using coordinated arms and legs.
- Cue participants, using the S.W.E.A.T. formula.
- Check body alignment.
- Check intensity using RPE and the talk test. Have participants adjust intensity as necessary.
- Cue participants to reduce intensity and change to a new move.

Regulate intensity by using the 4 S's:

TO DECREASE INTENSITY:

1. Slow down.
2. Make the move Smaller.
3. Stabilize with sculling.
4. Substitute a modified or different move.

TO INCREASE INTENSITY:

1. Stabilize with sculling.
2. Enlarge the Size of the move.
3. Push with more force, increasing the Speed.
4. Continue to work up the intensity progression using the S.W.E.A.T. formula.

When you add equipment, be sure to teach participants the purpose of the equipment and its proper use and safety.

Cue 1 Walking in Shallow Water
Cardiorespiratory Endurance and Body Composition

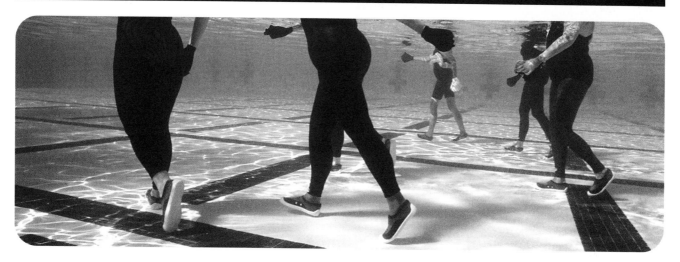

Balance the following muscle groups during walking:

LOWER BODY
Soleus
Tibialis and gastrocnemius
Quadriceps and hamstrings

UPPER BODY
Biceps and triceps
Deltoids
Latissimus dorsi

Check that participants perform all movements with balance and good alignment, balancing the following muscles:

LOWER BODY
Erector spinae
Abdominals
Gluteals

UPPER BODY
Pectorals
Latissimus dorsi
Rhomboids

Upper Body

- Cue participants to use flat hand sculling to stabilize.
- To assist or resist, have participants use a scull, push and pull the hands through the water, or do the breaststroke arm movement.

S.W.E.A.T. Intensity Variations

SURFACE AREA AND SPEED
Heel strike/toe strike
Toes in/out
Plantarflex/dorsiflex
Increase force

WORKING POSITION
Maintain navel to nipple water depth.
Extended position

ENLARGE
Gradually increase size of movement.

WORK AROUND BODY
Forward/backward
Sidestep, move diagonally

TRAVEL
Forward, backward, sideways, diagonally

Movement variations: Grapevine; "Smooth and Chunky" (move smoothly but lift knees higher); side step; "Step Out of the Tub" side step; lunge walk; ice skaters' stride; half-circle walk (trace a half-circle with the toe) forward, backward, and sideways

Cues and Coaching

- Refer to medical considerations in chapter 15.
- Tell participants to keep movements smooth, strong, and steady.
- Give very buoyant participants weight belts.
- Give the following cues for body alignment:
  ➤ Lift the chest.
  ➤ Keep the chin neutral, with ears and shoulders in alignment.
  ➤ Keep the lower back neutral. Get into the ready position and contract the abdominal and gluteal muscles.

Jogging in Shallow Water
Cardiorespiratory Endurance and Body Composition

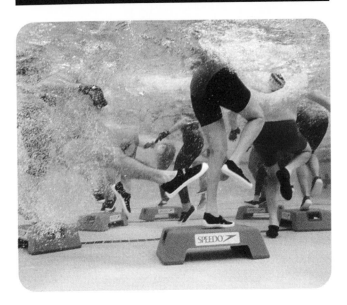

Balance the following muscle groups during jogging:

LOWER BODY
Quadriceps and
    hamstrings
Illiopsoas and gluteals
Gastrocnemius and
    tibialis
Soleus

UPPER BODY
Deltoids
Pectorals and rhomboids
Biceps and triceps
Latissimus dorsi

Check that participants perform all movements with balance and good alignment, balancing the following muscles:

LOWER BODY
Erector spinae
Abdominals
Gluteals

UPPER BODY
Pectorals
Latissimus dorsi
Rhomboids

Upper Body

- Cue participants to use flat hand sculling to stabilize.
- To assist or resist, have participants use a scull while traveling:
  - Scull with fingers up, push forward to assist travel backward.
  - Scull with fingers down, push back to assist travel forward.
  - Propeller scull to assist travel sideways.

S.W.E.A.T. Intensity Variations

SURFACE AREA AND SPEED
Dorsiflex/plantarflex
Toes in/out
Increase force

WORKING POSITION
Rebound, neutral, and suspended

ENLARGE
Gradually increase size of movement.

WORK AROUND BODY
Knees forward, knees wide, heels up behind

TRAVEL
Forward, backward, sideways, diagonally
Movement variations: Insteps (One foot points forward, the other is rotated and open to the side. Step sideways by pulling the heel of the rotated foot into the instep of the other foot.); reach for heels in back, then opposite heels; pigeon-toed jog; reach or clap under thigh. Refer to *Introduction to the Speedo Aquatic Fitness System* video.

Cues and Coaching

- Refer to medical considerations in chapter 15.
- Maintain the size of the movement.
- Coach participants in proper postural alignment:
  - Lift the chest.
  - Keep the chin neutral, with ears and shoulders in alignment.
  - Keep the lower back neutral. Get into the ready position and contract the abdominal and gluteal muscles.

Cue 3 Kicking in Shallow Water
Cardiorespiratory Endurance and Body Composition

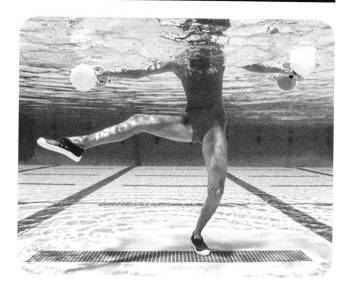

Balance the following muscle groups during kicking:

LOWER BODY	UPPER BODY
Quadriceps and hamstrings	Deltoids
Illiopsoas and gluteals	Pectorals, major and rhomboids
Peroneals and tibialis	Biceps and triceps
	Latissimus dorsi

Check that participants perform all movements with balance and good alignment, balancing the following muscles:

LOWER BODY	UPPER BODY
Erector spinae	Pectorals
Abdominals	Latissimus dorsi
Gluteals	Rhomboids

Upper Body

- Cue participants to use the following movements as stabilizers during stationary kicks:
  - ➤ For forward kicks, flat hand scull to the side.
  - ➤ For side-to-side kicks, flat hand scull in front. Increase to reaching out side to side in opposition to the legs.
  - ➤ For kicks to the back, flat hand scull in front or keep the arms in front, working in opposition to balance the kicking movement.

- To assist or resist during travel, have participants use a scull or push and pull the hands through the water.

S.W.E.A.T. Intensity Variations

SURFACE AREA AND SPEED

Dorsiflex/plantarflex
Lever length change by kicking from the hip or knee

WORKING POSITION

Rebound, neutral, and suspended

ENLARGE

Gradually increase size of movement.

WORK AROUND BODY

Kick forward, side to side, to the back.

TRAVEL

Forward, backward, sideways, diagonally
Movement variations: Point toe kick, cross kick, small soccer kicks, Cossack kicks (singles, double, wide legs). Refer to *Introduction to the Speedo Aquatic Fitness System* video.

Cues and Coaching

- Refer to medical considerations in chapter 15.
- Coach participants in proper postural alignment:
  - ➤ Lift the chest.
  - ➤ Keep the chin neutral, with ears and shoulders in alignment.
  - ➤ Keep the lower back neutral. Get into the ready position and contract the abdominal and gluteal muscles.
- Maximize leg movements. Have participants use arms for balance, stability, and lift.

Cue 4 Rocking in Shallow Water
Cardiorespiratory Endurance and Body Composition

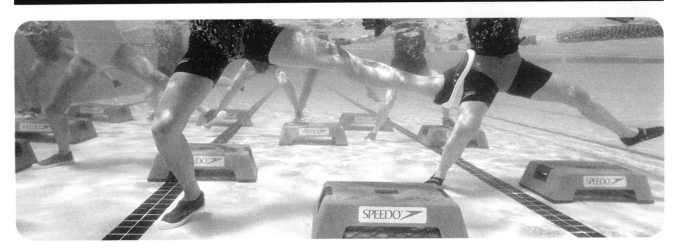

Balance the following muscle groups during rocking:

LOWER BODY
Gastrocnemius and
   tibialis
Illiopsoas and gluteals
Obliques and
   hamstrings
Soleus

UPPER BODY
Deltoids
Pectorals and latissimus
   dorsi
Biceps and triceps

Check that participants perform all movements with balance and good alignment, balancing the following muscles:

LOWER BODY
Erector spinae
Abdominals
Gluteals

UPPER BODY
Pectorals
Latissimus dorsi
Rhomboids

Upper Body

- Cue participants to use the following movements as stabilizers during stationary rocking:
  - ➤ For back-and-forth rocking, use flat hand sculling at the side.
  - ➤ For side-to-side rocking, push and pull the arms through the water.
- To assist or resist, have participants push and pull the hands through the water or use breaststroke arms.

S.W.E.A.T. Intensity Variations

SURFACE AREA AND SPEED
Lever length change by rocking with the knee flexed or the knee extended
Toes in/out
Increase force

WORKING POSITION
Rebound

ENLARGE
Gradually increase size of movement.

WORK AROUND BODY
Forward and back, side to side, diagonally

TRAVEL
Forward, backward, sideways, diagonally
Movement variations: Refer to *Introduction to the Speedo Aquatic Fitness System* video.

Cues and Coaching

- Refer to medical considerations in chapter 15.
- Maintain the size of the movement.
- Coach participants in proper postural alignment:
  - ➤ Lift the chest.
  - ➤ Keep the chin neutral, with ears and shoulders in alignment.
  - ➤ Keep the lower back neutral. Get into the ready position and contract the abdominal and gluteal muscles.

Cue 5 Jumping in Shallow Water
Cardiorespiratory Endurance and Body Composition

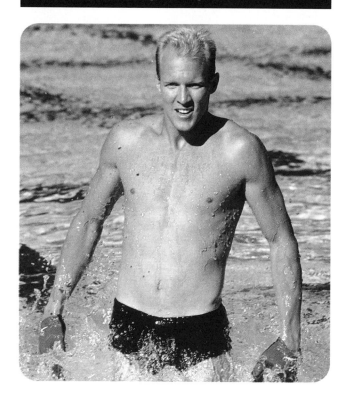

Balance the following muscle groups during jumping:

LOWER BODY
Soleus and gastrocnemius
Quadriceps and hamstrings
Illiopsoas and gluteals

UPPER BODY
Deltoids
Latissimus dorsi
Pectorals
Biceps and triceps

Check that participants perform all movements with balance and good alignment, balancing the following muscles:

LOWER BODY
Erector spinae
Abdominals
Gluteals

UPPER BODY
Pectorals
Latissimus dorsi
Rhomboids

Upper Body

- Cue participants to use flat hand sculling to stabilize.
- Have participants push down to lift upward.
- To assist or resist, have participants use a scull or push and pull the hands through the water.

S.W.E.A.T. Intensity Variations

SURFACE AREA AND SPEED
Lever length change (arms can work either close to body or extended to the sides)
Increase force

WORKING POSITION
Rebound, neutral, and suspended

ENLARGE
Gradually increase size of movement.

WORK AROUND BODY
Tuck (knees together in front of body)
Wide knees (frog jump)
Heels up behind

TRAVEL
Forward, backward, sideways, diagonally

Movement variations: Tuck jump stationary side to side (neutral slalom skier), hopscotch, single and double leg heels-up jumps, leaps, surfboard jumps (from lunge position, jump up with heels toward the buttocks, then return to lunge position). Refer to *Introduction to the Speedo Aquatic Fitness System* video.

Cues and Coaching

- Refer to medical considerations in chapter 15.
- Coach participants in proper postural alignment:
  - ➤ Lift the chest.
  - ➤ Keep the chin neutral, with ears and shoulders in alignment.
  - ➤ Keep the lower back neutral. Get into the ready position and contract the abdominal and gluteal muscles.

Cue 6 Scissors in Shallow Water
Cardiorespiratory Endurance and Body Composition

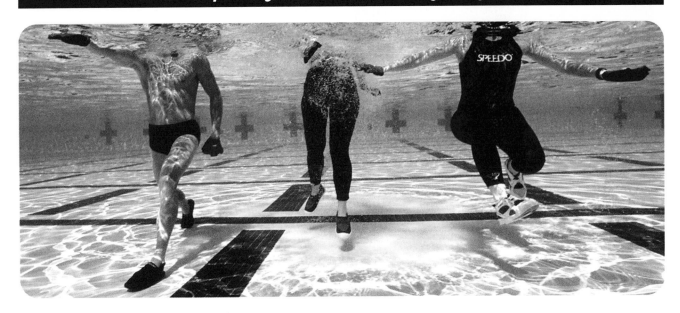

Balance the following muscle groups while performing scissors:

LOWER BODY
Soleus
Tibialis and gastroc-
    nemius
Quadriceps and
    hamstrings
Illiopsoas and gluteals

UPPER BODY
Biceps and triceps
Deltoids
Latissimus dorsi
Pectorals

Check that participants perform all movements with balance and good alignment, balancing the following muscles:

LOWER BODY
Erector spinae
Abdominals
Gluteals

UPPER BODY
Pectorals
Latissimus dorsi
Rhomboids

Upper Body

- Cue participants to use flat hand sculling to stabilize.
- To assist or resist, have participants scull, push and pull the hands through the water, or use breaststroke arms.

S.W.E.A.T. Intensity Variations

SURFACE AREA AND SPEED
Toes in/out
Increase force

WORKING POSITION
Rebound, neutral, suspended

ENLARGE
Gradually increase size of movement

WORK AROUND BODY
Cross-country
Jumping jax and diagonal lunge

TRAVEL
Forward, backward, sideways, diagonally

Movement variations: Refer to *Introduction to the Speedo Aquatic Fitness System* video.

Cues and Coaching

- Refer to medical considerations in chapter 15.
- Tell participants to keep movements smooth, strong, and steady.
- Coach participants in proper postural alignment:
  - ➤ Lift the chest.
  - ➤ Keep the chin neutral, with ears and shoulders in alignment.
  - ➤ Keep the lower back neutral. Get into the ready position and contract the abdominal and gluteal muscles.

Muscular Strength/Endurance and Flexibility and Range of Motion

The next set of cue cards contains movements for building muscular strength and endurance and increasing flexibility and range of motion.

Muscular Strength/Endurance

Use the following teaching progression:

- Identify the targeted muscle and joint.
- Have participants submerge their joints.
- Cue the stabilizers.
- Have participants adjust their stationary stance for stabilization or thermoregulation.
- Have participants practice the movement and breathing patterns.
- Use the **S.W.E.A.T.** formula to regulate exercise intensity.
- Examine current and buoyancy direction, and use it to help participants assist or resist work or to maximally engage the stabilizers during stationary work.
- Have participants perform sets and reps.
- Provide positive, specific, corrective feedback.
- Check intensity, using Rate of Perceived Exertion or muscle fatigue.
- Check body alignment.

Regulate intensity by using the 4 S's:

TO DECREASE INTENSITY:

1. Slow down.
2. Make the move Smaller.
3. Stabilize the body and working joints, and let go of the equipment.
4. Substitute lower-resistance equipment.

TO INCREASE INTENSITY:

1. Stabilize the body position and working joints (submerge the joints).
2. Practice and use the functional range or appropriate Size of the pattern for the muscle groups being targeted.
3. Adjust resistance by choosing the proper Surface area overload.
4. Add force and increase Speed for higher resistance.

When you add equipment, be sure to teach participants the purpose of the equipment and its proper use and safety.

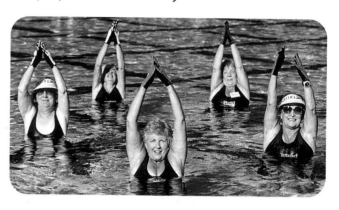

Flexibility and Range of Motion

Use the following teaching progression:

- Have participants practice moving through a functional range of motion for each joint.
- Check participants' balance, body alignment, and comfort.
- During static stretches, tell participants to stretch until they feel a pull, then back off and hold the stretch for 10 to 15 seconds. Repeat three to four times. Check for body warmth and to see if the stretch is being felt in the right place!
- Use the **S.W.E.A.T.** formula to increase the stretch or range of motion.
- Keep participants warm with "thermal" moves between static stretches.
- Include range of motion moves that use the entire body, such as leaping to stretch hamstrings.

Regulate intensity by using the 4 S's:

TO ADJUST INTENSITY:

1. Decrease the range of motion, make it Smaller.
2. Reduce the effects of additional Surface area or buoyancy assistance, enhancing the stretch and range of motion.
3. Substitute by slightly changing the plane of the stretch, moving the joints on a diagonal to feel the stretch differently and target slightly different fibers.
4. Apply the components of the **S.W.E.A.T.** formula that apply.

Cue 7 Elbow Joint (Biceps) in Shallow Water
Muscular Strength/Endurance and Flexibility and Range of Motion

Practice Movement Pattern With Full Range of Motion

Flex the elbow with the power phase on the flexion. Cue participants to power/open webbed gloves on the flexion and recover/slice on the extension.

Stationary Movement Patterns

Participants wear webbed gloves or use equipment that increases surface area.

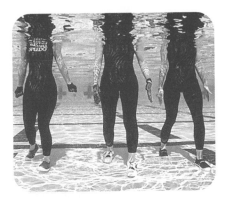

ELBOW FLEXION

"Power up"

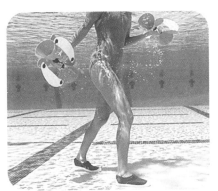

ELBOW FLEXION WITH POWER BUOYS

(single or double)

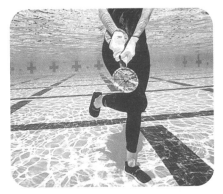

DIAGONAL CURL

"Shovels" shown with a paddle for overload.

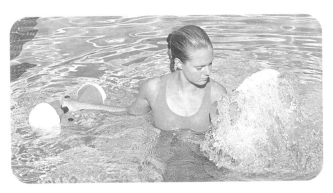

SINGLE ELEVATED CURLS PERFORMED WITH POWER BUOY

Variations

Stationary: Submerge the joint, stabilize, and adjust the surface area (hands slice, make a fist, open webbing) and speed.
Assisting with travel: Walk or jog backward or sideways with the current.
Resisting with travel: Walk or jog forward or sideways against the current.
Traveling vertically: Squat, then rebound upward.

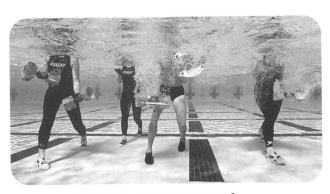

"BUBBLES" (SMALL RANGE ISOTONIC)

With power buoys and gloves "power up and down."

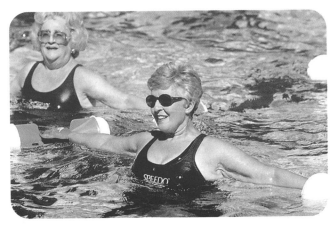

RANGE-OF-MOTION STRETCHES

Cue 8 Elbow Joint (Triceps) in Shallow Water
Muscular Strength/Endurance and Flexibility and Range of Motion

Practice Movement Pattern With Full Range of Motion

Extend elbow with power phase during extension and recovery on the flexion. Cue participants to power/open webbed gloves on elbow extension (hands supine or prone) and recover/slice on elbow flexion.

Stationary Movement Patterns

Participants wear webbed gloves or use equipment that increases surface area.

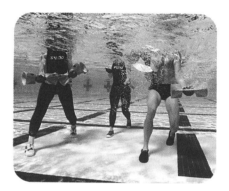

ELBOW EXTENSION
"Power down" shown with power buoys and webbed gloves.

SINGLE ARM IN FRONT AND (OR) IN THE BACK

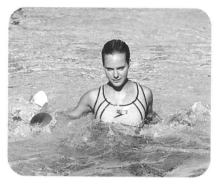

ELEVATED EXTENSION
Singles or doubles "power out"

SMALL RANGE EXTENSIONS TO THE BACK

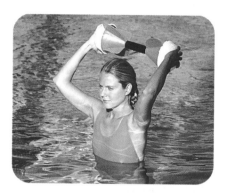

TRICEPS OVERHEAD ELBOW EXTENSION WITH WATER-FILLED POWER BUOY

Variations

Stationary: Submerge joint, stabilize, and adjust surface area and speed.
Assisting with travel: Walk or jog forward or sideways with the current.
Resisting with travel: Walk or jog backward or sideways against the current.
Traveling vertically: Move downward against buoyancy.

RANGE-OF-MOTION STRETCHES

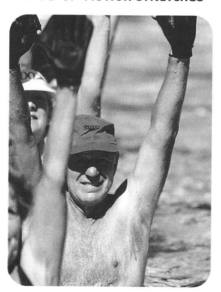

TRICEPS REACHING STRETCH

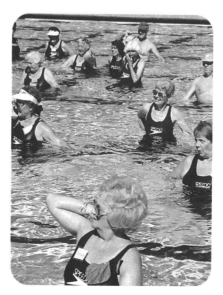

TRICEPS BACK SCRATCH STRETCH

Cue 9 Shoulder Joint (Rhomboids and Trapezius) in Shallow Water
Muscular Strength/Endurance and Flexibility and Range of Motion

**Practice Movement Pattern
With Full Range of Motion**

- Begin at the surface and horizontally abduct arms/elbows back, squeezing (adduct) the shoulder blades (trapezius) together.
- Begin at the surface, pull arms downward and back, squeezing the shoulder blades (rhomboids) together.
- Practice the power phase during scapular retraction and depression.

- Retract the shoulders, check for back cleavage, and adjust the length of the lever (arms) for safety and comfort.
- Cue participants to power/open webbed gloves on horizontal shoulder abduction and recover/slice to the starting position.

Stationary Movement Patterns

Participants wear webbed gloves or use equipment that increases surface area.

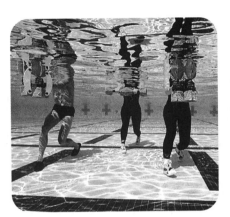
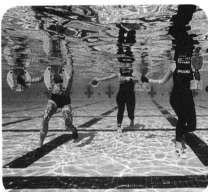
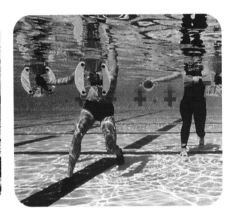

HORIZONTAL ABDUCT (TRAPEZIUS)
(singles or doubles)

SINGLE PULLS

> **CHALLENGE TIP**
>
> Combine fins, flotation belt, and gloves for a cardio-resistance combination. Kick to move backward, and work the trapezius by pulling the hands backward. Great trunk work, too!

Variations

Stationary: Submerge the joint; stabilize; straddle jog; use the squat or lunge stance.

Assisting with travel: Crab walk sideways; do arm pulls with the current (single arm abduct); walk/jog/tuck jump forward (double arm abduct).

Resisting with travel: Crab walk sideways; do arm pulls against the current; walk/jog/tuck jump backward against the current.

RANGE-OF-MOTION STRETCHES

Cross the hands and reach forward to stretch the upper back.

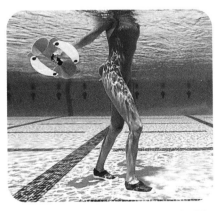

HORIZONTAL AROUND AND DOWN
(rhomboids)

Cue 10 Shoulder Joint (Pectorals) in Shallow Water
Muscular Strength/Endurance and Flexibility and Range of Motion

Practice Movement Pattern With Full Range of Motion

Practice with the power phase on the shoulder horizontal adduction. Cue participants to power/open webbed gloves on horizontal adduction (thumbs up) and recover/slice to the starting position.

Stationary Movement Patterns

Participants wear webbed gloves or use equipment that increases either surface area or surface area and buoyancy.

"PASS BALL UNDER LEG"

ELEVATED ADDUCTION

(add buoyancy)

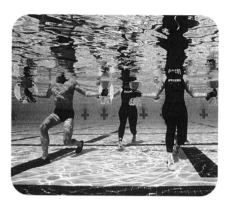
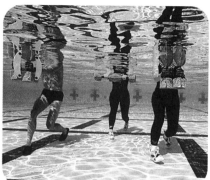

ELEVATED HORIZONTAL ADDUCTION
Singles and doubles, "power in"

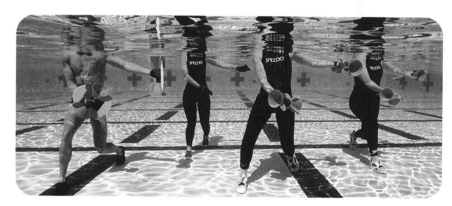

DIAGONAL PULL DOWN

RANGE-OF-MOTION STRETCHES

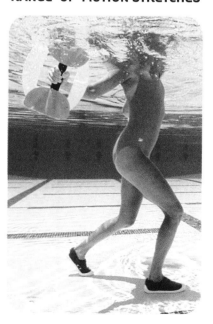

Walk forward with an open chest, drag hands or equipment, and stretch. Extend one arm to the right side, circle around to the left. Repeat on the other side.

Intensity Variations

Stationary: Submerge the joint; assume a stable position; use a lunge stance for stabilization, then jog to thermoregulate; adjust surface area and speed.

Assisting with travel: Walk or jog backward with the current; jog and circle in the direction of the current with a single arm movement.

Resisting with travel: Walk, jog, or rock forward against the current; jog and circle against the current with a single arm movement.

Practice Movement Pattern With Full Range of Motion

Note: Shoulder adduction then shoulder extension

Power phase on shoulder extension or adduction. Cue participants to power/open webbed gloves on shoulder extension or adduction and recover/slice to the starting position.

SHOULDER ADDUCTION OR SHOULDER EXTENSION (singles and doubles)

SHOULDER EXTENSION (singles)

Variations

Stationary: Submerge joint, stabilize, power downward webbed, slice up to recover.
Assisting with travel: Power the movement and allow the body to propel forward.
Resisting with travel: Power the adduction and squat down or power the extension and walk backward.

RANGE-OF-MOTION STRETCHES
Reach forward. Lean on buoyancy equipment, if possible, to enhance the stretch.

Stationary Movement Patterns

Participants wear webbed gloves or use equipment that increases either buoyancy or surface area and buoyancy.

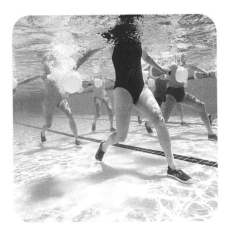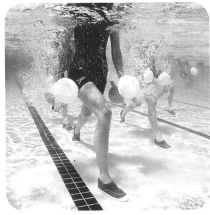

SHOULDER ADDUCTION
Doubles with a staggered stance position

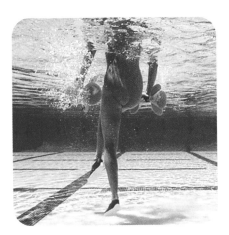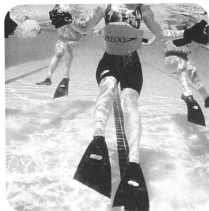

SHOULDER ADDUCTION WITH A KICK

SHOULDER EXTENSION (singles)

Cue 12 Wrist and Finger Joints (Forearms and Hand) in Shallow Water
Muscular Strength/Endurance and Flexibility and Range of Motion

Practice Movement Pattern With Full Range of Motion

- Practice wrist flexion and extension for forearm.
- Practice finger extension.
- Practice forearm supination and pronation.

Stationary Movement Patterns

Participants wear webbed gloves.

"S" PATTERN
Moving hand and fingers in front of body

FINGER POPS
Clench fist and open fingers wide underwater.

TURN THE DOORKNOB

PIANO HANDS

OPEN THE JAR

WRING OUT THE TOWEL

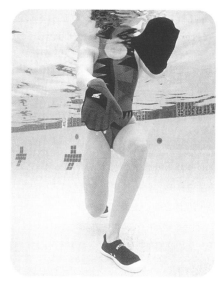

PIANO HANDS
(wrist flexion and extension)

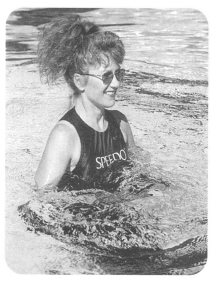

SCULLING

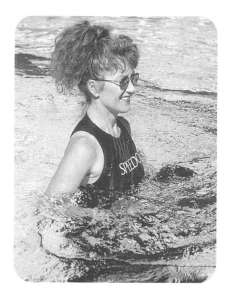

SCULLING FINGERS UP (FLAT HAND)

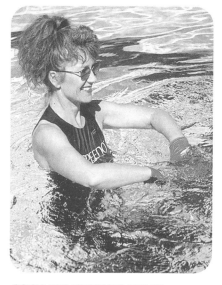

SCULLING FINGERS DOWN

Variations

Stationary: Stabilize; submerge the joint; move legs for thermal regulation.

Assisting with travel: Walk or jog, moving with the current.

Resisting with travel: Walk or jog sculling against the current.

RANGE-OF-MOTION STRETCHES

Open fingers and pretend to bat a ball from one hand to the other. Allow the water to stretch the fingers into extension.

Cue 13 Ankle Joint and Foot (Lower Leg and Foot) in Shallow Water
Muscular Strength/Endurance and Flexibility and Range of Motion

Practice Movement Pattern With Full Range of Motion

- Practice dorsiflexion and plantarflexion.
- Practice flexion and extension of the toes.
- Practice full rotation of the ankle.

Stationary Movement Patterns

Participants wear webbed gloves. They may use a flotation belt or buoyant barbells for stabilization, and may add an aquatic step for even more overload.

ANKLE POPS

Hop on two feet or on to one. Add a step for more work.

ANKLE CIRCLES

In neutral position, stand on one leg and circle ankles.

TOE CURLS

Squeeze toes (try to pick up a coin from the bottom).

JOG "S" FOOT

Jog and trace an "S" shape with the foot before landing.

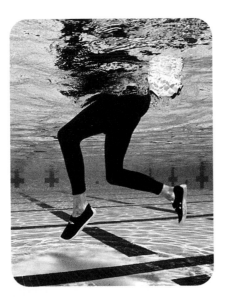

HOPPING/SKIPPING

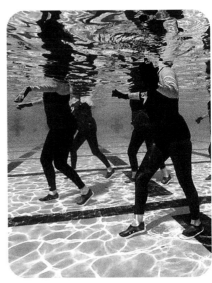

TOE/HEEL WALKING

Variations

Stationary: Stabilize and thermal regulate.
Assisting with travel: Travel forward or sideways with the current.
Resisting with travel: Travel backward or sideways against the current.

RANGE-OF-MOTION STRETCHES

Stand on one leg with the other leg back and the top of the foot on the bottom. Squat to feel a stretch on the top of the foot. Then extend the leg forward, heel on the bottom. Pull the toes up and back to stretch the calf and foot.

Cue 14 Knee Joint (Hamstrings and Quadriceps) in Shallow Water
Muscular Strength/Endurance and Flexibility and Range of Motion

Practice Movement Pattern With Full Range of Motion

Practice knee flexion with the power phase and knee extension slowly for the recovery phase for hamstrings. Practice knee extension with the power phase and knee flexion for recovery phase for quadriceps.

Stationary Movement Patterns

HAMSTRINGS

Jog heels up

Cossack kicks with power on flexion (singles/doubles)

Surfer repeaters

Single Cancan kick

Power in (knee extension)

Leap frogs

QUADRICEPS

Power out (kick extension)

Cossacks power on extension

Squats

Staggered stance

Clock squats

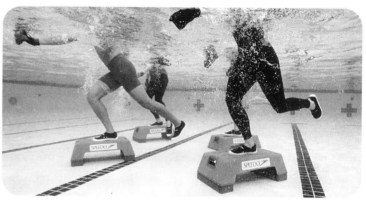

SKATEBOARD KNEE FLEXION AND HIP EXTENSION

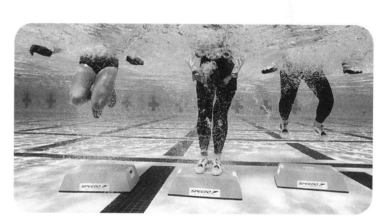

DOUBLE OR SINGLE HEEL UP JUMPS ON STEP

Variations

Stationary: Use arms for balance, stabilization, and lift.

Assisting with travel: Move forward for hamstrings and backward for quadriceps work.

Resisting with travel: Move backward for hamstrings and forward for quadriceps work.

Cue 15 Hip Joint (Gluteals) in Shallow Water
Muscular Strength/Endurance and Flexibility and Range of Motion

Practice Movement Pattern With Full Range of Motion

Power phase on hip extension. Cue participants to scull or use coordinated arm movement for stability.

Stationary Movement Patterns

Participants wear webbed gloves or use equipment that increases either buoyancy or surface area and buoyancy.

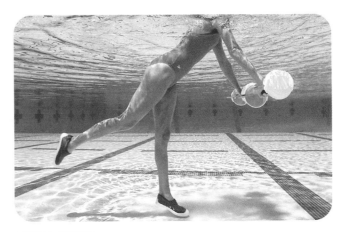

KICK BEHIND

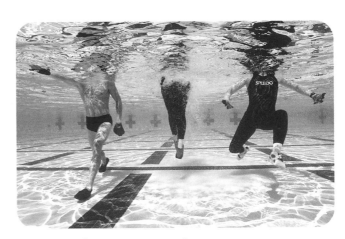

SCISSORS (CROSS COUNTRY)
(neutral, rebound, or suspended)

Variations

Stationary: Stabilize, then scull and kick downward, powering on the extension.
Assisting with travel: Lean forward, sculling for balance, then kick to the back and travel forward.
Resisting with travel: Travel backward.
(walking, cross country, kick)

RANGE-OF-MOTION STRETCHES

Stand on one leg and grab under the thigh. Stand tall and give the thigh a hug to feel the gluteals stretch.

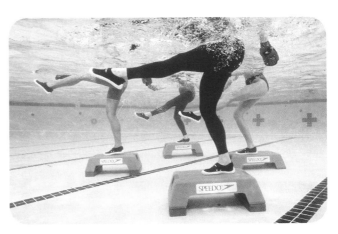

SKATEBOARD ON THE STEP "POWER DOWN AND BACK" TO HIP EXTENSION
(lower intensity by not using step)

Cue 16 Hip Joint (Adductors and Abductors) in Shallow Water
Muscular Strength/Endurance and Flexibility and Range of Motion

**Practice Movement Pattern
With Full Range of Motion**

Practice hip adduction/abduction, powering in to work adductors and powering out to work abductors.

Stationary Movement Patterns

SINGLE-LEGGED JAX

(with buoyancy equipment)

SIDE STEP

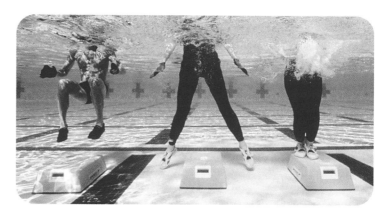

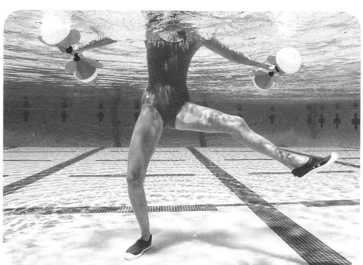

ONE LEG JAX

Variations

Stationary: Stabilize, do stationary jax, and add power to the correct phase.
Assisting with travel: Do single-leg jax, assisting the abductors, and travel in the direction opposite the leg movement.
Resisting with travel: Travel sideways against the power phase for overload.

RANGE-OF-MOTION STRETCHES

To stretch the adductors, stand in a wide stance (with legs apart). Crawl sideways and feel the stretch on the inner thighs. To stretch the abductors, extend one leg to the side and fall sideways toward the standing leg. Feel the stretch on the outside of the standing leg.

Cue 17 Trunk Stabilizers (Abdominals and Erector Spinae) in Shallow Water
Muscular Strength/Endurance and Flexibility and Range of Motion

Practice Movement Pattern With Full Range of Motion or Stabilization

Cue participants to check their posture and tighten their abdominals.

Stationary Movement Patterns

Stand on one leg and swish the water with the hands in front (like windshield wipers)

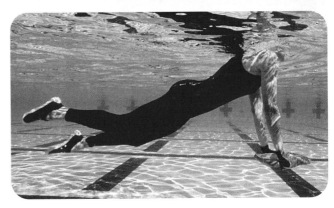

KICKBOARD KICK

Pull the shoulders down and back and tighten the abdominals as you kick.

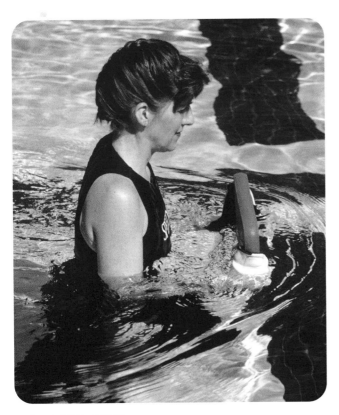

KICKBOARD WALK

Partially submerge a board and walk using good posture, forward and backward.

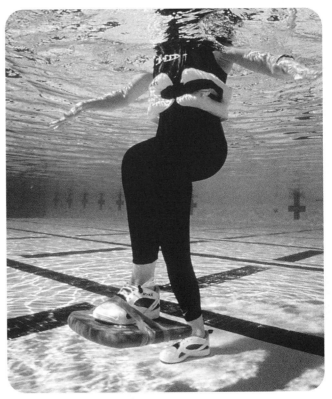

KICKBOARD BALANCE

Use a resistance band to secure a small kickboard to one foot. Contract the abdominals to balance. Move the leg away from the body for more work. Use a flotation belt for support.

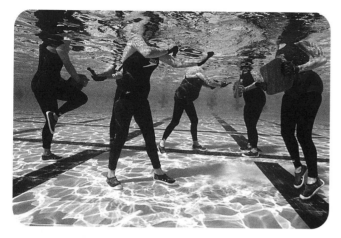

Variations

Stationary: Gradually increase the intensity by eliminating the bases of support.

Resisting with travel: Walk or jog forward, backward, or sideways, allowing the water current to challenge stability.

RANGE-OF-MOTION STRETCHES

With both hands on hips, stretch the torso up and slightly back. Feel the abdominals stretch. Walk forward through the water.

RUNAROUNDS

Push water against a partner's body or run around the partner to create currents. Hold a kickboard underwater or stand on one leg for more challenge.

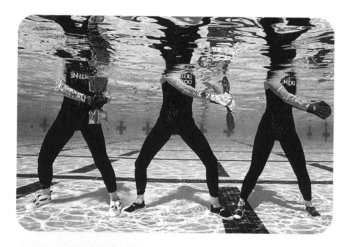

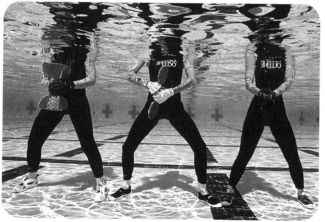

Stir it up wearing gloves or equipment to overload. Stir a big pot!

Functional Activities of Daily Living (ADL)

Use the following teaching progression:

- Demonstrate the basic move, thermal movements, and stabilization skills (such as flat sculling and jogging).
- Show participants how to keep proper alignment and neutral posture. Check and correct them as necessary.
- Tell participants the functional objective for each exercise, such as climbing stairs.
- Tell participants what the primary muscles will be that are involved in each exercise, and have them practice the pattern of movement:
  - ➤ Have participants adjust the size of the move as necessary, and check participants' functional range of motion.
  - ➤ Cue participants to use proper posture and biomechanics.
  - ➤ Cue participants in how to breathe during the exercise.
  - ➤ Check and correct them as necessary.
- Gradually increase resistance overload by applying the **S.W.E.A.T.** formula.

DURING CLASS, DO THE FOLLOWING:

- Observe participants and respond as needed.
- Remind participants to adjust exercise intensity using the 4 S's. Encourage participants to work at their own pace.

- Check that participants use proper biomechanics and correct them as needed.
- Encourage and celebrate their efforts!
- Ask if they are warm while they are working. If not, tell them how to get warmer.
- Provide personal, positive, and specific feedback.
- Remind participants to monitor their exercise intensity (Rate of Perceived Exertion or talk test).
- Give participants water breaks.
- After each set, reduce intensity and begin a new progression.

Regulate intensity by using the 4 S's:

TO DECREASE INTENSITY:

1. Slow down.
2. Make the move Smaller.
3. Stabilize position and check balance and posture.
4. Substitute a modified move if needed.

TO INCREASE INTENSITY:

1. Stabilize, using coordinated arms and legs.
2. Speed up.
3. Enlarge the Size (ROM) of the move.
4. Apply the **S.W.E.A.T.** formula.

Cue 18 Freeze Frame (Shallow Water)
Functional ADL Training

Objectives: Balance, trunk stabilization, and walking
Equipment: Aquatic step (optional)
Pattern of movement: Participants walk "purposefully" through the water. On cue, they stop and hold. They should feel the currents try to push them off balance and should have to work the trunk to hold steady.

PROGRESSION

Low Intensity............increasing the intensity........higher intensity..........

Freeze on both legs, use a flat scull.

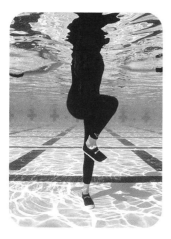

Freeze on one leg, using hands for balance.

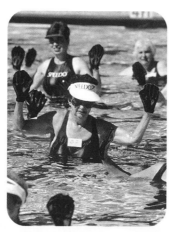

Freeze on one leg with hands out of water.

..........highest intensity

Freeze, hands overhead in diagonal.

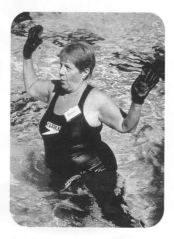

Add step and repeat progression.

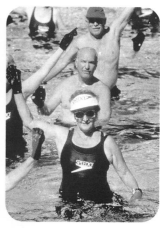

Step and hold hands on diagonal.

Cue 19 Clock Squats (Shallow Water)
Functional ADL Training

Objectives: Improving ability to stand from a sitting position, climb stairs, and balance
Equipment: Aquatic step
Patterns of movement: Participants balance on one leg and perform squats on top of the step, changing the position of the free leg like the hands of a clock. Have participants alternate the standing leg as they begin to fatigue.

PROGRESSION
Low Intensity

- Begin with no step, then add a step for more challenge.
- Use a flat scull for balance.
- Perform the skill with hands above the surface.
- Keep working while your partner runs circles around you to create turbulence!

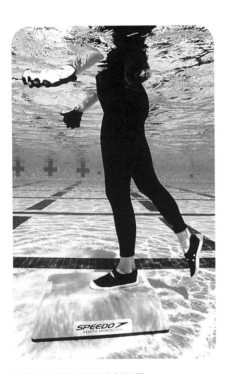

THE 6 O'CLOCK SQUAT

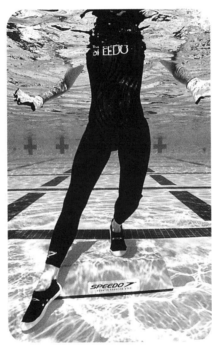

THE 12 O'CLOCK SQUAT

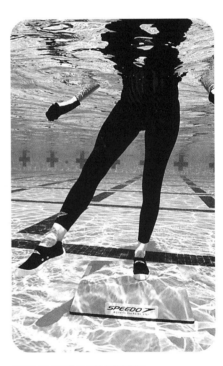

THE 3 O'CLOCK SQUAT

Use a flotation belt or ski poles to assist with balance if necessary.

Cue 20 Leash Me (Shallow Water)
Functional ADL Training

Objectives: For the person in the pair who walks, balance correction and increasing stride length. For the person in the pair who tugs on the resistance band, cardiorespiratory training and thermal work.

Equipment: Five-foot-long resistance band

Patterns of movement: Working in pairs, one partner leashes the other with a five-foot-long resistance band. The "walker" of the pair walks smoothly, strongly, and steadily with good posture. The "tugger" of the pair jogs vigorously from side to side, tugging on the band to the side to "surprise" his or her partner. Walkers should use their trunks to recover and avoid being pulled off balance. Check for proper posture and gaze (eyes forward). Tuggers should be sure to release the band tension between tugs and only pull during the brief tug.

PROGRESSION

Low Intensity

- Begin work in chest-deep water, sculling for balance.
- Walkers increase stride length; tuggers increase the frequency of tugs.
- Walk with hands above the water.

High Intensity

Repeat the activity in shallower water.
Variations: Walk backward, tuggers in front. Walk sideways, tuggers at the side following the walkers. They tug to the front and back.

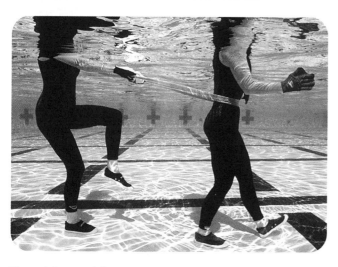

Tug side to side.

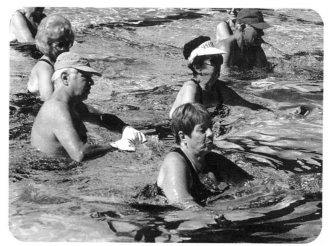

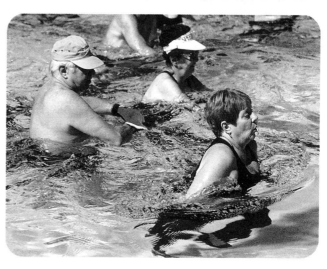

Cue 21 Vacuuming, Raking, and Shoveling (Shallow Water)
Functional ADL Training

Objectives: Improving the efficiency of pushing and pulling for "turbocharged" vacuuming

Equipment: Webbed gloves, paddles, or power buoys (used to increase the difficulty of the exercise)

Patterns of movement: Participants stabilize in a lunge position and push and pull using one arm.

PROGRESSIONS

Vacuuming

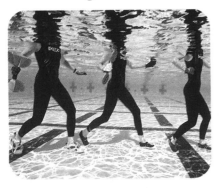 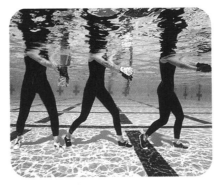 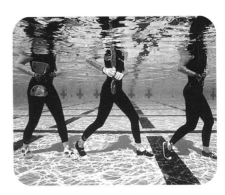

- Perform the skill without equipment, then add equipment that increases surface area for more challenge.

- Increase the ROM and the force of the pushes and pulls.
- Change the direction of the lunges.

Raking

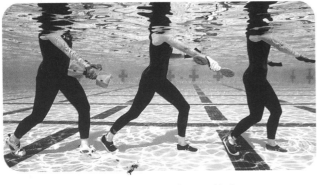 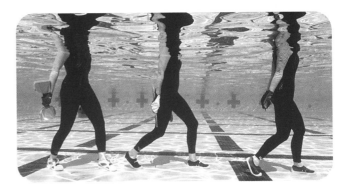

- Increase the force on the pull down.

Shoveling

- Scoop and shovel. Use the legs to assist lifting the load.

Note: Three levels and types of surface-area equipment are shown in the progression: webbed gloves, paddles, and power buoys.

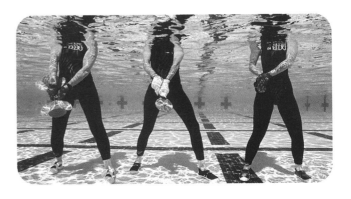

Cue 22 Getting On and Off a Bus (Shallow Water)
Functional ADL Training

Objectives: Improving stair climbing and bus entry and exit skills

Equipment: Aquatic step

Patterns of Movement: Participants step up and down from a step.

PROGRESSION

Low Intensity:

- Step up and slowly down, using balance aids as needed. Aids might include ski poles (with tennis balls on the tips), power buoys with caps on for buoyancy, or webbed gloves for sculling assistance.

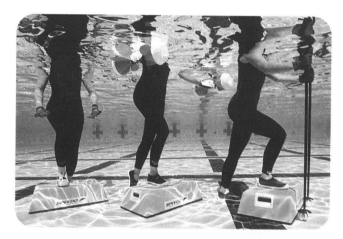

Increasing Intensity

- Keep hands above the surface.

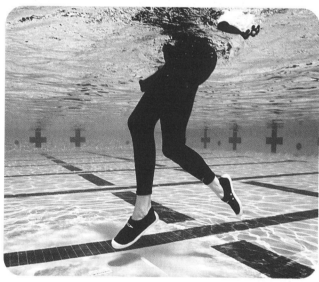

High Intensity:

- Power push off the bottom onto the step (use a flotation belt or buoyant barbells if needed for balance).
- Create a circle with steps, some stacked (bus steps are different heights), and work in a circle, changing directions occasionally for trunk work.

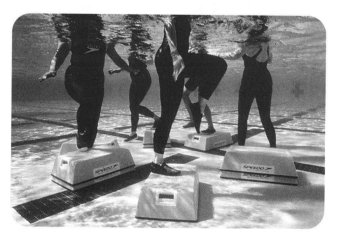

Cue 23 Get a Grip and Go! (Shallow Water)
Functional ADL Training

Objectives: Strengthening and stretching finger flexors; reaching and walking

Equipment: Foam balls

PATTERNS OF MOVEMENT

Strengthening
Walk forward, backward, and sideways while squeezing water from the foam ball as you reach in various planes, above and through the water.

Stretching
Alternate squeeze exercises with pushing the ball back and forth at the surface, allowing the water to assist with stretching your fingers into extension during the pushes.

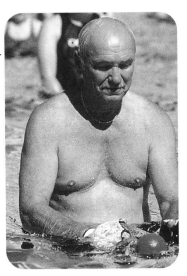

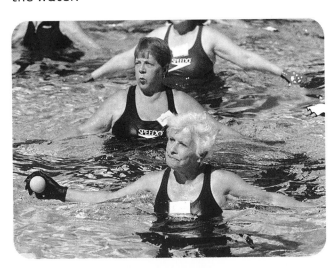

PROGRESSION

Low Intensity

- Begin with a small, soft ball.
- Then increase the number of repetitions.
- Then add an increase in the speed of walking.
- Finally, add an increase in the power of fingers pushing through the water.

High Intensity

- Use a denser ball and repeat the progression.

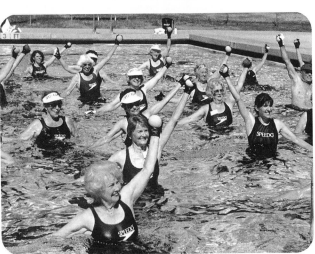

Cue 24 Jump Rope Tag (Shallow Water)
Combination Conditioning

Objectives: Partners work together to target cardiorespiratory conditioning, muscular endurance, and range of motion in a run, jump, and catch combination.

Equipment: Five-foot-long resistance band

Group Formation: Groups of three to four people, one or two of whom are "runners" and two of whom are "holders"

Patterns of Movement: The holders stabilize themselves as they hold the ends of the resistance bands. The runners step or jump sideways over the resistance bands and jog around the holders, repeating the jump from the other side, creating a figure-eight current in the water. Roles are changed often to let everyone play!

PROGRESSION

Low Intensity:
Runners step over the bands and walk around the holders.

Increasing Intensity
- Runners progress from a walk to a jog.
- Runners use a different walk or jog to push against the current.
- Runners jump and jog.

High Intensity:
Add a second runner, creating more turbulence and a chase!

Glossary

Abduction To move laterally away from the midline of the body, drawing AWAY from the midline of the body.

Activities of Daily Living (ADL) Tasks that one uses in order to take care of oneself, be mobile in the environment, and care for all daily needs (Lewis, 1995).

Adduction To move medially toward the midline of the body, drawing INTO the midline of the body.

Aerobic With, or in, the presence of oxygen (Study, 1991).

Anaerobic Without the presence of oxygen; not requiring oxygen (Study, 1991).

Anterior Front or belly side.

Arteriovenous oxygen difference (a-v̄)O₂ The difference in oxygen content of arterial and mixed venous blood (McArdle, Katch, and Katch, 1991).

Athletic stance See *ready position*

Body composition The total body mass, fat weight, and fat free weight. Total body mass and fat weight are generally reduced with cardiorespiratory endurance training programs that include greater frequency and duration of training at an adequate level of overload, coupled with proper nutrition.

Cardiorespiratory conditioning The ability to perform large-muscle movements over a sustained period of time; the capacity of the heart-lung system to deliver oxygen for sustained energy production (Study, 1991).

Cardiorespiratory endurance Conditioning of the heart and lungs for an aerobic cardiorespiratory training effect. This type of exercise improves the efficacy of the heart, lungs, and the ability of the body to meet the skeletal demands for oxygen. Oxygen consumption or V̇O₂max measures the ability of the body to maximize oxygen uptake, and it describes the arterial venous difference, which is an indicator of cardiorespiratory endurance capacity.

Center of buoyancy This is the center of balance in the water. It is usually around the chest when the lungs are submerged.

Center of gravity This is the point of intersection of the three planes—sagittal, frontal, and transverse—where the body can move in balance on the land. It is usually at the hips or pelvic girdle area, where the bones are the heaviest. In water, this center is about the same place due to bone density; however, if enough buoyancy is present to overcome the density of the hips, the body may need to balance around a center where buoyancy is greatest, especially if buoyancy equipment is worn around the waist or chest.

Cha-Cha-Cha A neutral posture cue that stands for chin, chest, check the back. (Sanders and Rippee, 1993)

Concentric contraction A contraction in which a muscle exerts force, shortens, and overcomes a resistance (Study, 1991).

Core stabilizers/stabilization The primary muscles that stabilize the "core" or center of the trunk, which also support and protect the spine from stressful movement. Primary core muscles that need to be strengthened include the abdominals, obliques, spinal extensors, and trapezius. (Sanders and Rippee, 1993)

Critical thinking Exploration of a situation, question, or problem to arrive at a conclusion by integrating all information. It involves seeing multiple points of view on complex issues or analyzing.

Deep muscles Farther from the surface of the body, inside near the bones.

Deep water Water depth measured on the individual "standing" in a vertical position, when the lungs are submerged. It is usually about armpit depth or deeper. At this depth, the feet may be touching the bottom lightly or not at all. (Sanders and Rippee, 1993)

Depression Returning from elevation, pulling downward.

Distal Farther from the attached end. It is the opposite of proximal.

Dynamic flexibility Resistance to motion at the joint involving speed during physical performance (Study, 1991).

Eccentric contraction A contraction in which a muscle exerts force, lengthens, and is overcome by a resistance (Study, 1991).

Elevation Raising a body segment, pulling upward.

End range Taking a joint to the end of its normal range of motion and sustaining that position during the exercise or stretch.

Exercise intensity Is how hard a person is working. A specific level of maintenance of muscular activity, which can be measured as power or the amount of work that is being performed.

Extended position Neutral posture or functional stance, standing tall.

Extension To straighten or increase the angle between two joints, to return to anatomical position (or neutral position) from flexion.

Fartlek training Interval training in which the participant chooses the rest/work interval times based on how he or she feels, rather than on systematically timed intervals chosen by a coach or trainer (Study, 1991).

Fitness The ability to perform moderate-to-vigorous levels of physical activity without undue fatigue and the capability of maintaining this capacity throughout life (ACSM, 1998).

Fitness program Organized actions or activities that are aimed at promoting an improved state of health and behavior, enabling a person to have the highest quality of life. (Howley and Franks, 1989)

F.I.T.T. principle When designing an exercise program consider Frequency (how often to work out), Intensity (how hard to work out), Time (how long to work out) and Type of activity to determine if the program will meet suggested guidelines for training by the ACSM or your health care provider.

Flexibility The range of motion possible about a joint or group of joints (Study, 1991).

Flexion To bend or decrease the angle between two parts, the drawing of two body parts together.

Flexuous Elastic, lacking rigidity, supple.

Four S's (4 S's) A simple reminder of how participants can regulate their own exercise intensity. It stands for: Slow down, reduce the Size of the move, Stabilize by finding a balanced position, and Substitute a similar, more comfortable move if necessary. (Sanders and Maloney-Hills, 1998)

Frontal plane of motion This plane divides the body into the front and back portions (on your tummy, on your back), running from head to toes.

Functional ADL exercise Exercises designed to most closely simulate the individual's identified functional activities. The exercise must be specific to the task. (Lewis, 1995)

Functional ADL water fitness training Exercises performed in the pool that target improvements of ADL on the land, such as walking, getting up and down from a chair, climbing stairs, and lifting items.

Functional fitness/exercise Exercise designed to improve targeted activities that the participant wants to be better adapted to perform. For older adults, it may be activities such as walking with more balance. Athletes may exercise with the objective of improving their capacity to perform a specific sport or play a game. Any exercise performed safely should improve a person's functional capacity.

Functional position/neutral spinal position The least painful, most stable position of the spine for each particular activity or exercise (Morgan, 1988).

Glenohumeral and scapular muscles The muscle group that provides full range of motion of the scapulohumeral bones and scapular motion for normal overhead elevation of the arm in flexion or in abduction. These muscles include the pectoralis major and minor, latissimus dorsi, teres major and minor, and subscapularis for full range lateral rotation; and the teres minor, infraspinatus and posterior deltoid for full range medial rotation. (See chapter 5 for descriptions of bones and muscles.)

Heart rate max reserve (HRR) The result of subtracting the resting heart rate from the maximal heart rate; represents the working heart rate range between rest and maximal heart rate within which all activity occurs (Study, 1991).

Hydrophobia Fear of water.

Hydrostatic pressure The pressure exerted by a fluid on any object immersed in a fluid. Hydrostatic pressure exerts a multidimensional force that is proportional to the depth. The deeper into the water we go, the more pressure is exerted at the bottom of the object. The net result is an upward force on the object, which results in the buoyant force upward (Brancazio, 1984).

Hyperextension Extension of a limb or part beyond the normal limit (Stedman, 1976).

Inferior Farther from the head end.

Intensity The physiological stress on the body during exercise. Indicates how hard the body works to achieve a training effect (Study, 1991).

Intensity progression A method of increasing or decreasing the workload by varying a component or components of an exercise in order to change the degree or level of physical demand or intensity.

Isometric contraction A contraction in which a muscle exerts force but does not change in length.

Joints Place of union, or junction, between two or more bones of the skeleton (American Academy of Orthopaedic Surgeons, 1991).

Kilocalorie (kcal) A measure of heat used to express the energy value of food (McArdle, Katch, and Katch, 1991).

Lactate (lactic acid) A waste product of anaerobic energy production known to cause local muscle fatigue (Study, 1991).

Maximal heart rate (MHR) The highest heart rate a person can attain (Study, 1991). Also referred to as *Heart rate max* (HRmax). The maximal heart rate declines with age to the same extent for both men and women (McArdle, Katch, and Katch, 1991). It is estimated as 220–age (in years).

Maximal oxygen consumption ($\dot{V}O_2$) The highest volume of oxygen a person can consume during exercise: maximum aerobic capacity (Study, 1991).

Medial Nearer the midline.

MET METs, or the metabolic energy cost of activities, is a means of measuring physical energy expenditure. A MET is a unit of oxygen expended, with one MET being the energy (measured as kilocalories) needed while the body is in a resting state (Study, 1991). A kilocalorie (kcal) is a measure of heat used to express the energy value of food (McArdle, Katch, and Katch, 1991). For example, an activity that uses seven METs requires seven times more energy (and kcals) than does a state of rest.

Muscular endurance According to ACSM (1995), it is the time limit of a person's ability to maintain a specific force or power level while performing muscular work. This type of training is best developed by using lighter weights with a greater number of repetitions.

Muscular strength training Training by using heavy weight (that requires maximum or nearly maximum tension development) with few repetitions.

Neutral posture The most biomechanically correct, neutral posture from which stabilization can begin (Cole, Moschetti, and Eagleston, 1992).

Neutral spine or neutral joint position The least painful, most stable position of the spine or joint for each particular activity or exercise (Morgan, 1988).

Neutral working position The body is submerged to about shoulder depth. Feet lightly tap or touch the bottom for support, light impact, and balance.

Overload principle (overload) You must perform an exercise in greater than normal amounts (overload) to get an improvement in physical fitness.

Pattern of movement Is defined by listing the body part involved and the direction of movement to meet a specific objective. For example, reaching items on the top shelf requires patterns of movement that include shoulder flexion. The shoulder is the body part and flexion is the direction (Styer-Acevedo and Cirullo, 1994).

Physical activity Any bodily movement produced by skeletal muscles that results in energy expenditure (Blair et al., 1995).

Physical fitness A subset of physical activity defined as planned, structured, and repetitive bodily movement done to improve or maintain one or more components of physical fitness (Blair et al., 1995).

Piriformis syndrome A term to describe a condition in which the piriformis muscle (embedded deep within the gluteal group) causes sciatic pain. Two opinions on the reasons for this irritation exist. Freiberg and Vinke (1934) claim the associated sciatic pain is due to a *contracted* piriformis, while Kendall, McCreara, and Provance (1993) attribute the pain to a stretched piriformis. During standing, the piriformis acts as an external rotator of the femur and helps tilt the pelvis down laterally and posteriorly. If the body is in poor position (leg in postural adduction, internal rotation with anteriorly tilted pelvis), the *stretched* piriformis muscle and sciatic nerve are thrust into close contact.

Plyometric Explosive jump training. Overload is applied to a muscle so that it is rapidly placed on stretch (eccentric or lengthening phase), immediately followed by the concentric phase or contraction (McArdle, Katch, and Katch, 1991).

Posterior Back side.

Power Rate of doing work, or work done, divided by time interval (work/time). Power is a combination of speed and strength, the capacity to do a given amount of work as rapidly as possible (Brancazio, 1984).

Primary muscle mover The muscle that contracts concentrically to accomplish the movement in any given joint action (Study, 1991).

Principle of progression Overload should not be increased too slowly or too rapidly if fitness is to result. Gradually increase overload to achieve optimal benefits.

Principle of specificity To develop a certain aspect of fitness, you must overload specifically for that particular fitness component.

Properties of water The unique characteristics of water that affect the body during exercise in water, including inertia; buoyancy; action/reaction; and form, frictional, and wave drag resistance.

Range of motion (ROM) The number of degrees that a joint will allow one of its segments to move (Study, 1991).

Rating of Perceived Exertion (RPE) Developed by Borg, this scale provides a standard means for evaluating a participant's perception of his or her physical exertion.

Ready position The body position in which the ears, shoulders, and hips are aligned and the legs are flexed for movement in any direction. Also known as the *athletic stance.*

Responsive teaching A teaching method that requires instructors to understand the health objectives of participants and their individual challenges. A responsive instructor is able to provide instruction that addresses individual health and fitness goals by teaching participants how to modify exercises for their special conditions or limitations. The instructor provides tips so students can be responsible for their own success. Responsive teaching might include teaching participants how to adjust the intensity at which they perform exercises (students are encouraged to work at their own level) and giving positive corrective feedback (Sanders and Maloney-Hills, 1998).

Resting heart rate A person's heart rate, or beats per minute, when he or she is at rest, preferably before rising from bed in the morning but also after at least four or five minutes either sitting or lying down (Study, 1991). Heart beats per minute can be calculated by counting heart beats for 30 seconds, then multiplying by 2 or by counting the number of beats in 60 seconds. To take a heart rate, use a heart rate monitor or measure the pulse with two fingers either at the carotid site (side of the neck) or at the radial pulse site (at the wrist).

Rotation Movement around a longitudinal axis in a transverse plane (Kendall, Kendall-McCreara, and Provance, 1993). With lateral or external rotation, the anterior surface of the extremity is turned away from the midline of the body. With medial or internal rotation, the anterior surface of the extremity is turned toward the midline of the body.

Sagittal plane of motion This plane divides the body into the right and left sides (to your right, to your left) extending from head to toes.

Sarcopenia An overall weakening of the body caused by a change in body composition in favor of fat and at the expense of muscle (Evans and Rosenberg, 1991).

Sculling A figure-eight motion using the hands and arms to help stabilize the body or assist with travel through the water.

Shallow water depth Water that is navel to nipple depth, measured with the individual standing on the bottom of the pool.

Specificity of training Specific exercises will elicit specific adaptations creating specific training effects (McKardle, Katch, and Katch, 1991). When training for an activity such as running, swimming, or cycling, participants must use the specific muscles used for the skill and overload the cardiorespiratory system if improvements in performance are to occur. For example, to improve a participant's ability to climb stairs, the muscles used need to be strengthened and stretched appropriately for the task and the cardiorespiratory system needs to be trained to provide the energy to perform the task.

Stabilizer muscles (stabilizers) Muscles that stabilize one joint so a desired movement can be performed by another joint (Study, 1991).

Superficial Nearer the surface.

Superior Nearer the head end of the body.

Thermoregulation Maintenance of core body temperature by establishing a balance between metabolic heat production and heat loss.

Threshold of training The minimum amount of exercise that will improve physical fitness. This level may be different for each individual, so progressions should be taught to ensure that participants can reach their own threshold.

Training response Responses to training are complex and individual; however, training responses for fitness usually are changes in $\dot{V}O_2$ max, muscular strength and endurance, flexibility, and body composition.

Transitional depth water Nipple to neck depth, where the lungs are submerged and the feet can touch the bottom.

Transverse plane of motion This plane divides the body into upper and lower portions (upper body and lower body), crossing approximately at the waist.

Trunk corset Primary muscles that stabilize the center of the trunk or body core. They also support and protect the spine from stressful movement. They include abdominals, obliques, spinal extensors, trapezius, and latissimus dorsi.

$\dot{V}O_2$ **max** See *maximal oxygen consumption*

$\dot{V}O_2$ **reserve** See *heart rate maximum reserve*

Water fitness or water exercise program Exercises performed primarily in a vertical orientation in shallow or deep water. This type of exercise program usually does not include swimming skills, which are based on efficient propulsion horizontally through the water. Water exercise instead uses movements that amplify drag by unstreamlining the body to create resistance. The goal of this program is to create sufficient intensity to provide fitness training adaptations in oxygen consumption ($\dot{V}O_2$), muscular strength/endurance, flexibility, and body composition.

Water specific Movements, exercises, or equipment designed to amplify the properties of water by changing the water's effect on the body.

References

American Academy of Orthopaedic Surgeons. 1991. *Athletic training and sports medicine.* Rosemont, IL: American Academy of Orthopaedic Surgeons.

American College of Sports Medicine. 1998. The recommended quantity and quality of exercise for developing and maintaining cardiorespiratory and muscular fitness, and flexibility in healthy adults. *Medicine and Science in Sports and Exercise* 30(6): 975–991.

American College of Sports Medicine. 1995. *Guidelines for exercise testing and prescription* (5th ed.). Phildelphia: Lea & Febiger.

Blair, S., H. Kohl, C. Barlow, R. Paffenbarger, L. Gibbons, and C. Macera. 1995. Changes in physical fitness and all-cause mortality. *JAMA* 273(14): 1093–1098.

Brancazio, P. 1984. *Sport science, physical laws and optimum performance.* New York: Simon & Schuster.

Cole, A., M. Moschetti, and R. Eagleston. 1992. Getting backs in the swim. *Rehabilitation Management* (August/September): 62–70.

Evans, W., and I.H. Rosenberg. 1991. *Biomarkers, the 10 keys to prolonging vitality.* New York: Simon & Schuster.

Freiberg, A.H., and T.H. Vinke. 1934. Sciatica and sacro-iliac joint. *Journal of Bone Joint Surgery* 16: 126–136.

Howley, E.T. and B.D. Franks, 1989. *Health Fitness Instructor's Handbook.* Champaign, IL: Human Kinetics.

Kendall, F., E. Kendall-McCreara, and P. Provance. 1993. *Muscles, testing and function* (4th ed.). Baltimore: Williams and Wilkins.

Lewis, C. 1995. *Aging, the health care challenge: An interdisciplinary approach to assessment and rehabilitation of the elderly.* Philadelphia: Davis.

McArdle, W., F. Katch, and V. Katch. 1991. *Exercise physiology, energy, nutrition and human performance.* Philadelphia/London: Lea & Febiger.

Morgan, D. 1988. Concepts in functional training and postural stabilization for the low-back injured. *Topics in Acute Care and Trauma Rehabilitation* 2(4): 8–17.

Sanders, M. and C. Maloney-Hills. 1998. Golden Waves Functional Water Training for Health Program, WaterFit/Wave Aerobics, Reno, NV.

Sanders, M., and N. Rippee. 1993. *Speedo aquatic fitness system, instructor training manual.* London: Speedo International.

Stedman's Medical Dictionary. (23rd ed.). 1976. Baltimore, MD: Williams & Wilkins.

Study, M., ed. 1991. *Personal trainer manual, the resource for fitness instructors.* San Diego, CA: American Council on Exercise.

Styer-Acevedo, J. and J.A. Cirullo. 1994. Integrating land and aquatic approaches with a functional emphasis. Orthopaedic Physical Therapy Clinics of North America. 3(2): 165–178.

Index

About the Editor

Mary E. Sanders, MS

Has a master's degree in exercise science and is adjunct professor at the Department of Health Ecology, University of Nevada, Reno, where she conducts research in water exercise. She is the founder of Wave Aerobics®, training water fitness instructors in over 20 countries, and she has taught Wave Aerobics® for years at the Reno Family YMCA. Mary chairs the Water Fitness Advisory Committee for IDEA, The Health & Fitness Source, and she presents for IDEA. In 1997 she received the "Instructor of the Year" award from IDEA. She has served on the certification committee for the American Council on Exercise (ACE), was a contributing author to the *Aerobics Instructor's Manual,* and is currently a Continuing Education Specialist for ACE. She also authored the Water Exercise section of the *Exercise Standards and Guidelines Manual* for the American Fitness Association of America (AFAA). Mary is a member of and presenter for the American College of Sports Medicine (ACSM) and is an associate editor for *ACSM's Health & Fitness Journal.* She also is an ACSM Health/Fitness Instructor and ACE certified. Mary is the recipient of the Aquatic Exercise Association 2000 Global Award, Lifetime Achievement in Aquatic Fitness, and was named Fitness Educator of the Year, 2001, by the Fitness Educators of Older Adults Association. She developed the Speedo® Aquatic Fitness System and served as education director/fitness consultant with Speedo® International for over six years. In the past, Mary was an instructor trainer of water safety and lifeguard training for the American Red Cross and a competitive swimmer for the University of Wyoming. Mary can be reached at **www.waterfit.com.**

Contributing Authors

Shirley Archer, JD, MA

Associate Director of the Health Promotion Resource Center at the Stanford Center for Research in Disease Prevention, Stanford University School of Medicine. Shirley is a licensed attorney in California, New York, and Washington, DC, and is an ACE-, ACSM-, and YMCA-certified health and fitness instructor with more than 15 years' experience. Shirley is a committee member for IDEA, The Health & Fitness Source, and a continuing education provider for ACE and the YMCA. Shirley's previous positions include Association Group Exercise Coordinator for the YMCA of the Mid-Peninsula in northern California; research administrator and financial manager for the Division of Cardiovascular Medicine at Stanford University; and consultant to the State Bar of California in continuing education.

Mary Curry

Adjunct faculty at the College of St. Catherine, St. Paul, MN., and a YMCA Faculty Trainer; coordinator of water fitness programs and regional training in St. Paul. She is a member of the IDEA Water Fitness Committee and an IDEA presenter and a faculty member of the Water FIT School at the University of Nevada, Reno. Mary teaches water fitness classes to a number of YMCAs in the St. Paul area.

Ellen Evans, PhD

Earned her BS at Western Illinois University in physical education and fitness instruction; her MS at the University of Illinois, Urbana in kinesiology/exercise physiology; and her PhD at the University of Georgia in exercise science/exercise physiology. She currently is a postdoctoral research fellow at Washington University School of Medicine, Division of Geriatrics and Gerontology. Ellen is an experienced fitness instructor who has taught exercise classes to a wide variety of people.

Carol Kennedy, MS

Program Director of Fitness/Wellness in the Division of Recreational Sports at Indiana University, as well as a water fitness instructor at the university. Carol is a water fitness researcher and the author of numerous articles on both the physiology of water training and the management of water fitness programs. She is a member of the American College of Sports Medicine (ACSM) certification committee and was the first chair of the Water Fitness Advisory Committee for IDEA, The Health & Fitness Source.

Tatiana Kolovou, MBA

Assistant Director of Fitness/Wellness at Indiana University, Bloomington. Tatiana has been a fitness instructor trainer to staff over 100 sessions offered at the university. She is a presenter at water fitness and management workshops at IDEA conferences and other international events. Tatiana has a bachelor's degree in exercise science and is certified by ACSM and ACE. She is a former swimming and water polo competitor.

Cathy Maloney-Hills, RPT

Licensed physical therapist with over 15 years of diverse clinical experience. Cathy has developed a community-based aquatic exercise program for older adults called Master's Aquatics, and she co-developed the Golden Waves™ aquatic functional ADL program with Mary Sanders. She currently provides aquatic rehabilitation for patients at the Courage Center of Golden Valley, Minnesota.

Debbie Miles-Dutton

Aquatic director and instructor trainer for the University of California, Santa Barbara. Debbie is the co-founder of Land & Sea Fitness and Aquamotion. She is a member of the IDEA Water Fitness Advisory Committee, and she received the Five Star Award from IDEA, The Health & Fitness Source, for excellence in teaching. Debbie has 15 years' experience in competitive swimming, lifeguarding, water safety instruction, and group fitness instruction.

Ghada Muasher

The Red Sea and the sea animals are home and friends of Ghada's. She created a unique program blending her love of the animals with the joy of moving in the pool. She is a water exercise enthusiast who learned to blend the science and mind/body aspects with her water fitness moves, bringing it all to you on video and in her book. She is an author and champion of the essence of the pure joy of moving in the water!

Nicki Rippee, PhD

Associate professor of physical education at the University of Nevada, Reno, where she is also a faculty member for the Water Fitness Instructor Training (FIT) course. She conducts research in water fitness and was co-investigator for the Golden Waves study. She is co-author of the book Is Your Aerobics Class Killing You?

Laura J. Slane

Associate Director for Aquatics, YMCA of the USA. Laura earned her bachelor's degree in recreation from Central Missouri State University, Warrensburg, Missouri. She has been a YMCA professional for more than 20 years, working in local Ys at St. Louis, Fort Worth, and Dallas as an aquatic director, physical director, program director, branch executive, and district executive. She holds YMCA certification in many areas, including health and fitness, aquatics, and management. As the Associate Director for the YMCA of the USA, Laura has developed the YMCA Splash and YMCA Swim Lessons programs and materials, as well as the book On the Guard II and Principles of Aquatic Leadership.

Additional Resources

See the current YMCA Program Store Catalog for details about these additional items for your water fitness programs, or contact the Program Store, PO Box 5076, Champaign, IL 61825-5076, phone (800) 747-0089, 7:00 a.m. to 7:00 p.m. (CST). To save time, order by fax (217) 351-1549.

Water Fitness & Exercise

0-99-004208-1	Introduction to Waterfit Aquatic Fitness System (video)	$25.00
0-99-001999-3	Specificity of Training & Deep Water Exercise Program (video)	$25.00
0-99-002003-7	Tidal Waves (video)	$25.00
0-99-002000-2	Aquatic Step Program (video)	$25.00
0-99-002001-0	Golden Waves 1 (video)	$25.00
0-99-002002-9	Golden Waves 2 (video)	$25.00
0-88011-792-3	YMCA Fun and Fitness Activity Chart	$6.00

Arthritis Foundation YMCA Aquatic Program and AFYAP PLUS

0-99-003189-6	Instructor's Guide/Guidelines and Procedures Guide (booklet + 3-ring binder)	$22.00
0-99-003190-X	Trainer's Guide/Recertification Guide	$13.00
0-99-003191-8	Deep Water Instructor's Guide	$5.00
0-99-003192-6	Deep Water Trainer's Guide	$4.00
0-99-003193-4	Juvenile Arthritis Instructor's Guide	$4.50
0-99-003194-2	Juvenile Arthritis Trainer's Guide	$4.50

All prices shown are subject to change.